DON'T LET YOUR MORNING PICK-ME-UP TEAR YOU DOWN

- Caffeine can't provide energy, only chemical stimulation, an induced emergency state that can lead to irritability, mood swings, and panic attacks.

- Caffeine's ultimate mood effect can be letdown, which can lead to depression and chronic fatigue.

- Caffeine gives the illusion of heightened alertness by dilating pupils, quickening heart rate, and raising blood pressure. In fact, caffeine does not increase overall mental activity.

LET *CAFFEINE BLUES* BRING YOU BETTER HEALTH

CAFFEINE
BLUES

WAKE UP TO THE HIDDEN DANGERS OF AMERICA'S #1 DRUG

STEPHEN CHERNISKE, M.S.

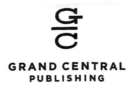

GRAND CENTRAL
PUBLISHING

New York   Boston

Grand Central Publishing
Hachette Book Group
237 Park Avenue
New York, NY 10017

www.HachetteBookGroup.com

First Edition: December 1998

Grand Central Publishing is a division of Hachette Book Group, Inc.
The Grand Central name and logo is a trademark of Hachette Book Group, Inc.

The publisher is not responsible for websites (or their content) that are not owned by the publisher.

Library of Congress Cataloging-in-Publication Data
Cherniske, Stephen.
    Caffeine blues : wake up to the hidden dangers of America's #1 drug / Stephen Cherniske.
        p. cm.
    Includes index.
    ISBN 978-0-446-67391-4
    1. Caffeine—Health aspects. 2. Caffeine habit. 3. Coffee—Health aspects. 4. Coffee habit. I. Title.
QP801.C24C47 1998   98-24372
                                                                      CIP

Book design and text composition by L&G McRee
Cover design by David Reinhardt

For the children, who need to be
nourished and protected.

ACKNOWLEDGMENTS

I would like to acknowledge my mother for her commitment to health and good nutrition more than fifty years ago, and all of the teachers, researchers, and scientists who over the years instilled in me a love of scientific inquiry. Particularly, I would like to thank Robert Garvin and Allan Watts for showing me that truth is most often found by looking beyond the conventional viewpoint.

I have also benefited tremendously from many scientists who paved the way. Jack E. James and Keryn Stirling produced a valuable analysis of the harmful effects of habitual caffeine use in 1982. Annette MacKay Rossignol and Linda Massey conducted groundbreaking research concerning caffeine and women's health. Roland R. Griffiths was an early researcher into caffeine's addictive properties, and Dr. Richard M. Gilbert published *Caffeine as a Drug of Abuse* in 1976, long before anyone else caught on. Thanks to Dr. Eric Strain and his colleagues who finally proved the existence of a caffeine dependence syndrome.

Thanks also to G. Alan Smith for showing the world that caffeine reduction is a critical step in the treatment of anxiety, headache, sleep disturbance, and abdominal symptoms, and to Dr. Milton Krisiloff for illuminating the caffeine connection to urinary and prostate problems. I am grateful for the inclusion of material concerning caffeine abuse from the clinical experience of Drs. Michael Liepman and Jesse Hanley, and for perspectives gained from the work of Drs. Michael Murray, Dean Ornish, Jeffrey Bland, and Ralph Golan.

In the process of creating this book and program, I was assisted greatly by Caroline MacDougall, a pioneer in the creation of caffeine-free beverages. Her insight, word-smithing, inspiration, tireless support, and criticism were essential to the project. The editorial and writing assistance of Cynthia Anderson was once again crucial and greatly appreciated. Special thanks to Cindy Latham, Wendy McClure, Robert Gangwer, and research assistants Grace Molonai, Catherine Rhodes, and Elliott MacDougall.

I am grateful for research provided by the Natural Resources Defense Council, the Smithsonian Migratory Bird Center, and for the remarkable work of Marcus Colchester and Larry Lohmann exploring the issues of human rights and rain forest destruction.

Warmest gratitude to Robert Stricker, my literary agent, who found the very best home for this manuscript. To Warner Books for having the courage to take a stand at this critical point in time. To Vice President and Hard-cover Publisher Jamie Raab, John Aherne, editor, and Heather Kilpatrick, deputy general counsel.

Thanks also to B. William Lee, H. Y. Sung, Stuart Ochiltree, and the staff of Univera Pharmaceuticals for resources, time, encouragement, and the ability to create solutions where others see only problems.

And finally, I am indebted to my wife, Deborah, for holding the family together while Daddy worked late; for her unending support on every level and her many contributions from concept to final draft.

CONTENTS

FOREWORD

As a physician, I prescribe drugs with great care, because all drugs have effects and side effects. In addition, some can create a state of dependence. Clearly, caffeine is such a drug, and I find that very few people are aware of its side effects and dangers. In fact, most people do not even know how much caffeine they are consuming, and what concerns me is that this information is purposely withheld from consumers.

Caffeine is clearly addictive, completely unregulated, and its presence in our foods and beverages is often hidden! Almost daily I see a patient whose symptoms are made worse by the consumption of caffeine. The drug contributes to palpitations, panic attacks, hypoglycemia, gastritis, fatigue, insomnia, and PMS, to name a few. Some people are so sensitive to caffeine that they don't realize a fruit drink with hidden caffeine can cause their symptoms.

Although I know a few people who use caffeine prudently, most people I meet report drinking what you will discover are dangerous amounts of caffeine. Perhaps an occasional cup is safe, but by the time you realize that you can't make it through the day without caffeine, you're in trouble. Coffee, tea, soft drinks, caffeine-spiked beverages, and the other hidden forms of caffeine are promoted as harmless, energizing treats. I consider this deceptive and false advertising. And what concerns me most is the dramatically increasing use of caffeine by children, accompanied of course by large amounts of sugar or artificial sweeteners, which add to beverages' deleterious and addictive effects.

I find *Caffeine Blues* to be an extraordinary and important book. Knowledge is power, and this book will empower you to regain and protect your health. Finally, you have in your hands all the information you need to make an informed choice regarding caffeine use. Everyone needs to know the short- and long-term effects of caffeine. Everyone, including doctors, needs to become more aware of caffeine's role in cardiovascular disease, anxiety, depression, gastrointestinal disorders, and women's health. I've looked forward to this exposé for years, and I'm pleased that it is so well documented and readable. I recommend it to my patients and keep a copy in the waiting room.

I've known and learned from Stephen Cherniske for many years. His in-depth knowledge, experience, and scientific research on numerous topics in health and nutrition make him a natural to tell this shocking and critical story. I encourage you to trust his information and insight, as I do.

Caffeine Blues will make my job a great deal easier. I suggest that you take the book seriously, and discover the truth that's been hidden from you for far too long. This book not only blows the whistle on the caffeine industry, but it also provides you with a proven strategy to kick the habit without suffering through weeks of withdrawal. For many of my patients, kicking caffeine has been an important step on the road to optimum health. Enjoy the journey.

—JESSE LYNN HANLEY, M.D.

INTRODUCTION

"Coffee?" she intoned. "Thank you," I replied, taking a cup from the hostess in the airport lounge. I was waiting for an early-morning flight to Anchorage to give a weekend seminar on clinical nutrition. The flight was delayed, so I had another cup as I read the newspaper. I didn't notice when she refilled my cup.

When we finally boarded, a flight attendant had a cup of coffee in my hand before I had my seat belt fastened. Breakfast was served twenty minutes later, along with another cup of coffee. Looking back, it seems extraordinary how all this took place, but at the time it appeared perfectly normal. The entire five-hour flight was punctuated with "Coffee?" "Cream and sugar?" "Can I warm that up for you?" "Coffee, sir?"

Here I must tell you that I love coffee, and at that time was in the habit of drinking two cups every day. I also love to fly, because there are no clients, no charts, and, until recently, no phone. It's usually one of the most relaxing times of my busy schedule. But this flight was a nightmare. I felt anxious. Instead of "zoning out," thoughts raced through my mind with surprising intensity. I felt flushed and heated; I loosened my tie but could not get comfortable. Finally, lunch was served, which provided a brief diversion—and another cup of coffee.

By midflight, I was nearly panicked. For the first time in my life, I felt claustrophobic and fearful. I tried to figure out what was wrong, but I couldn't put my finger on it. I tried to organize my lecture notes, but couldn't concentrate. "Coffee?" the stewardess chimed. "Do you need a refill, sir?" I looked at my watch every fifteen minutes as the time dragged on.

Finally, the Anchorage area came into view. But as we approached the airport, the captain announced that weather conditions would delay our landing. Thirty minutes later, we were *still* circling the airport, and I did something I'd never done before: I yelled at the flight attendant.

"When the *hell* are you going to land this plane?" I snapped. Slightly taken aback, she placed a hand on my shoulder and answered as if she were speaking to a three-year-old. I felt like an idiot. "I'm really not feeling myself," I muttered.

Flying north for these seminars is usually not a problem. I gain an hour from Pacific Standard Time, and normally arrive for my presentation refreshed and well prepared. This time was different. Nothing seemed to go right. The hotel van was crowded. The university had neglected to reserve a room near the lecture hall. A box holding my slides had opened inside my suitcase, and it took me over an hour to put them back in order.

I walked up to the speaker's podium feeling frazzled and disconnected, and my lecture proved to be just as bad. For the first time in my professional career, I had lapses of memory and omitted important information. A number of slides were upside down. The usual flow of my presentation was completely gone.

I consoled myself with the thought that I would do better the following day. Walking to the elevator, I was approached by a student who had taken a number of my previous classes. "Are you all right?" he asked. "You look terrible." Back in my room, I had to admit he was right. Instead of my usual healthy glow, there were dark circles under my eyes and deeply etched wrinkles. I felt old.

Still, I reasoned, after a good night's sleep, I'd be back to my energetic, positive self. Instead, I tossed and turned for hours until it hit me: insomnia. How many cups of coffee had I had that day? I couldn't remember, but it had to be at least six, maybe more. Strange as it may sound, I was relieved that I finally had an explanation for my terrible experience. Firmly resolved to quit coffee, I fell asleep around 2 A.M.

I arose four hours later, feeling like I'd been hit by a bus. The first lecture began at 8 A.M., and I wanted to prepare well to make up for the previous day. A cold shower served to rouse my tired body, and I managed to arrive at the lecture hall looking half decent.

I carefully avoided the coffee urns that dotted the back and side aisles of the auditorium and, with a pitcher of water by my side, began the morning topic. By 10 A.M., I had a splitting headache. I announced a thirty-minute break and retreated to my room.

Ice did nothing. Aspirin did nothing. My hands were shaking. I felt nauseous and was suddenly afraid that if I blew the second day, student evaluations would be dismal. A single thought pounded in my head: "Have a cup of coffee. There's too much at stake."

One large cup of coffee later, the headache was gone. Within an hour, I was a new man, pain free and alert. It was hard for me to admit that I was addicted to coffee, but the hell I had been through the day before was clearly a drug overdose, and the worse hell I had faced that morning was clearly a drug withdrawal. Quite simply, I was feeling better because I had had my fix. This realization was frightening and unacceptable to me, so I decided then and there to kick the caffeine habit.

I also left the conference resolved to research carefully the effects of caffeine. During six years of college, I had been told only that caffeine was a mild stimulant and its association with health disorders was unproven. I was also told that caffeine is not addictive. Since I knew from my own painful experience that the opposite was true, I reasoned that perhaps I had been snowed on the whole topic.

What I quickly learned was that *everyone has been snowed*—researchers, doctors, journalists, and especially the public. The deception has been well coordinated by an industry whose goal is quite simple: to get as much caffeine into your body as possible. If the caffeine industry can accomplish that, they have you as a customer for life. They know caffeine saps your natural sense of vitality, leaving you dependent on their products to get through the day. They know that you actually crave their products and, more importantly, that you suffer when you don't consume them.

It's a marketing dream, and it's legal. No wonder more and more companies are jumping on the caffeine bandwagon, churning out products from specialized coffees and teas to "herbal" caffeinated energy pills, caffeine-laced fruit beverages, "supercharged" soft drinks, caffeinated beer, and even caffeinated bottled water.

A Clear and Present Danger

Cardiologists report that caffeine raises blood pressure. Endocrinologists acknowledge that it contributes to adrenal exhaustion. Neurologists document changes in brain biochemistry. Researchers identify correlations between caffeine intake and certain types of cancer. Internists say that coffee (even decaf) increases ulcer risk, and gynecologists say that caffeine intake contributes to hormone imbalance and a long list of health disorders in women.

Why aren't health warnings required on coffee cans? Why, in the face of this mountain of data, are physicians not warning their patients? Because there is no comprehensive view of the problem. Everyone is looking at their own little piece of the puzzle. In 1993, a study published in the *Journal of the American Medical Association* found that regular drip coffee (the kind most people drink) raises blood cholesterol levels. Nevertheless, the authors conclude that the increased risk to heart disease is small. Apparently, they're not talking to their colleagues who have found that caffeine also raises blood pressure, increases homocysteine (a biochemical that damages artery walls), promotes arrhythmias, and constricts blood vessels leading to the heart.

Viewed together, these effects present a clear picture of caffeine's contribution to the nation's leading cause of death. But in countless newspaper articles, the issue is presented in pieces, and the truth is diluted by "experts" who are unwilling to take a stand and instead qualify their findings by saying, "There's not enough evidence."

Caffeine Myths Debunked

In the pages of *Caffeine Blues*, I present the full scope of caffeine's effects on physical, mental, and emotional well-being, and debunk the following popular misconceptions about caffeine:

1. *Caffeine gives you energy.* Wrong. Caffeine does not provide energy—only chemical stimulation. The perceived "energy" comes from the body's struggle to adapt to increased blood levels of stress hormones. In most cases, this induced emergency state leads to well-defined side effects collectively known as caffeinism. Ironically, caffeinism is characterized by fatigue.
2. *Caffeine gives you a "lift."* Wrong. Using coffee for mood enhancement is a short-term blessing and a long-term curse. While the initial adrenal stimulation may provide a transient antifatigue "lift," caffeine's ultimate mood effect is a letdown, either subtle or profound. Advertisers and coffee "institutes" have kept this side of caffeine from public view. In Chapter 4, you'll find clear and unequivocal evidence of caffeine's role in depression and anxiety. What's more, caffeine is positively linked to panic attacks, a psychiatric disorder affecting an estimated 5 million Americans.
3. *Caffeine sharpens your mind.* Wrong. While caffeine users may feel more alert, the experience is simply one of increased sensory and motor activity (dilated pupils, increased heart rate, and higher blood pressure). The quality of thought and recall is improved no more than the quality of music is improved when played at a higher volume or speed. In Chapter 4, you will find a convincing argument, backed by clinical research, that caffeine actually *decreases* overall mental acuity.

The Dark Side of Caffeine

There are plenty of people who don't want you to know the truth about caffeine. If it were just a matter of "coffee jitters," it wouldn't be such an issue. But as you will see, the effects of caffeine are far-reaching and can be quite serious. Importantly, women are at higher risk than men, and children are the most vulnerable to caffeine because of their limited ability to detoxify the drug. Caffeine stays in a child's brain and bloodstream much longer than an adult's, and subsequent doses produce a cumulative increase in stress and addiction. Is it any wonder that soft drinks, to which manufacturers add caffeine, have become the most widely consumed beverages in America? The truth is, Americans of all ages are *addicted* to the caffeine in soft drinks!

It's a fact that young children consume alarming amounts of caffeine, entering the cycle of dependency and nervous system dysfunction early in life. One study identified peak consumption periods at three, thirteen, and seventeen.[1] These children are set up for a lifetime addiction with serious health consequences. In the following chapters, we'll explore caffeine's connection to hyperactivity, learning and behavior disorders, fatigue, cancer, heart disease, ulcers, headache, allergy, PMS, birth defects, and more.

Caffeine Is Literally a Pain in the Neck

You'll learn that many of our physical experiences of tension and pain are directly related to the level of stress hormones in our bodies—and that caffeine acts as a pain trigger because it elevates blood levels of these biochemicals. Susan M., for example, came to me as a last-ditch effort to help with her neck and shoulder pain. She'd been to doctors, chiropractors, and acupuncturists, but the pain was relentless.

Susan listed four cups of coffee per day on her diet diary, and I soon learned that her "cup" was a sixteen-ounce mug. She was thus consuming over 900 milligrams of caffeine per day from coffee and, ironically, another 190 milligrams in her over-the-counter painkiller. Using the Off the Bean program outlined in Chapter 10, she gradually reduced her caffeine intake to almost zero. Three weeks later, she was pain free for the first time in twenty years.

This case is not an isolated incident. Over the years, I have counseled hundreds of patients who could trace the beginnings of their chronic pain to a time when they started drinking large amounts of coffee. Often, it was during their college years, or when they started working in an office. And usually there was the vicious cycle of coffee and stress. Perhaps you have found yourself in a similar situation.

Unsafe at Any Speed?

Newspaper and magazine articles appear every week identifying some health risk associated with caffeine. Invariably, however, they conclude with the absurd statement that "moderate intake" is no problem. The fact is that no scientist can tell you how much caffeine is safe for you to ingest because the effects of caffeine differ significantly from person to person. A multitude of individual differences enter the picture, including age, weight, sex, and numerous biochemical, psychological, and emotional factors. What is tolerable for one person may be excessive for another. Moreover, what is tolerable caffeine intake at one point in your life may actually cause health problems just a few years later.

If this sounds strange, remember that caffeine is a drug with cumulative effects over time. Also keep in mind that of all of the thousands of research papers that have been published on caffeine, *none have concluded that caffeine is good for you.* Rather, the continuing debate in the popular and scientific press focuses entirely on the degree to which caffeine is injurious.

Caffeine Blues will help you understand how your body works. With the right care, the human body is designed to last 100 years or more, but most of us fall apart after age sixty and die in our mid-seventies. I have drawn upon thirty years of clinical and research experience and will give you graphic case histories culled from thousands of client files. But in the final analysis *you* are the only scientist who matters, and the only laboratory you need is your body.

Health risks are rarely self-evident. For a cigarette smoker, the destruction of lung tissue occurs silently over many years—until one day it's too late. Likewise, the first overt consequence of a high-fat diet is often a fatal heart attack. As a society, we therefore make education about such health issues a priority. We put warnings on cigarettes and encourage sensible eating. But I would like to remind you of a sobering fact. Cigarette companies fought successfully for years against warning labels, and only recently admitted that nicotine is addictive. The caffeine industry has refused even to disclose the amount of caffeine in their products. Big business watches bottom-line profits, and addiction to any substance means higher levels of consumption and more product sales. The caffeine industry knows this better than anyone.

Caffeine Alternatives: There *Is* Hope

Caffeine Blues presents a credible and carefully researched argument against the habitual consumption of caffeine, but, unlike other health exposés, it will not leave you feeling helpless. This book will give you a new view of life after caffeine as seen through the eyes of former coffeeholics. I am keenly aware that coffee plays a major role in most people's lives. Without their morning "wake-up" cup and their midmorning and midafternoon jolts, most of my clients were concerned that they would not be able to function effectively.

These concerns led to my next research project: finding safe and effective alternatives to caffeine. I scrutinized botanical texts, ran hundreds of Medline computer searches, and ultimately traveled to three continents researching every legal substance purporting to have energy-enhancing effects. This research was a real eye-opener. There was a tremendous amount of misinformation, especially concerning so-called herbal energizers. Most, like guarana, kola nut, yerba maté, and ma huang (ephedra), turned out to be nothing more than plant sources of caffeine and other stimulant drugs. Their mode of action is exactly the same as coffee: stimulation of the central nervous system resulting in adrenal stress. The fact that these stimulant products are found in health-food stores and claim to be "all natural" is simply part of the hype that fills the energy market. These "alternatives" to coffee are thoroughly debunked in Chapter 7.

Let me state this clearly: *A substance that purports to give you energy by stimulating your nervous system isn't giving you anything.* It's harming you! Using stimulants is like whipping a horse. They work for a short time, but prove disastrous when used repeatedly. My goal was to find substances that would nourish the body, not stress the adrenals, substances that would enhance the metabolic efficiency of the body in order to fulfill our inherent potential for vitality and wellness.

Eventually, I discovered a group of substances with true energizing properties. Just as a tune-up can enhance the efficiency of your car's engine, this group of vitamins, minerals, herbs, coenzymes, and organic acids can dramatically improve your body's production of energy. And I'm not just talking about energy in the sense of strength, stamina, and endurance. Imagine every cell in your body operating at a higher level of efficiency, including your immune system, brain, and nervous system. This "tune-up" has already changed countless lives, and you too can experience the exhilaration of peak vitality and what I call *high-level wellness*.

It's ironic that all the things you thought you could get from caffeine can in fact be obtained only by getting off it. These breakthrough alternatives are presented in detail and supported with abundant scientific and medical references in Chapter 10. I'll show you how to quit coffee by drinking delicious, satisfying, healthful alternatives and rebuild your natural abundant energy supply without harmful stimulants.

Beating the Caffeine Blues

Perhaps you've already thought about reducing your caffeine intake. But to make that decision, you need accurate information, and the facts on coffee have been slow in getting out. And you also need more than just information, since facts alone are not enough to motivate change. *Caffeine Blues* is designed to lead you through a discovery process that will increase your health awareness. For some people, awareness begins when they add up how much caffeine they consume every day. Then they connect their caffeine intake to the tired feeling they have when they wake up, or the roller-coaster mood and energy swings they experience throughout the day.

The challenge, of course, is to discover just how addicted you are to caffeine, and how that addiction affects the quality of your life. I suggest that you try kicking the habit for sixty days—the minimum amount of time you'll need to evaluate the benefits of a caffeine-free body and mind. For some people, I know that's asking a lot. But don't worry. Chapter 10 will give you an effective, clinically proven, and pain-free method for reducing or eliminating caffeine. This step-by-step Off the Bean program will enable you to free yourself from dependence on caffeine without the headaches, irritability, fatigue, and depression normally associated with caffeine withdrawal.

This program is not theory or conjecture. Thousands of people have already taken this important step, and are right now experiencing greater vitality, greater energy, and better health than they ever felt when they were addicted to caffeine. You can also enjoy these blessings if you really want them. The choice is up to you!

A Word about Notes

In compiling this manuscript, I initially handed my editor over 700 footnotes. "Take out these footnotes," he said. "They make it look like a textbook."

I protested. "I'm asking readers to consider a very controversial subject," I argued, "one that purports to show beyond the shadow of a doubt that most everything they've heard about caffeine is wrong. How can I expect them to believe me if I don't provide legitimate scientific support?" I also wanted the health-care community to pay attention to this material, and they would of course require careful documentation.

So we compromised. The key controversial statements are referenced, and notes are listed at the end of the book. This level of scientific integrity means that you can share the book with your doctor without the fear of being labeled a "health nut." The research cited here can be found in any medical library. You can skip the notes or use them for further study.

CHAPTER 1

Coffee and Caffeine: A Dose of Reality

We have seen several well-marked cases of coffee excess. . . . The sufferer is tremulous, and loses his self-command; he is subject to fits of agitation and depression; he loses color and has a haggard appearance. The apatite falls off, and symptoms of gastric catarrh may be manifested. The heart also suffers; it palpitates, or it intermits. As with other such agents, a renewed dose of the poison gives temporary relief, but at the cost of future misery. . . . By miseries such as these, the best years of life may be spoilt.

—SIR T. CLIFFORD ALLBUTT and
DR. WALTER ERNEST DIXON in *A System of Medicine*, vol. II, London, 1909

Goatherds, Monks, and the Rest of Us

The origins of coffee are lost in legend, although the most popular tale traces its discovery to a goatherd dwelling in Ethiopia. According to the story, the goatherd watched his flock eat the bright red berries from a wild evergreen bush—and was subsequently amazed to see the animals leap about with wild abandon. He tried some of the berries himself, and soon he was leaping too.

By around the sixth century A.D., the plant had reached Arabia, where it was used as a food and medicine. Coffee berries were either fermented to make wine, or dried, crushed, mixed with fat, and eaten. It was not until the thirteenth century that Arab monks made a revolutionary discovery: Roasted coffee beans could be made into a drink. No more falling asleep at prayers! The news spread from monastery to monastery, then hit the streets with the world's first coffeehouses.

Everyone who tried coffee wanted more—and if they were travelers, they wanted to take it home with them. With lightning speed, coffee became a valuable trading commodity and spread to the world at large: first to Turkey, then to Italy and France, and finally to the rest of Europe by the mid-seventeenth century.

The Arabs maintained strict control of the coffee trade until smugglers from other countries got hold of the seeds. The Dutch brought coffee to Java and Ceylon, the French transported it to the West Indies, and a Brazilian obtained coffee for his homeland. Today coffee is cultivated widely in regions between the Tropics of Cancer and Capricorn: Central and South America, Java, Sumatra, India, Arabia, equatorial Africa, Hawaii, Mexico, and the West Indies.

Most American colonists drank tea, a caffeine-containing leaf from the *Camilia senensis* bush, until the boycott against King George's tea tax climaxed with the Boston Tea Party in 1773. From that point forward, coffee grew in popularity as America's national drink. Americans are now the largest consumers of coffee in the world, drinking over 420 million cups per day, or about one-fifth of the world's total annual supply. In America, coffee wins hands down as the most popular substance containing caffeine, with soft drinks, tea, and chocolate as runners-up.

From Plant to Percolator

The word *coffee* comes from the Arab word *qahwah*. The botanical name of the original species discovered in Africa whose beans are grown around the world today is *Coffea arabica*. There are three general groupings of coffee: Brazils (all *Coffea arabica* grown in Brazil), Milds (all *Coffea arabica* grown outside of Brazil), and *Coffea robusta*, a variety of coffee grown at lower elevations and generally considered to be inferior in quality to *Coffea arabica*. Robusta beans contain nearly twice the caffeine of arabica and are also more acidic. Mass-marketed brands of coffee contain primarily robusta, whereas specialty coffees tend to be made primarily from arabica beans.

One reason coffee spread so quickly around the globe is because it's an exceptionally hardy, self-pollinating plant. Though it's usually referred to as a tree, coffee is actually an evergreen shrub that, when cultivated, is pruned to a height of twelve feet or less. An arabica tree produces only about one to two pounds of coffee beans per year, so supplying worldwide demand requires an incredible amount of space. We'll discuss the problems associated with coffee cultivation in Chapter 7.

Coffee berries—the fruit of the plant, which contains the beans—are usually harvested by hand and undergo a lengthy processing procedure. Once removed from the berries, the beans are fermented, washed, dried, hulled, and peeled before they are roasted. After roasting, the beans are ground and then they are ready to perk, brew, or drip into your favorite cup of java.

A Cupa Cupa Cupa Cupa Chemicals

Caffeine has received a great deal of attention ever since it was identified as the principle stimulant in coffee (1820). But it seems that every year, even more noxious ingredients are isolated in coffee. In 1992, researchers found another stimulant compound distinctly different from caffeine that may be responsible for coffee's gastrointestinal effects.[1] To date, over 700 volatile substances in coffee have been identified, including more than 200 acids and an incredible array of alcohols, aromatic compounds, carbonyl compounds, esters, hydrocarbons, heterocyclic compounds, and terpenoids. Nonvolatile substances in coffee include caffeine and other purines, glycosides, lipids, melanoidins, caffeic acid, and chlorogenic acid.

And that's just the stuff that's *supposed* to be there. Coffee often contains a raft of pesticide residues and other contaminants such as nitrosamines, solvents, and mycotoxins. These carry well-defined health risks, and some are carcinogenic.[2]

Survival of the Bitterest

Caffeine is produced by more than eighty species of plants, and the reason may well be survival. As it turns out, caffeine is a biological poison used by plants as a pesticide. The caffeine gives seeds and leaves a bitter taste, which discourages their consumption by insects and animals. If predators persist in eating a caffeine-containing plant, the caffeine can cause central nervous system disruptions and even lethal side effects. Most pests soon learn to leave the plant alone.

Which is not to say that coffee is impervious to insects. On the contrary, the modern agricultural practice of growing coffee plants in dense plantations fosters the development of insect infestations. Enormous amounts of chemical pesticides and herbicides are then applied to control those infestations. In fact, coffee is the most heavily sprayed food or beverage commodity on the face of the earth.

Caffeine: Romancing the Drug

When coffee was first brought to European cities in the seventeenth century, people were repelled by its color and taste. They complained that it smelled and looked like roofing tar. But after they experienced its stimulating effect, the beverage was quickly proclaimed to be one of nature's miracles. Historians record this phenomenon without noticing the irony of what they are writing. Caffeine is, after all, a psychoactive drug, and human beings tend to crave substances that alter their state of mind—among them caffeine, morphine, nicotine, and cocaine. Indeed, all of these alkaloids are chemically related and, while they produce widely different effects, all are poisonous.

Caffeine is considered harmless simply because it is so widely used. Obviously, from a scientific perspective, that is not valid reasoning. What's more, if caffeine were proposed today as a new food additive, the FDA would never approve it. Any substance that causes such extreme reactions—heart palpitations, anxiety, panic, insomnia, and even birth defects—would be treated by the FDA as a new drug and denied status as a food additive. Yet amazingly, even health-conscious people, many of whom try to minimize their use of additives, preservatives, and drugs, consume high amounts of caffeine with no thought to the consequences.

My goal in *Caffeine Blues* is to provide you with the facts you need to make informed choices about your own caffeine consumption. Until now, reliable information about caffeine has been unavailable, and there are some intriguing reasons for that. First of all, most people are generally unaware of the amount of caffeine they are ingesting. Manufacturers can add caffeine to any food or beverage they want without disclosing the amount. (More about that in Chapter 7.) Few people know how much caffeine is in a cup of coffee or a can of soda, so they have no way of evaluating the danger. Instead, they rely on what they hear and read in the media, and that information is rarely accurate.

In his landmark review of caffeine and human health, R. M. Gilbert concludes: "If more were known about caffeine's effects, and if what is known were known more widely, the damage done by caffeine might very well appear to be intolerable."[3]

Industry Feathers in the Academic Nest

The caffeine industry has generated a tremendous amount of propaganda and disseminated it successfully throughout the scientific, medical, and public arenas. But you won't see SPONSORED BY THE CAFFEINE INDUSTRY stamped across the top. This material is invariably published by foundations and institutes with very academic-sounding names. But the fact is that many of these august bodies are heavily influenced by the caffeine industry, and so are the reports you read and hear.

The International Life Sciences Institute, for example, has been churning out studies and information to government, academic, and public institutions for decades. Few know that it is supported by the caffeine industry. In 1985, the ILSI merged with the prestigious Nutrition Foundation, an organization whose mission statement includes the acknowledgment that it is "created and supported by leading companies in the food and allied industries." Prominent among the trustees of the combined ILSI/Nutrition Foundation are executives from the Coca-Cola Company, PepsiCo, Hershey Foods, NutraSweet, and Procter & Gamble.

A Case in Point

If you were curious about the dangers of caffeine, you would undoubtedly come across a brochure entitled *What You Should Know about Caffeine.* You would find this ubiquitous brochure on information racks in hospitals, pharmacies, public health offices, or in your doctor's office. It's available through the mail and on the Internet. *What You Should Know about Caffeine* is published by the very official-sounding International Food Information Council in Washington, D.C. The brochure does not list sponsors or disclose an industry affiliation. When I requested specific details of industry sponsorship, I received another glossy color brochure that mentioned nothing about which organizations supply the funds to disseminate all this information.

After pressing the issue through several phone calls, I finally received a list of IFIC "supporters," including Pepsi-Cola, Coca-Cola, M&M/Mars Candy, NutraSweet, Nestlé, Hershey Foods, Frito-Lay, Procter & Gamble, and the Arco Chemical Company. Oddly enough, the IFIC "partners" also included the Association of Women's Health, Obstetric and Neonatal Nurses; the National Association of Pediatric Nurses Associates and Practitioners; and the Children's Advertising Review Unit of the Council of Better Business Bureaus, Inc.

This strategy perfectly illustrates the approach of the caffeine industry: aligning itself with professional health organizations and scientific foundations. What better way to head off criticism that its products are harming the American public?

Is the Information Accurate?

What You Should Know about Caffeine states: "Caffeine does not accumulate in the bloodstream or body and is normally excreted within several hours following consumption." *In fact, only about 1 percent of caffeine is excreted.* The remaining 99 percent must be detoxified by the liver, and the removal of the resulting metabolites is a slow and difficult process. In Chapter 3, you will learn that it can take up to twelve hours to detoxify a single cup of coffee.

In fact, the matter of accumulation has never been resolved. Evidence suggests that it may take up to *seven days* to decaffeinate the blood of habitual coffee drinkers.[4]

Plus, it can take three weeks or more for the body's levels of stress hormones to return to normal. If that's not accumulation, what is?

All the News That Fits, We Print

Prominent on the first page of *What You Should Know about Caffeine* is a colored box that states:

> Research in relation to cardiovascular disease, reproduction, behavior, birth defects, breast disease and cancer has identified no significant health hazard from normal caffeine consumption.

When I inquired as to exactly what "normal" consumption was, I was told 200 to 300 milligrams per day. As you will soon find out, most American adults ingest that amount before noon.

What about ingestion of more than 300 milligrams of caffeine? The IFIC doesn't say a word about that, but in the following chapters you will learn exactly how that much caffeine can damage and even destroy your health. This information has been withheld from you because until now, the loudest voices in the caffeine debate have been connected directly or indirectly to the caffeine industry.

Digging Deeper

When I asked the IFIC for scientific support for their assertion that 300 milligrams of caffeine was perfectly safe, they sent me a report published in *Food and Chemical Toxicology*. The authors of this report are both employees of the Coca-Cola Company and members of the National Soft Drink Association.[5] As you might expect, the report downplays the effects of caffeine in the American diet, using some interesting techniques.

When Is a Cup Not a Cup?

Answer: When it's a "standard" five-ounce serving. For some reason, the above authors state that a standard serving of coffee equals five fluid ounces. That way they can list the caffeine content as eighty-five milligrams per cup. (Most studies claim that a standard cup of coffee equals six fluid ounces, the amount held by a teacup—which is still far less than almost anyone actually drinks at one time.)

Likewise the "standard" soft drink serving is listed as six ounces, when all sodas come in twelve-ounce cans—and soft drink manufacturers are now heavily pushing the twenty-ounce bottle. The caffeine content of soft drinks is listed as eighteen milligrams per six-ounce serving. In reality, soft drinks contain anywhere from forty-five to seventy-two milligrams per twelve-ounce can.

"What Caffeine Problem?"

Caffeine consumption is also downplayed in the study cited above by using per capita figures, which is simply the gross amount of caffeine consumed divided by the total population. The problem, of course, is that not everyone consumes caffeine in equal amounts. Per capita figures may be useful for a discussion of economics, but not of health. If you are supposedly reviewing the safety of a substance, it is absolutely critical to consider the individuals most vulnerable to possible adverse effects.

You'll find, however, that none of the caffeine industry reports take that approach. Instead, they constantly refer to "mean" values, "average" people, and "normal" consumption. Remember the statistician who drowned trying to wade across a lake with an average depth of three feet? You have to look at reality, which is what you're going to do in Chapter 2 when you calculate the amount of caffeine you consume.

For a scientist, the word *average* raises a red flag because average figures are often useless. Even worse, the use of averages is the easiest way to manipulate data. In the coffee research reported in newspapers and magazines, you will invariably see "average consumption figures." But in a group of people with an average consumption of three cups per day, you'll find some people who drink no coffee at all, some who drink one to three cups, and some who drink six to ten cups a day. Now this might average out to three cups per person, but what good is this information? The effects of caffeine are very much dose related, and, as you have probably already guessed, the effects of one cup of coffee are quite different from the effects of four or six.

It is important to understand that the caffeine industry's "average" consumer *does not exist.* This mythical person, upon whom all their conclusions are based, is neither male nor female, weighs approximately 150 pounds, never experiences excessive stress, has perfectly functioning adrenals and liver, does not use birth control pills or any other caffeine-interacting drugs, consumes less than 300 milligrams of caffeine per day, and eats a well-balanced diet including a variety of foods high in B vitamins, calcium, magnesium, and zinc. Anyone who has a disorder that would be aggravated by caffeine is either dropped from caffeine industry studies or buried under the mountain of "mean" values.

The Search for Truth

For the past eight years, I have conducted a systematic review of the world scientific literature on caffeine. This research has taken some real detective work. It's difficult to tell what's *really* going on at first. After all, I drank coffee for over twenty years, simply because I believed like everyone else that coffee, and caffeine, had no adverse health effects.

I was in for the surprise of my life. The first thing I noticed was that much of the research on coffee was imprecise. The majority of researchers refer to the standard coffee cup as a six-ounce serving, but most people drink from mugs, which contain twelve to fourteen ounces or more. That's not to mention convenience-store coffee cups, which contain anywhere from twenty to thirty-two ounces. If you're like most people, you probably consume far more caffeine than you think you do.

Likewise, many reports on coffee failed to specify the brewing method. Six ounces of drip-filtered coffee contain about 100 milligrams of caffeine, but the same amount of percolated coffee gives you 120 milligrams, and European-style boiled coffee packs in 160 milligrams of caffeine per cup.

I began to see that the caffeine issue is rarely taken seriously. Nearly every researcher starts from the assumption that caffeine is okay. Why? Because, consciously or sub-consciously, they are influenced by the fact that they themselves depend on coffee. I have visited the offices of hundreds of scientists, professors, and clinicians. The coffee machine is as much a part of their environment as test tubes and computers. Likewise, the journalists who report health news to the public are usually heavy coffee drinkers. I'm not saying that these people are dishonest, only that information can be biased by the habits of those who make and break the news.

The Great Chain of Caffeine

It is also important to look at the chain of biochemical and behavioral events that caffeine creates, not just the immediate effects. Scientists rigorously adhere to this rule when looking at other drugs, but ignore it when studying caffeine. This error is illustrated graphically by one study on the effects of caffeine on schizophrenic patients, where regular coffee was replaced with decaf.[6] The researchers postulated that if caffeine produces detrimental psychoactive effects, the patients should improve when decaf is used instead of regular coffee. They made the switch, the patients did not improve, and so the researchers concluded that caffeine has no effect on psychiatric patients.

What's wrong with this conclusion? The study ignored the chain of events that result from caffeine withdrawal. Here a group of hospitalized schizophrenic patients, who are used to drinking three to eight cups of coffee a day, are switched to decaf without their knowledge. These people are going to have serious withdrawal reactions, including disorientation, irritability, anxiety, and depression. Obviously, they will not show signs of improvement. How could they? Most of them probably had splitting headaches from caffeine withdrawal! Yet the research was published and is frequently used to support the erroneous view that caffeine produces no negative psychoactive effects.

It gets worse. These same researchers introduced decaf a second time and *did* see behavioral improvements. Did they recognize the likelihood of a decreased withdrawal reaction? No way—instead, they stated that these improvements were probably a result of coincidence.

A Matter of Interpretation

I must say right away that I also found investigators who did an excellent job at analyzing the behavioral effects of caffeine ingestion by schizophrenics. One extremely well-designed study documented significant increases in thought disorder and psychosis after caffeine administration. The investigators also found that caffeine increased blood pressure and stress hormone levels in the patient group.[7]

This is important information for anyone involved in psychiatric care, but how the issue of caffeine and mental health is resolved depends upon which study is read and how the reader wishes to interpret the information. When I brought the latter study to the attention of a leading psychologist, he acknowledged that caffeine can cause significant increases in stress hormone levels but concluded, "A cup of coffee is no more stressful than watching a suspense thriller on TV."

Can you see the profound error of this response? It

looks blindly at the short-term consequences of caffeine use and ignores the real issue, which is *the effects of long-term use*. After all, what psychologist would condone the viewing of five suspense thrillers every day, year after year? Yet that analogy accurately describes the body's hormonal response to regular caffeine consumption.

More Flawed Research: Caffeine and Hypertension

Another common mistake in caffeine research has to do with the relationship of caffeine to hypertension (high blood pressure). I found numerous studies in which hypertensive patients were taken off coffee. After a week or two, when blood pressure did not drop, investigators concluded that caffeine has no significant effect on blood pressure. This is absurd because it may take three weeks or more after withdrawal from caffeine before stress hormones return to normal. Evaluating blood pressure over the first one or two weeks is meaningless.

What's Real for You?

If you look at the way real people consume coffee and soft drinks, you find, first of all, that most consume a great deal more than 300 milligrams of caffeine per day. There have been studies that measure the caffeine content of beverages as people actually consume them. One such study, published in *Food and Chemical Toxicology*, found that the caffeine content of a six-ounce cup of drip, filtered coffee (the type most people drink) ranged from 37 to 148 milligrams.[8] A survey conducted by the Addiction Research Foundation found that a "cup" of coffee, as defined by the individual drinker, could contain as much as 333 milligrams of caffeine.[9]

This conflicting data once again demonstrates that the idea of "normal" caffeine consumption is meaningless. Some scientific studies suggest that a 170-pound man could successfully detoxify 300 milligrams of caffeine over the course of a day without serious damage to his body. Theoretically, this may be possible—but not if he is under any significant degree of stress. Moreover, a 110-pound woman is almost certain to experience significant adverse effects from that amount of caffeine. And for anyone under a great deal of stress, even one cup may be enough to trigger the negative effects of caffeine.

Obviously, caffeine intake needs to be evaluated on an individual basis. In the chapters that follow, you will see that the effects and dangers of caffeine depend upon a host of variables, including gender, weight, age, stress level, general health, and medications. What's more, caffeine may affect the same person differently at different times. The only way to safeguard your health and the well-being of your family is to inform yourself. A great place to start is by taking the "Are You Addicted?" tests in the next chapter.

CHAPTER 2

Are You Addicted?

How Much Is Too Much?

In the old days, coffee was served in teacups that sit on saucers. That size cup holds six ounces of beverage, which is considered the standard-size cup by researchers and the coffee industry. However, when I ask patients how much coffee they drink and they say, "Oh, no more than three cups a day," I invariably find that means three *mugs* a day at fourteen ounces apiece, or the equivalent of seven cups of coffee. In most coffee shops, a "normal" cup of coffee is fourteen ounces and a large cup is twenty ounces. Thus, one large cup equals 3.3 cups of coffee.

One of my clients told me that he only drank one cup of coffee a day. It turned out to be one of those giant thirty-two-ounce convenience-store mugs with the vented cover for drinking while you drive. This man (and millions like him) consumed nearly 500 milligrams of caffeine on his way to work on an empty stomach. No wonder there's so much conflict and tension at the office. By the time they get to work, these coffee-inhaling employees are wired and ready to fly off the handle.

There's no doubt that the damage done by caffeine is very much dose related. But it's impossible to make general, blanket statements about how much caffeine is okay and how much is dangerous, since caffeine's effects are different for each person. Understanding the effects of your own caffeine ingestion requires self-knowledge and experimentation. As you reflect on the material presented here, most likely you will see yourself in one of the examples or case histories. As you read, keep an open mind and consider the possibility that how well you live, *and even how long you live,* depend to a significant degree on the amount of caffeine you consume. This book provides the information you need, but the rest is up to you.

Obviously, there are many factors affecting longevity and health, but none is easier to modify than caffeine intake. In my clinical practice, I have counseled more than 9,000 patients and kept careful records regarding their compliance and level of success. Of all my recommendations—including weight loss, dietary change, exercise, and stress management—no single factor matched the impact of caffeine reduction.

Again, it's not that all those other things are unimportant. On the contrary, I believe that exercise and a balanced diet are critical to optimum health, and I've devoted my career to making those goals obtainable. But the truth is, getting people to make significant changes in diet or exercise is extremely difficult. Research shows that even with careful supervision, compliance is well below 30 percent. On the other hand, getting off caffeine (at least with my Off the Bean program) is relatively easy, and the rewards are often immediate and dramatic. Over 80 percent of the people who've tried the Off the Bean program have stuck with it—and have experienced tremendous health benefits as a result!

What Your Doctor Doesn't Know Can Hurt You

Until now, people had no way of evaluating their caffeine intake and the harm it can do. Remember that the initial stages of caffeine damage are often silent—just like lung damage from smoking or cardiovascular disease from a high-fat diet. Also be aware that the information you need about caffeine is not likely to come from your doctor.

Consider the guidelines given to physicians in the medical literature. A typical example appeared in *Postgraduate Medicine*, in which doctors were advised that caffeine can cause abnormal heart rhythm.[1] The article, citing a report entitled "Caffeine and Arrhythmias: What Are the Risks?" stated that "about 80% of American adults drink three to four cups of coffee each day." It then went on to explain that each cup contains between 60 and 150 milligrams of caffeine. The logical conclusion from this information is that many American adults are consuming 500 to 600 milligrams of caffeine from coffee per day. The bullet points of the article inform doctors that:

Point 1: "Consuming less than 300 mg of caffeine per day does not seem likely to produce significant arrhythmias."

Comment: We've already learned that most Americans consume more than 300 milligrams of caffeine per day from coffee alone (remember the six-ounce cup?), not to mention additional caffeine from soft drinks, medications, and other sources. And what exactly is significant arrhythmia? If your heart fails to maintain normal beats, you are in mortal danger, period.

Point 2: "People with underlying heart disease probably should avoid consuming more than 300 mg of caffeine per day since significant increases in arrhythmias have been reported after consumption of higher amounts."

Comment: Good advice, but (A) people with underlying heart disease often do not know that they have heart disease; (B) people have no way of following this advice since manufacturers are not required to list the amount of caffeine in their products.

Do you see the folly of this approach? First of all, most people already consume over 300 milligrams of caffeine per day. What's more, the 300-milligram level does not take into consideration the myriad factors that influence how caffeine affects individual people. One person who consumes 300 milligrams of caffeine might only experience disturbed sleep, while another person might experience severe anxiety, depression, or dramatically increased risk for heart disease. Women are affected by caffeine far more than men. Age, overall health, weight, and a host of other lifestyle factors also enter the picture. How can you determine your own personal risk level? You can start by figuring out your caffeine quotient—exactly how much caffeine you presently consume, and how it is affecting your life.

Is Caffeine Hurting You?

If you are a regular caffeine user, chances are high that the drug is affecting the quality of your life right now. You probably depend on the stimulating "lift" to energize your body and clear your mind. Your total daily intake of caffeine comes from a variety of sources—not just coffee, but also tea, cocoa, soft drinks, medications, and chocolate. In fact, if you're like most Americans, you find it hard to get through the day without multiple hits of caffeine. You are probably addicted.

If you object to that statement, take a few minutes to complete the following self-tests. You have nothing to lose. If caffeine's not a problem for you, great. But if it is, confronting the addiction is the only way to do something about it. This book will help you evaluate the effects caffeine has on your life and, most importantly, show you how to achieve far greater levels of energy and vitality without the drug.

Test I: Your Caffeine Intake

In the first column, enter the number of servings, then multiply to get your total caffeine intake from each source. Figures given for coffee and tea are based on a six-ounce serving. *Remember that most coffee mugs or cups hold twelve to fourteen ounces. A "large" coffee cup holds twenty ounces or more, so be sure to calculate accordingly.* Amounts of caffeine listed for each type of beverage are averages; variations may occur from product to product.

The amount of caffeine in common medications may surprise you. However, according to the FDA, nearly 1,000 prescription drugs and 2,000 over-the-counter medications contain caffeine—anywhere from 30 to 200 milligrams per tablet or capsule.[2]

Servings per day	Item	Mgs. Caffeine	Total
Coffee	Drip brewed	100 mg. per 6 oz.	_____
(6-oz. cup)	Percolated	120 mg. per 6 oz.	_____
(*A mug holds*	Instant	90 mg. per 6 oz.	_____
12–14 oz.; a	Brewed decaf	5 mg. per 6 oz.	_____
large cup holds	Instant decaf	3 mg. per 6 oz.	_____
20 oz. or more.)			
Tea	Green	35 mg. per 6 oz.	_____
(6-oz. cup)	(5-minute steep)		
	Black	70 mg. per 6 oz.	_____
	(5-minute steep)		
	Canned ice tea	35 mg./12-oz. can	_____
Cocoa	Cocoa beverages	13 mg. per 6 oz.	_____
Soft Drinks	Leading colas	45 mg.	_____
(12-oz. can)	(diet and reg.)		
	Mountain Dew	54 mg.	_____
	Josta (PepsiCo)	58 mg.	_____
	Surge (Coca-Cola)	51 mg.	_____
	Jolt cola	72 mg.	_____

ARE YOU ADDICTED?

Servings per day	Item	Mgs. Caffeine	Total
Medications per tablet)	Anacin	32 mg.	_____
	Dristan	16 mg.	_____
	Dexatrim	200 mg.	_____
	Excedrin	65 mg.	_____
	Midol	32 mg.	_____
	No-Doz (reg.)	100 mg.	_____
	Vivarin	200 mg.	_____
	Vanquish	33 mg.	_____
Chocolate[*]	Milk chocolate	6 mg. per ounce	_____
	Baking chocolate	35 mg. per ounce	_____
	Small candy bar	25 mg. per bar	_____
Total Daily Caffeine Intake			_____

[*]Although chocolate does not contain a great deal of caffeine, it contains high amounts of a related compound known as theobromine. If you add the stimulant effects of both caffeine and theobromine, chocolate has the stimulating power of forty milligrams of caffeine per one-ounce piece.

Sources: FDA, Industry publications, J. J. Barone and H. Roberts, "Human Consumption of Caffeine," in P. D. Dews (ed.), *Caffeine: Perspectives from Recent Research* (New York: Springer-Verlag, 1984), pp. 59–73; and R. M. Gilbert, "Caffeine Consumption," in G. A. Spiller (ed.), *The Methyl-xanthine Beverages and Foods: Chemistry, Consumption and Health Effects* (New York: Alan R. Liss, 1984), pp. 185–214.

YOUR CAFFEINE QUOTIENT

"Caffeinism" is a state of chronic toxicity resulting from excess caffeine consumption. Caffeinism usually combines physical addiction with a wide range of debilitating effects, most notably anxiety, irritability, mood swings, sleep disturbance, depression, and fatigue. Use your "Total Daily Caffeine Intake" from the previous page to determine if you are a victim of caffeinism.

- If your caffeine quotient is less than 100 milligrams per day, it is highly unlikely that you are a caffeine addict.
- If your total is between 100 and 300 milligrams per day, you're in the "danger zone." Disruption of sleep patterns begins at this level, and certain heart disease risk factors may be increased.
- If your total is 300 to 600 milligrams per day, you are undoubtedly experiencing some degree of mental and physical addiction to caffeine. Research shows an almost 200 percent increase of risk for ulcers and fibrocystic disease at this level.
- Intake of 600 to 900 milligrams per day indicates almost certain addiction. At this level, your mood and energy levels are severely affected. Research suggests that your risk of heart attack may be twice that of non–caffeine users. If you are a premenopausal woman, your chance of maintaining optimal iron levels is slim.
- At 900 milligrams or more per day, you're a caffeine addict—hook, line, and sinker. At this level of dependency, all heart disease risk factors are significantly increased, as are the risks for stroke, psychological disorders, and gastrointestinal disease. You may need medical help to kick the habit.

"Although infrequently diagnosed, caffeinism is thought to afflict as many as one person in ten of the population."

Source: Jack E. James and Keryn P. Stirling, "Caffeine: A Summary of Some of the Known and Suspected Deleterious Effects of Habitual Use," *British Journal of Addiction*, 1983;78:251–58.

Test II: Caffeine's Effects on Your Body

Do you experience any of the following on a recurrent or frequent basis?

	YES	NO
1. Energy swings or periods of fatigue during the day	___	___
2. Mood swings or periods of depression during the day	___	___
3. Headaches	___	___
4. Gastrointestinal distress; cramping, diarrhea	___	___
5. Constipation and/or dependence on caffeine for bowel movement	___	___
6. Tension or stiffness in your neck, shoulders, jaw, hands, legs, or stomach	___	___
7. Premenstrual syndrome; menstrual irregularity, cramps, sore breasts	___	___
8. Painful/sensitive lumps in the breast	___	___
9. Insomnia	___	___
10. Clenching the jaw or grinding teeth during sleep	___	___
11. Anxiety	___	___

	YES	NO
12. Irritability, including inappropriate "fits" of anger	___	___
13. Involuntary movement in the leg (restless leg syndrome)	___	___
14. Irregular or rapid heartbeat	___	___
15. Light-headedness/dizziness	___	___
16. Wake up feeling tired	___	___
17. Generalized pain (back pain, stomach pain, muscle aches)	___	___
18. High blood pressure	___	___
19. Ulcers	___	___
20. Anemia	___	___
21. Shortness of breath	___	___
22. Difficulty concentrating and/or memory loss	___	___
23. Ringing in the ears	___	___
24. Coldness in the extremities, especially fingertips	___	___
25. Hand tremor	___	___

If you have 6 to 7 "yes" answers, caffeine is a problem for you. Decreasing or eliminating caffeine intake will significantly improve your health.

If you have 8 to 10 "yes" answers, caffeine is a serious problem. Decreasing or eliminating caffeine is an urgent need.

If you have 12 or more "yes" answers, your caffeine intake represents a critical health risk that may actually decrease your life expectancy. Act now to take control of your life and health.

Dr. Fred Sheftell, director of the New England Center for Headache, states: "It's not unusual for us to find people who are taking 1,000 mg of caffeine or more per day." He notes that adverse side effects have been reported from as little as 250 milligrams per day.[3]

Test III: Caffeine's Effects on Your Nervous System

Caffeine has been found to impair motor steadiness in neuropsychological tests.[4] Here is a simple way to evaluate this effect without expensive laboratory procedures:

Sitting up in a chair, extend your arm straight out in front of you, locking the elbow, palm down. Look at the tips of your fingers. If there is any noticeable trembling, chances are that caffeine has already damaged your nervous system.

In Chapters 3 and 4, we will discuss how caffeine disrupts biochemical message centers in the brain known as receptors. Human and animal data suggest that dopamine and benzodiazepine receptors are involved in hand tremor,[5, 6] and the condition is common in both habitual and casual coffee drinkers.[7, 8] The good news is that this damage can be repaired, but not until you get your caffeine intake under control. In Chapter 10, you'll see that it's not as difficult as you might think.

Test IV: Caffeine's Effects on Your Muscles

Muscle tension is hard to evaluate. Many times, we don't even know we're tense until we get a headache, or someone places their hands on our shoulders and we wince. Tension in the jaw muscles, however, is fairly easy to measure.

1. Open your mouth as wide as you can, then close slowly. Do you hear any popping or cracking? This is often a sign of problems with jaw alignment known as temporomandibular joint dysfunction (TMJD). TMJD affects millions of Americans, contributes to headache and a raft of other disorders, and is positively associated with stress and caffeine intake.[9] That's because caffeine and stress cause a tightening of the jaw muscles that contributes to misalignment of the jaw on the skull. Teeth clenching and grinding (bruxism) at night are also related to stress and caffeine.[10]

2. Now open your mouth wide again, and this time try to insert your first three fingers held vertically. (Or use a wine cork.) This is another simple test to see if you are holding significant tension in your jaw muscles. Reduced jaw mobility is a classic sign of chronic tension exacerbated by caffeine.

The Four Warning Signs of Caffeine Dependence

The most common response I hear from people who have eliminated caffeine from their lives is their surprise at how much better they feel. I know what you're thinking: "How could they feel better? Every time I try to quit coffee I feel like I've been hit by a truck." That's because caffeine is an addictive drug with a very well-defined withdrawal syndrome.

I'm not going to split hairs about whether people are truly addicted or just dependent on the drug. Studies have found conclusively that caffeine produces classic signs of addiction.[11] And you don't have to consume huge amounts of coffee to become addicted. In one recent study, the median daily intake of the caffeine-dependent group was 357 milligrams, and 19 percent of them consumed less than the U.S. daily average.[12] Here is how the scientists conducting that study made the diagnosis of caffeine dependence. See if it describes how you feel.

1. WITHDRAWAL

Reducing the dose or stopping the drug altogether produces well-defined symptoms, which may include:

- Headache
- Depression
- Profound fatigue
- Irritability
- Disorientation
- Increased muscle tension
- Nausea
- Vomiting

Ninety-four percent of the caffeine-dependent subjects experienced some of these withdrawal symptoms.

2. DEPENDENCE

Researchers defined dependence as consuming the beverage "despite knowledge of a persistent or recurrent physical or psychological problem that is likely to have been caused or exacerbated by caffeine."

Ninety-four percent of the caffeine-dependent subjects experienced this behavior.

3. INABILITY TO QUIT

This was defined as a "persistent desire or unsuccessful efforts to cut down or control use."

Eighty-one percent of the caffeine-dependent group found that they were unable to reduce or discontinue drinking caffeine-containing beverages.

4. TOLERANCE

The body develops a tolerance for caffeine so that greater amounts are required to produce the same level of stimulation.

Seventy-five percent of the caffeine-dependent group reported tolerance.

Source: E. C. Strain et al., "Caffeine Dependence Syndrome: Evidence from Case Histories and Experimental Evaluations," *Journal of the American Medical Association,* 1994;272:1043–48.

Caffeinism: It Could Happen to You!

In over a decade of practice as a clinical nutritionist, I have seen firsthand, with thousands of clients, that caffeine is a health hazard. Anxiety, muscle aches, PMS, headaches, heartburn, insomnia, and irritability are the most common symptoms, and they can usually be lessened or eliminated simply by avoiding caffeine. That's good news for most people.

However, if that's all caffeine has done to you, you're lucky. Others are not so fortunate. Like the woman whose baby was born with a heart defect because no one told her to avoid caffeine during pregnancy. Or the man who underwent three surgical operations and nearly had his stomach removed because his ulcers would not heal. No one told him to avoid coffee. And what about people misdiagnosed as neurotic or even psychotic, who spend years and small fortunes in psychotherapy—all because no one asked them about their caffeine intake?

To those who claim that caffeine is harmless, I say look at the facts—and, more important, look at your life. Your health is your most valuable possession, and life is short. I am convinced that to enjoy life to its fullest we must maintain health on three levels: physical, mental, and emotional. At each one of these three levels, caffeine is an adversary.

Caffeine versus Physical Vitality

On the physical level, we need a steady source of energy to accomplish our goals. Nothing is more frustrating than to be motivated, to have a great plan, but no energy to carry it out. When I ask patients about their reasons for drinking coffee, the most common response is: "I need the energy." The irony, as you will see in Chapter 3, is that caffeine is a major cause of fatigue. Depending on caffeine to get you through the day might work for a while, but in the long run it will make your dreams harder and harder to achieve.

To see what I mean, try this experiment. Clench your fist tightly. Hold it closed and very tight for thirty seconds. What happens to your arm and hand? They get tired. This exercise illustrates what happens to your body when you ingest caffeine. First you feel strong, but soon afterwards you feel weak. That's because caffeine doesn't give you energy—*it creates tension,* and the ultimate result of tension is always fatigue. You felt the result of squeezing your fist, which only involves a few muscles. Imagine the energy drain created by muscle tension throughout your body after ingesting caffeine.

Caffeine versus Mental Vitality

On the mental level, we need to be consistently alert and aware to function effectively in our daily lives. As you will see in Chapter 4, caffeine puts you on a roller-coaster ride where mental clarity alternates with periods of confusion, depression, and lethargy. You'll also learn that caffeine does nothing to enhance learning, but actually impairs memory and cognition.

When patients relate their coffee stories to me, a common pattern usually emerges. They started drinking coffee occasionally, either as a morning "wake-up" or to stay up late. Gradually, they found themselves reaching for coffee or cola beverages throughout the day just to stay alert. In time, the habit became an addiction, with their only dependable mental energy coming from the coffeepot. This is sad, because the coffee habit has a steep downside. We pay dearly for those "borrowed" periods of clarity by sacrificing our true mental vitality.

"There is no doubt that the excitation of the central nervous system produced by large amounts of caffeine is followed by depression."

Source: J. Murdoch Ritchie in *The Pharmacological Basis of Therapeutics*, Goodman and Gilman eds.

Vitality Is Our Birthright

What we must remember is that vitality is not something that disappears in adulthood. We throw it away by becoming sedentary and damaging our bodies and minds with caffeine. We set ourselves up for a life of ups and downs, when each of us is capable of maintaining a high level of physical and mental vitality well into our advanced years. A healthy child doesn't require caffeine to get out of bed in the morning, and there is no reason why you can't experience the same boundless energy of your youth!

But first you must stop punishing your body and mind with caffeine. Is it worth it? The answer is an unqualified *yes*. Patients who have followed the Off the Bean program outlined in Chapter 10 have found their bodies healthier and minds sharper at fifty-five than they were at twenty-five.

Of course, total health also requires emotional stability, peace of mind, and an optimistic attitude. The effects of caffeine diminish these qualities. Relationships with friends, partners, and co-workers depend on harmony, which is destroyed by anxiety, irritability, and tension. Caffeine not only intensifies the stress in our lives, but makes us less able to cope.

If I had a magic wand, I would instantly remove the stress from my clients' lives. Until that magic wand appears, I will do everything I can to help them control their caffeine intake. For some, regaining mental vitality after caffeine means learning a relaxation technique such as those described in Chapter 10. For others, psychological counseling is recommended. But everyone needs to start by taking a close look at their caffeine intake.

Caffeine and Anxiety

For five years, I worked in a team practice with physicians and psychotherapists. Often, the psychological evaluation would include one or more anxiety syndromes and the recommendation was for counseling. I would point out that the person was consuming excessive amounts of caffeine and request a trial month off caffeine prior to therapy sessions. In about 50 percent of cases, the anxiety syndrome would resolve with caffeine withdrawal alone.

Of course, I recognize that counseling can play a vital role in restoring wholeness and peace of mind. It's just that counseling a patient for anxiety who is drinking coffee is like trying to fill a leaky bucket.

Caffeine and Alcohol: Psychoactive Cousins

The undeniable fact is that caffeine is a psychoactive drug, affecting mind, mood, and behavior. While the effects of caffeine are obvious but not always recognized, the effects of alcohol, another psychoactive substance, are easy to spot. We all know how intoxicated individuals behave. When they are involved in automobile accidents, their blood alcohol is measured and they may face criminal charges. No one would think of measuring blood caffeine levels after an accident because there is no data to suggest that caffeine impairs performance.

I would like to suggest, however, that the biochemical and behavioral changes brought about by caffeine may very well contribute to auto accidents. In the following chapters, I will present clear evidence that caffeine disturbs normal decision-making processes. Is it far-fetched to assert that ill-advised lane changes, tailgating, speeding, rage, and stress contribute to auto accidents? Watch your driving the next time you're "wired" on caffeine and tell me I'm wrong.

There *Is* Life after Caffeine

Life after caffeine does not have to be dull. In fact, there are delicious and very satisfying alternatives, and I'm not talking about pallid teas, decaf, and instant coffee "substitutes." You'll learn about rich, robust, and healthful beverages that brew like coffee but contain no caffeine. Likewise, life after coffee does not have to be lethargic. Breakthrough research in human metabolism and brain biochemistry has made it possible for you to enjoy greater energy and alertness without coffee than you ever experienced when you were "on the drug."

You'll read about natural alternatives to caffeine that actually enhance metabolic energy production while decreasing the tension in your body. The difference, once you make the switch, is astounding. You'll also learn how to repair your nervous system, manage stress, and improve your energy production naturally. Finally, you'll learn how to obtain the quantity and quality of energy you need for the rest of your long, healthy life. You'll discover that life without caffeine has the potential to be better than you ever dreamed possible!

CHAPTER 3

Caffeine and Your Body

If five million people do a foolish thing, it is still a foolish thing.

—Ancient Chinese proverb

Ageless Wisdom Is Sometimes Unwise

Today nearly 90 percent of American adults drink caffeinated beverages. This includes the scientists who explore caffeine's effects and the journalists who report the scientists' findings. The result is that Americans are misinformed because no one is willing to say, "This is a foolish thing." In this chapter, we are going to look at the science of caffeine. Before we begin, I'd like to remind you that no scientific study has ever shown that coffee is *good* for you. The discussion only concerns the degree to which it will harm you.

The scientific method is an extraordinary systematic process for discovering what is real. In other areas of human endeavor, exactly the opposite is true. Take advertising, for example. Here is an entire system of communication designed not to reveal the truth, but to manipulate behavior. Sometimes it's absurd. A cigarette brand, for example, is advertised as being "alive with pleasure" even though everyone knows that cigarettes are the leading cause of preventable death.

Isn't it interesting, then, to learn that most people are influenced far more by advertising than they are by science? In other words, we tend to make decisions that affect our lives and the lives of our children based not upon what is real, but upon habit, or upon what other people want us to think. When it comes to coffee, the most common reaction I hear is, "How can it be bad for you? People have been drinking coffee for centuries."

To a scientist, this observation is meaningless. History is filled with cases where millions of people made serious mistakes. There are herbs in China, for example, that have been used medicinally for thousands of years, and are still being used to treat sinus congestion. But repeated use of these herbs over time can cause cancer of the nose and throat. Epidemiologists (scientists studying the distribution of disease in populations) have estimated that this habit has caused premature and painful death for millions of Chinese people. Clearly, great numbers of people *can* be wrong, especially when they don't know the facts.

Facing Reality

Today, nearly 100 million American adults drink three or more cups of coffee each day.[1] So what is reality? Is coffee "good to the last drop," or is it a powerful drug with dangerous side effects that needs to be used with caution and moderation? To discover the truth you need science, and you need to be willing to dismiss the advertising and hype surrounding the beverage. Forget the schmaltzy pictures of two female friends sharing a special moment over coffee. Those two women are increasing their risk for heart disease, osteoporosis, anemia, PMS, panic attacks, and fibrocystic breast disease.

You should also question the sanity of common statements that we hear from friends, celebrities, and co-workers. In the movie *Shadow of a Doubt,* Joseph Cotten's famous line was, "I can't face the world in the morning. I must have coffee before I can speak." Now, substitute for the word *coffee* any other drug, say amphetamines. If a person said he or she can't face the world without amphetamines, we'd call him or her an addict. We'd whisk the person off to rehab and maybe even throw him in jail. But because coffee is a drug we consume ourselves, we wink and nod and say, "Yeah, ain't it the truth!"

Biochemical Individuality

When it comes to nailing down the precise effects of a drug, scientists always run up against the fact that people are different. Because of what is termed "biochemical individuality," the appropriate dose of a drug for one person may be an overdose for someone else. Physicians need to make educated guesses when prescribing many of their medications, taking into account the patient's size and age in order to arrive at the optimal dose. Often, further adjustments are made during treatment.

This is especially true with caffeine. We know that a single 100-milligram dose (about six ounces of regular coffee) can cause palpitations and ringing in the ears in one person, while another may experience only a pleasant boost in alertness. This is because caffeine, like all drugs, has to be detoxified by the body, and the organs responsible for that feat perform their jobs at varying rates of speed and efficiency. We know that caffeine is rapidly and completely absorbed by everyone. Getting rid of the toxin, however, is another story.

Caffeine's Cumulative Effect

Scientists measure the rate of which a drug is eliminated or broken down by its "half-life": the time it takes the body to remove one-half of the dose. With caffeine, this varies widely from person to person, depending on age, sex, general health, weight, metabolic rate, and current medications. Genetic factors also affect the rate at which the body eliminates caffeine.[2] Thus, the half-life of a single dose of caffeine can range from three to twelve hours. Obviously, then, in real life, there is a very important cumulative effect, since most coffee drinkers have additional cups before the first dose wears off.

This cumulative phenomenon is overlooked by most researchers. They take a group of people, give them a quantity of caffeine, and administer various tests. When the people don't have heart attacks, they make the absurd statement that coffee is safe. Or they report various side effects, but conclude that coffee in "moderation" is safe. *In reality, no one—not a scientist, your doctor, or your psychic aunt—can tell you how much coffee is safe for you.* Nor can you rely on symptoms like sweaty palms and rapid heartbeat. These symptoms tend to go away as the body adjusts to the drug. What does not go away, however, is the damage being done to your adrenals, blood vessels, breasts, brain, gastrointestinal tract, DNA, immune system, and bones. And all of that is silent.

In the remainder of this chapter we take a close look at twelve critical points—organs, glands, and processes in the body where the cumulative effects of caffeine become most evident over time.

Critical Point #1: Your Liver

The liver performs an enormous range of tasks. On physiology exams, it was a common joke among my colleagues that for any question, you could simply write "the liver" and be correct most of the time. The liver is in charge of collecting and distributing nearly every nutrient from every bite of food you will ever eat. It's also primarily responsible for removing anything from the bloodstream that you don't want. Sometimes that takes real ingenuity. Faced with a substance it cannot chemically reduce or eliminate (like DDT), the liver breaks up the dangerous material into tiny fragments and distributes it to remote areas of the body in order to decrease the concentration of the poison in any one site.

Fortunately, the caffeine we consume is also distributed throughout the body and, unlike DDT, the liver *does* have the machinery to break it down. When we drink a cup of coffee, however, an enormous amount of the toxin is dumped in the bloodstream all at once. Caffeine is rapidly absorbed by every organ and tissue in the body and diffuses into body fluids, including saliva, semen, breast milk, and amniotic fluid. Caffeine goes everywhere and easily crosses the blood-brain barrier. Only then does the liver begin the task of reducing this troublesome toxin, and it's not easy.

Usually, drug detoxification is a job shared by the liver and kidneys. The kidneys remove what they can and excrete it in the urine. Not so with caffeine. The kidneys try to get rid of the molecule, but it is reabsorbed into the bloodstream before it reaches the urinary tract. Thus, the burden falls entirely on the liver.

Remember that coffee contains a host of chemicals, not just caffeine, among them a group of extremely toxic compounds known as polycyclic aromatic hydrocarbons (PAHs). You might remember them as the cancer-causing agents isolated from barbecued meat. The liver also has to deal with all the aldehydes, alcohols, and sulfides found in coffee. Caffeine alone is broken down into more than twenty-five by-products or metabolites, the primary ones being paraxanthine, theobromine, and theophylline. Interestingly, each of these metabolites has its own biochemistry and effect on the body.

A DEADLY DUO: CAFFEINE AND YOUR MEDICINE CABINET

At any one time, more than 36 percent of American adults are using some prescription or OTC (over-the-counter) medication. Among the elderly, that percentage is much higher. Hundreds of these drugs contain caffeine but, more important, many of them, like birth control pills and cimetidine (brand name Tagamet), interfere with the liver's ability to detoxify the chemicals found in coffee.[3] Common antibiotics such as ciprofloxacin (brand name Cipro) also inhibit the detoxification of caffeine,[4] and researchers warn that ingestion of caffeine while taking such drugs can increase risk for liver disease, cardiac arrhythmias, and even epilepsy.[5]

Other pharmaceutical drugs have been shown to increase blood levels of caffeine by more than 600 percent.[6] Later in this chapter you will learn just how dangerous and damaging this can be to the body. In turn, coffee can drastically affect the metabolism, blood level, and detoxification of pharmaceutical drugs, including a laundry list of commonly consumed medications.[7-9] When your doctor prescribes a drug for *any* condition, it is important to ask about possible interactions with caffeine.

What's more, even moderate liver disease can remarkably reduce caffeine clearance. Individuals with disorders involving the liver (e.g., alcoholic cirrhosis, hepatitis) can have elevated blood levels of caffeine for two to six days from a single cup of coffee.[10]

For cigarette smokers, on the other hand, caffeine clearance is accelerated. Apparently, in a heroic effort to rid the body of the potent carcinogens delivered by tobacco smoke, the liver produces more enzymes capable of detoxifying caffeine. This interaction of powerful toxins has two important results. First, smokers will tend to drink more coffee than nonsmokers in an effort to achieve the same level of stimulation. And second, smokers who drink coffee have the deck stacked against them when they try to quit. That's because without the cigarette stimulation, their caffeine detox system slows down, resulting in enormous increases in blood caffeine levels (up to 200 percent).[11] As you can imagine, this produces severe anxiety, nervousness, irritability, and insomnia. Added to the symptoms of nicotine withdrawal, it's enough to send even a highly motivated person running back to Marlboro country.

The take-home message here is: If you're going to quit smoking (the most positive step you can take to improve your health), it is highly advisable that you decrease your caffeine intake at the same time. In fact, I recommend that you quit coffee altogether (see Chapter 10, "Off the Bean") because studies show that removing caffeine will greatly increase your chance of quitting cigarettes for good.

RESEARCH CAPSULE
Caffeine Does Not Help Weight Loss

There is a popular belief, most likely derived from the inclusion of caffeine in diet pills, that caffeine is an aid to weight loss. This notion is debunked in Chapter 8, but I mention it here in order to clear up yet another popular myth: drinking coffee when you quit cigarettes does not help prevent weight gain, either. This concept was carefully tested in a controlled scientific experiment, and caffeine (even when combined with another stimulant known as ephedrine) provided no benefit. There was no difference in success rate, weight gain, cravings, or withdrawal symptoms between the caffeine and placebo groups.

Source: J. Norregard, S. Jorgensen, K. L. Mikkelsen et al., "The Effect of Ephedrine Plus Caffeine on Smoking Cessation and Postcessation Weight Gain," *Clinical Pharmacology and Therapeutics*, December 1996;60(6):679–86.

Critical Point #2: Your Adenosine Receptors

Caffeine and its breakdown products (collectively called methylxanthines) have a number of effects on the body.

First, they disrupt the normal function of adenosine receptors, biochemical control switches found throughout the brain, kidneys, gastrointestinal tract, cardiovascular system, and respiratory system. Now stay with me here; this sounds complicated, but it's important, and by the time you finish this page, you'll know more about the biochemistry of coffee than most MDs.

Have you ever inserted the wrong key in a door and found that the key fit just fine but it wouldn't unlock the door? That's what caffeine does in an adenosine receptor. It fits, but does not perform the adenosine function. Now imagine that you're standing there and you can't get the wrong key *out* of the lock. You are thus prevented from entering the room. Likewise, when caffeine plugs an adenosine receptor, an important biochemical message that was supposed to be sent to the cell is not delivered.

In the brain, adenosine dampens or slows down neuron firing. It acts like a fuse box to prevent your circuits from getting overloaded. When caffeine inactivates this control mechanism, your neuron circuits keep firing, and you feel alert. The problem is, your circuits keep firing, and firing, and firing. . . .

Critical Point #3: The Stress Response

It doesn't take a genius to see that there might be a downside to all of this neuron activity. In fact, uncontrolled neuron firing creates an emergency situation, which triggers the pituitary gland in the brain to secrete ACTH (adrenocorticotrophic hormone). ACTH tells the adrenal glands to pump out stress hormones—the next major side effect of caffeine. A single 250-milligram dose of caffeine (the equivalent of about 2½ six-ounce cups of coffee) has been shown to increase levels of the stress hormone epinephrine (commonly known as adrenaline) by more than 200 percent.[12] Caffeine also stimulates the production of norepinephrine, another stress hormone that acts directly on the brain and nervous system. Epinephrine and norepinephrine are responsible for increased heart rate, increased blood pressure, and that "emergency" feeling. In fact, the emergency is quite real. Caffeine can trigger a classic fight-or-flight stress reaction with all of the results listed in Illustration 1.

ANATOMY OF THE FIGHT-OR-FLIGHT RESPONSE

Caffeine can produce a cascade of physical and emotional changes as a result of increased stress hormones. This fight-or-flight response is hardwired into all animals as a survival mechanism.

NOWHERE TO RUN

Take a moment to consider a "then and now" scenario. Remember that the fight-or-flight reaction was in great part responsible for our survival as a species. For 1.6 million years, this neuroendocrine response gave us increased strength, stamina, and speed when we needed it. But today, the same trigger mechanism is killing us. That's because even though our bodies haven't changed *at all* in the last 25,000 years, everything else has.

Our ancestors needed every ounce of energy their bodies could produce to deal with sudden danger (a saber-toothed tiger, for example). Today stress is different: a crammed schedule, looming deadlines, lost car keys, or an unfair boss. And while we may have excellent coping

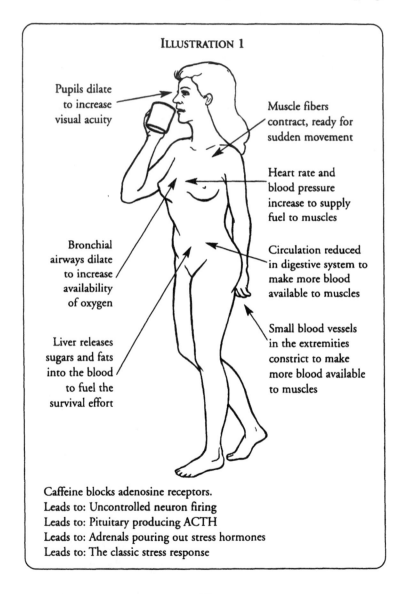

ILLUSTRATION 1

Pupils dilate to increase visual acuity

Muscle fibers contract, ready for sudden movement

Heart rate and blood pressure increase to supply fuel to muscles

Bronchial airways dilate to increase availability of oxygen

Circulation reduced in digestive system to make more blood available to muscles

Liver releases sugars and fats into the blood to fuel the survival effort

Small blood vessels in the extremities constrict to make more blood available to muscles

Caffeine blocks adenosine receptors.
Leads to: Uncontrolled neuron firing
Leads to: Pituitary producing ACTH
Leads to: Adrenals pouring out stress hormones
Leads to: The classic stress response

skills, there is one factor that tips the balance toward panic, and that is caffeine. It lowers the stress threshold so that events we would normally handle suddenly become insurmountable. Not only that, you will soon see that caffeine reduces the brain's problem-solving ability. As part of the ancient survival response, stress stimulates neuron activity in the primitive part of the brain known as the limbic system. However, the vast majority of problems we face today require reason, imagination, and creativity: all functions of the "higher brain" or cerebrum.

The fight-or-flight response was designed for stress that was episodic. Everything was fine, then there was a tiger, our adrenals pumped out epinephrine, and we ran like the dickens. Today, however, stress tends to be chronic, and when you consider that most people typically consume caffeine at regular intervals during the day, you begin to understand the magnitude of the problem. Our bodies are in a constant state of "emergency alert," and the results can be devastating.

For most of us, the appropriate response to stress is not fight or flight at all. You may be sitting at a desk or driving in your car when the stress mechanism is triggered. If that's the case, the sugar and fat that are dumped into your bloodstream go unused. The sugar creates additional metabolic stress, and the fat clogs your arteries. Your muscles tense, but to no useful purpose (after all, you can only grip the steering wheel so hard). And since blood flow has been diverted from the gastrointestinal tract, the food you just ate is converted to a fermenting and putrefying mass.

Caffeine Impairs Digestion

Impaired digestion is more of a problem than most people realize—and it gets worse with caffeine (see Chapter 5). That jumbo thirty-two-ounce soft drink or the double espresso we have with meals is a major contributor to the bloating, pain, and gas that roughly 50 percent of American adults experience after they eat. And these symptoms are only the physical signs of maldigestion. Unseen are the harmful by-products of fermentation and putrefaction. Some of these by-products are absorbed back into the bloodstream, and the toxins that stay in the gut increase your risk of gastrointestinal disease.

David Morgan, director of the University of South Florida's Institute on Aging, puts stress-induced maldigestion into an evolutionary perspective when he states, "There's no reason to digest your breakfast if you are about to become lunch. . . . [Under stress] a whole series of maintenance and repair activities just stop."[13]

Caffeine's Icy Grip

Have you ever noticed your fingers getting cold after a cup of coffee? That's another part of the stress response known as vascular resistance, in which peripheral blood vessels constrict. This response is great if you're fighting for your life—if you're cut, you'll lose less blood and your blood will clot faster. But if you're sitting at breakfast reading the morning paper, vascular resistance will only raise your blood pressure and significantly increase your chances of having a heart attack or stroke.

Of course, vascular resistance affects blood vessels

throughout the body, not just in your fingertips. The coldness in your hands and feet indicates that billions of cells are suffering from reduced metabolic efficiency. That means less oxygen is getting to those cells and less carbon dioxide and other wastes are being removed. It means that fine blood vessels in the brain are constricting and cerebral blood flow is reduced. And because caffeine increases brain activity at the same time, a situation known as relative brain hypoperfusion results.[14] In this condition, the brain is deprived of oxygen, and the consequences, when repeated day after day, can be quite serious.

Critical Point #4: Cortisol, the Long Burn

Epinephrine, it turns out, is only half the story. With daily caffeine use, another stress hormone known as cortisol becomes elevated.[15] The important thing to remember about cortisol is that it tends to remain in the bloodstream much longer than epinephrine or norepinephrine. In fact, people who consume more than 300 milligrams of caffeine per day may have elevated serum cortisol for eighteen out of every twenty-four hours. And that sets them up for countless health problems.

You don't really "feel" cortisol the way you feel adrenaline. It's hard to pinpoint exactly what's wrong, and after a while, most people don't even realize that they're different. The quality of their sleep is diminished, their immune system is adversely affected, age-related deterioration is accelerated, and there is a gradual but significant change in mind, mood, and behavior.

One client who kicked the caffeine habit recently told me, "It's as though a cloud has been lifted from my body and mind. I had no idea that I was such an angry and frustrated person." That's because cortisol has a powerful effect on personality.

Critical Point #5: Your Dopamine Levels

As neurobiologists unravel the mechanism of addiction, it becomes more and more clear that not only is caffeine addictive, but it also encourages other addictions to substances like nicotine. The key factor in this interaction appears to be a brain chemical known as dopamine.

Dopamine belongs to a class of biochemicals known as neurotransmitters. As the name implies, these remarkable substances, produced by the brain and nervous system, help control the transmission of information from neuron to neuron. Some neurotransmitters (called excitory neurotransmitters) speed up this information exchange. Inhibitory neurotransmitters slow neuron firing.

But these biochemicals do not merely control the speed of the brain; they also affect (some would even say determine) our feelings. They are therefore a powerful influence on behavior. Dopamine is associated with feelings of pleasure and elation, and scientists now believe that all addiction involves the ability of a substance to raise dopamine levels in the brain. Some substances, like amphetamines, do this by stimulating the brain to release greater amounts of dopamine, while cocaine and others block the brain's ability to clear dopamine from nerve endings. Either way, greater amounts of dopamine are available to stimulate receptor sites in the brain, thus producing the drug "high."

In May 1997, *Time* magazine ran a cover story on

addiction and listed caffeine with other addictive drugs. But they only stated that caffeine "may trigger release of dopamine."[16] In reality, the evidence for the caffeine-dopamine connection is unquestionable. A decade ago, scientists confirmed that caffeine raises dopamine levels. One study even noted that the mechanism by which this occurs is "similar to that observed during amphetamine administration."[17] In the last two years no less than twenty-six scientific studies have described the ways that caffeine interacts with dopamine to alter feelings and behavior. Research shows that caffeine also interacts with opiate receptors, and this may very well strengthen the addictive quality of the compound.[18]

Now, I know what you're thinking. There's no comparison between coffee and opium, cocaine, and amphetamines. Those drugs drive people to destructive behavior, while coffee merely produces a sense of stimulation. But that is precisely the point. We now know that *all* of these drugs act along similar biochemical pathways, in the same areas of the brain. It turns out that there is a continuum of addiction, and just because one substance is incredibly harmful does not mean that we should ignore other substances that are only moderately harmful. Moreover, it is not just the positive dopamine and adrenal stimulation that coffee drinkers are after. As in all truly addictive behaviors, coffee and cola drinkers need their fix in order to avoid the negative experiences of headache, fatigue, irritability, and depression.

Caffeine in some form is consumed by nearly 200 million Americans every day. The harmful effects of this drug are extremely well documented. It's time we all woke up to the truth about the addictive nature of caffeine, as well as its potential for great bodily and mental harm.

The good news is that you can free yourself from caffeine addiction by using the clinically tested Off the Bean program presented in Chapter 10. And if facing life caffeine free is too frightening a thought, rest assured that you will find many healthful suggestions for increasing your own natural energy and restoring your adrenals and nervous system.

BUT WHERE WILL I GET THE ENERGY?

The fact is that caffeine never gave you energy. It stimulated your nervous system and adrenals, and that's not energy, it's stress. To get this point across to my clients, I ask them to imagine going to a bank for a loan. The loan officer is superfriendly and readily agrees. But as you're leaving the bank, you read the fine print, which lists the interest rate at 75 percent! Would you be interested in such a loan? Likewise, the "energy" you receive from caffeine is really just a loan from your adrenals and liver, and the interest is extremely high. At some point (referred to as adrenal exhaustion) you may find yourself "bankrupt" and unable to repair the damage.

Stress—and by that I mean unresolved or unmanaged stress (perhaps more properly called distress)—is a silent saboteur of health. Every da,; 1 million Americans are absent from work because of stress-related disorders. Experts agree that stress is a factor in most diseases, and a major factor in disorders such as anxiety, insomnia, depression, ulcers, rheumatoid arthritis, headache, hypoglycemia, asthma, herpes, hypertension, and heart disease. And yet, if you walk into most hospital waiting rooms, you'll find a coffee machine. Perhaps that's because we don't understand how stress ruins our health. If you ask the average person, he or she will certainly tell you that stress causes tension. He or she may even know that this tension can increase blood pressure and give you headaches. But to make informed decisions about your caffeine intake, it's important to know all the facts—and in this case, it's fairly easy, because they all relate to your adrenal glands.

Critical Point #6: Your Adrenal Glands: Overworked and Underpaid

You don't gain much appreciation for the adrenal glands in physiology class. The focus is too much on memorizing their structure and function. Besides, the adrenals are rather small (smaller than your thumb) and easy to overlook (many anatomy charts don't even include them). So it wasn't until I got into clinical practice that I realized how extremely important they are. I was seeing patients every day with serious health problems that strong, healthy adrenals could have prevented. Why were these people vulnerable to allergy, inflammation, hypertension, infection, and fatigue? What was it that weakened their adrenals? To find the answer, you must learn something about these amazing glands. (A discussion of specific disorders associated with adrenal dysfunction is found in Chapter 5.)

The center of the adrenal gland, called the medulla, produces two major biochemicals: epinephrine and norepinephrine. As I mentioned, these are the fight-or-flight hormones that create the stress response listed in Illustration 1. But we need these hormones for more than the occasional emergency. Epinephrine and norepinephrine are also required for any stressful activity, including sports and recreation.

Surrounding the medulla is the adrenal cortex, which produces a variety of other hormones that help regulate blood pressure, blood sugar, mineral levels, immune activity, inflammation, and cell growth and repair. In all, more than 150 hormones are produced by the adrenals or metabolized from adrenal hormones.

One group, known as glucocorticoids (including cortisol), act as a brake on the immune system. This is an essential function that prevents overenthusiastic immune cells from attacking the body's own healthy tissues. But scientists have recently learned that excess glucocorticoid production (caused by stress and caffeine) can profoundly suppress immunity.[19, 20] The important point to understand is that caffeine combined with emotional stress has been shown to raise glucocorticoid production far more than either caffeine or stress alone.

Critical Point #7: Immunity and Aging

The vaccine response is one of the wonders of modern medicine. By exposing the body to a weakened (or even dead) strain of a disease, the body "remembers" the enemy so that any future encounter with the microbe will result in a swift and strong immune response. Obviously, the effectiveness of a vaccine depends upon the production of these memory cells, called antibodies.

A research team led by Dr. Ronald Glaser gave a hepatitis vaccine to forty-eight students, half of whom were in the midst of final exams (and drinking more coffee). A month later, it was found that the students with elevated stress hormones developed the least protection (produced the lowest number of antibodies) against hepatitis.[21]

But the stress-immune response is not always characterized by suppressed function. The other side of the coin is called immune dysregulation, a condition in which the immune system attacks healthy tissue. There is an intriguing but not fully understood connection between stress, caffeine, and autoimmune disorders such as rheumatoid arthritis, lupus, and MS. Now we know that the onset of autoimmune disease is very frequently preceded by a period of severe stress or depression, but it's not simply that stress weakens the adrenals and leads to poor immune control. Continued research has led to a very exciting breakthrough related to another hormone known as DHEA.

THE DHEA CONNECTION

DHEA (dehydroepiandrosterone) can accurately be called the vitality hormone. The adrenals produce it in abundance during youth, helping to create the energy, optimism, sex drive, and high level of immunity we enjoy in our twenties. DHEA is the precursor to other essential sex and youth hormones such as testosterone and estrogen. At about age twenty-five, DHEA levels start to drop, and this decline continues until at age seventy, most people are only producing about 15 percent of prime peak. The effects of low DHEA are unfortunate and far-reaching: decreased energy, decreased immune competence, and immune dysregulation contributing to autoimmune disease. Low DHEA obviously contributes to decreased sex drive, as well as reduced ability to repair and rebuild tissues.

Since such effects normally accompany aging, researchers thought the decline in DHEA production was just one of the inevitable effects of growing old. As it turns out, however, decreased DHEA production is also a *cause* of the aging process. In fact, some experts believe that declining production of DHEA is not inevitable at all, but simply reflects the declining health of the adrenal glands. Today, endocrinologists are using the term *adrenopause* to describe this phenomenon, and a growing number of health professionals (including myself) believe that much of the degeneration associated with aging can be avoided by maintaining high levels of DHEA. That, of course, is going to be terribly difficult if you're drinking a lot of coffee— since caffeine elevates cortisol, which leads to DHEA deficiency.

WHAT CAUSES ADRENOPAUSE?

Again, it's tempting simply to ascribe it to the aging process, but facts do not support that position. Looking at a population of sixty-year-olds, you'll find some with DHEA blood levels of 200 nanograms per deciliter and others with three times that amount. There are numerous factors that contribute to the spread, but mainly it reflects the differing ability of human beings to withstand the effects of stress.

Research is revealing that cortisol and DHEA, both produced in the adrenal cortex, hold an inverse relationship. As serum cortisol increases, DHEA levels fall. It may be that stress and caffeine create such a high need for cortisol that the exhausted adrenals simply cannot maintain production of DHEA at optimal levels. This results in the double whammy of degeneration: elevated cortisol and DHEA deficiency.

The importance of DHEA in maintaining peak immunity is clearly illustrated in the progression of HIV infection to full-blown AIDS. In this case, deterioration is marked by declining levels of an important immune cell known as the T helper (medical term: CD4 cell). Researchers have found a striking correlation between blood levels of DHEA and CD4 counts of AIDS patients.[22] The investigators in one study stated, "There is a relationship between the circulating sex hormone levels, particularly DHEA, and the progression of immune depression in HIV, whatever the risk factor." A 1996 editorial in the *Journal of Laboratory and Clinical Medicine* suggests that serum DHEA be used as a marker for progression of HIV,[23] and at least one clinical trial has found DHEA supplementation to be effective in reducing the amount of HIV virus in the body.[24]

The important point for this discussion is that cortisol has been found to accelerate HIV infection, while DHEA slows the virus down. There appears to be a "tug-of-war" in the bodies of HIV-positive individuals between these two adrenal hormones. To the degree that cortisol wins, the disease progresses. We would all do well to remember that this scenario is certainly not limited to AIDS, but most likely plays a role in every disease we suffer.

Critical Point #8: Your Stress Threshold

Life is an unpredictable mix of pleasant and unpleasant events. Unpleasant events can be divided into two categories: not getting what you want, and getting what you don't want. Either can create stress, but not necessarily distress, which suppresses immunity and increases risk for disease. The determining factor is the individual's emotional response to the event. Two people, for example, can experience the same stressful situation (traffic ticket, final exam, fight with spouse), but one of them is mildly annoyed while the other "flies off the handle" into distress. Psychologists look at this response as part of the Type A/Type B personality picture, but they have failed to look at the caffeine factor.

We now know that caffeine can lower the stress threshold (the point where stress becomes distress) in virtually anyone, whether they are Type A, Type B, or anything in between. And the amazing thing is that this "short-fuse" phenomenon occurs *either* when blood levels of caffeine rise, *or* (in habitual coffee drinkers) when blood caffeine levels fall. One eye-opening study looked at behavioral changes that occur when habitual coffee drinkers were deprived of their morning coffee. Compared to controls, the coffee drinkers reacted to situational challenges with a far greater number of negative mood effects, including anger, violence, frustration, and depression.[25]

CAFFEINE VERSUS GABA

As I mentioned, the brain uses adenosine receptors to keep neuron firing within safe limits. Neurotransmitters comprise another very powerful control system. Remember that excitatory neurotransmitters speed communication between neurons. The hormone norepinephrine is an excitatory neurotransmitter that is stimulated by the ingestion of caffeine.

The primary inhibitory neurotransmitter is known as GABA, or gamma aminobutyric acid. GABA has a unique ability to calm the mind without putting you to sleep. The researchers who discovered GABA took mice and taught them to find their way through a maze. Once this was accomplished, they stressed the mice by immobilizing them (mice hate that). Interestingly, the stressed mice could no longer find their way through the maze. But when GABA was injected into their brains, they waltzed right through. Seeing the obvious parallel between that experiment and the way most of us live, other researchers scurried to their labs to synthesize GABA for human consumption. This was accomplished in record time, and scant months later, GABA appeared on the shelves of health-food stores.

There are two reasons why I am telling you this story. First, it's a good "nutrition detective" lesson. In the mice study, the GABA was injected directly into the brain. The health-food store products are oral capsules. As it turns out, you cannot raise brain levels of GABA by eating it. The fragile molecule is completely digested in the stomach. So much for the idea of popping a few GABA capsules with your double espresso.

The second point is that the mice research revealed yet another reason to decrease your intake of coffee. Caffeine, it turns out, disrupts the normal metabolism of GABA.[26] Here's this wonderful brain biochemical that increases the "filter mechanism" of the brain, helps you to step back and see clearly even under stress, and caffeine screws it up. Thus, in the maze of life you never make it to the cheese.

GABA IN YOUR GUT

New research tells us that GABA is also produced in the intestinal tract, where it serves a similar purpose: calming anxiety and stress. Since caffeine disrupts the normal metabolism of GABA, investigators now believe they have found the smoking gun to implicate coffee with ulcers and irritable bowel syndrome. What's more, this anti-GABA action is powerfully amplified by other drugs, including commonly prescribed antibiotics. These medications interfere with the action of GABA and at the same time decrease the body's ability to detoxify caffeine.[27] This combination can produce anxiety, irritability, hyperactivity, and even epilepsy-like convulsions[28]—all the more reason to ask your physician if your medication has any interactions with caffeine.

RESEARCH CAPSULE
Habitual Caffeine Use Is No Protection

Coffee promoters are fond of claiming that the drug's negative side effects somehow "wear off" as you develop a tolerance to caffeine, but research does not support that claim. In fact, major scientific reviews agree that, while the diuretic effect may decrease with habitual use, humans do not develop "tolerance" to the far more dangerous central nervous system effects.[29–31]

Still, caffeine apologists can cite research where coffee drinkers were given caffeine and their blood pressure did not increase. But this is not a real-world experiment. In the real world, we are faced with numerous challenges as we go through the day. Some of these challenges are mental (like taking a final exam), some are emotional (dealing with a difficult relationship), and some are physical (sports and exercise). Research with real people shows conclusively that caffeine accelerates and magnifies the damage that we experience from stress. In fact, it is often the critical fac-

---

tor that pushes us over the stress threshold into distress, disease, and degeneration.

Here are three studies that debunk the idea that habitual coffee drinkers are somehow immune to caffeine-induced stress damage. Note that all three are well-designed, placebo-controlled experiments.

1. In this study, healthy students were selected to evaluate the combined response to caffeine and a difficult laboratory task. All of the students were coffee drinkers. Some were habitual consumers and others were light consumers. On the test day, they were given a moderate dose of caffeine based on their weight. A 150-pound man, for example, was given 238 milligrams, or the equivalent of a mug of strong coffee.

Caffeine administration more than doubled epinephrine and cortisol levels from baseline, and the magnitude of this increase was not different between the habitual and light coffee drinkers. The study authors concluded that: "Caffeine can potentiate both cardiovascular and neuroendocrine stress reactivity, and the habitual use of caffeine is not necessarily associated with the development of tolerance to these effects."

Source: J. D. Lane, R. A. Adcock, R. B. Williams et al., "Caffeine Effects on Cardiovascular and Neuroendocrine Responses to Acute Psychosocial Stress and Their Relationship to Level of Habitual Caffeine Consumption," *Psychosomatic Medicine*, May–June 1990;52(3):320–36.

2. Another study looked at the combination of caffeine and exercise. Again, the subjects were healthy young men with normal blood pressure. This time the dose of caffeine was even smaller, roughly the equivalent of one mug of coffee.

We know that exercise by itself increases blood pressure, so measurements were taken twice: once on the day when caffeine was administered and once on the day when subjects received a placebo. Dangerous elevations of blood pressure were recorded more than twice as often on caffeine days as compared to placebo days. In addition, caffeine impaired circulation due to the constriction of blood vessels and elevated stress hormones.

Source: B. H. Sung, W. R. Lovallo, G. A. Pincomb et al., "Effects of Caffeine on Blood Pressure Response during Exercise in Normotensive Healthy Young Men," *American Journal of Cardiology*, April 1, 1990;63(13):909–13.

3. In the third study, students were given either caffeine (the equivalent of one mug of coffee for a 150-pound person) or placebo during periods of low stress (no exams) or high stress (final exams). Over a period of eight days, heart rate and blood pressure were measured. As you would expect, the stress of exams increased blood pressure slightly. But when caffeine was added, blood pressure shot up in many of the subjects to the borderline hypertensive range. What's more, caffeine increased blood cortisol and cholesterol levels.

Source: G. A. Pincomb, W. R. Lovallo, R. B. Passey et al.; "Caffeine Enhances the Physiological Response to Occupational Stress in Medical Students," *Health Psychology*, 1987;6(2):101–12.

Because this is a real-world scenario, this study brings up an important point. In the real world, if a person were to go to the doctor with the symptoms created by exams and caffeine, he or she would likely be placed on blood pressure medication—which would be completely inappropriate and possibly dangerous. Do you think doctors routinely survey their patients to determine caffeine ingestion? Did your doctor ask you about caffeine at your last physical exam?

THE STRESS-FATIGUE-DISEASE CYCLE

It has been said that actions become habits and habits determine our lives. That is especially true when it comes to what we eat and drink. The problem with the caffeine habit is that it's very hard to be moderate or even sensible. That's because it sets up a cycle of alertness followed by fatigue. You might start with one cup in the morning, but most people find that they soon need a second cup at mid-morning, and another caffeine hit (coffee or cola) in the afternoon. Over time, adrenal weakness leads to deeper fatigue, more caffeine, and a spiral of increasing stress and decreasing health that can be devastating. The good news is that once you understand this cycle, you can break free. And only when you break free you can begin the task of repairing the damage.

ILLUSTRATION 2

THE STRESS-FATIGUE-DISEASE CYCLE

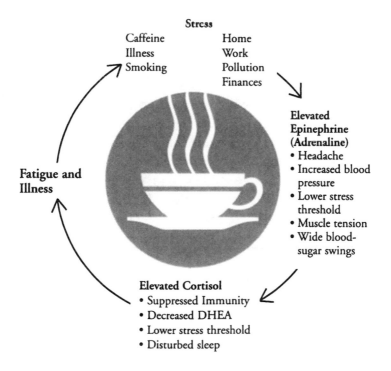

Stress
Caffeine
Illness
Smoking
Home
Work
Pollution
Finances

Elevated Epinephrine (Adrenaline)
• Headache
• Increased blood pressure
• Lower stress threshold
• Muscle tension
• Wide blood-sugar swings

Fatigue and Illness

Elevated Cortisol
• Suppressed Immunity
• Decreased DHEA
• Lower stress threshold
• Disturbed sleep

Clinical evidence suggests that at a certain point, stress and caffeine-induced alterations of hormone and metabolic functions may not be reversable. The following case history will give you a glimpse of how far this downward spiral can go.

Linda A. was a moderate coffee drinker until she started a very demanding job right after college. Working long hours meant an additional mug of coffee around 3 P.M. that would keep her going until six or seven. But the quality of her sleep began to suffer and, unlike her rise-and-shine past, she found that she had to drag herself out of bed. She even had to move her alarm clock out of reach to prevent herself from hitting the snooze button and being late for work. When she complained about this to her doctor, he told her that the afternoon coffee was not likely to be causing the insomnia and restlessness. He blamed it on the stress of her job.

As the months went on, however, she found that she could not function without two or three cups of coffee in the morning. She looked forward to a 10 A.M. cup at work, and usually had a cola beverage with lunch. Eventually, there was a steady stream of caffeine throughout her day; always a mug of coffee or a can of cola at her desk. She started getting headaches, and the only thing that seemed to help was a cup of coffee. She knew that she was, as she explained, "in trouble," but she thought she could hold everything together until things in her life "settled down." Unfortunately, that never happened. Instead, she came home one night and her husband announced that he was leaving her.

He told her that her entire personality had changed since they met. She was no longer a fun-loving, easygoing woman, but an irritable, anxious, and unhappy person.

She became defensive, blaming the stress of her career. When he pointed out that their sex life was next to nonexistent, she blamed her headaches and the fact that her periods literally knocked her out of commission for ten days out of every month. She had never told him about the painful lumps in her breasts that made intimacy a less than pleasurable experience.

The stress of her broken marriage got her to seek help, but all she received was a prescription for a tranquilizer and an antidepressant. At the age of thirty-three, she started experiencing painful swollen joints, but was given only painkillers.

Linda came to my office with the diagnosis of rheumatoid arthritis, cystic breast disease, PMS, migraine, and depression. Her food and beverage survey revealed that she was ingesting over 1,000 milligrams of caffeine each day, and my suggestion that caffeine was causing many of her troubles was at first met with disbelief and alarm. After all, she was convinced that without caffeine she could not function. It was only after I showed her research proof associating caffeine with *every one* of her disorders that she agreed to start cutting back. It took Linda four months to get down to two cups of coffee per day, and at that point, she switched to tea.

After one year on my Off the Bean program, including nutritional therapy to help repair her adrenals and nervous system, Linda was completely free of headaches. The painful lumps in her breasts disappeared, her mood swings evened out, her energy dramatically improved, and her PMS was a thing of the past. But three years later, she was still battling the arthritis. As her rheumatologist explained, something in her body just went "haywire," causing her immune system to attack her joint tissue. Aside from steroid drugs and other powerful immune-suppressing agents, he offered no hope for relief.

I believe that Linda will one day be free of rheumatoid arthritis, but it may take years. For so long her body had been held in a perpetual state of near panic. Stress hormones ravaged her immune system, destroyed muscle fibers, drove her DHEA levels down to those of a seventy-year-old, and left her adrenals exhausted and weak. The road back is not easy, but she has seen tremendous improvement.

By the way, Linda was using birth control pills when she first noticed that her sleep was disturbed. These drugs decrease the body's ability to detoxify caffeine, and as it turns out, that 3 P.M. mug of coffee was keeping caffeine coursing through her blood until 2 A.M. It was all downhill from there.

Critical Point #9: Your Sleep Cycle

Few people understand the importance or the function of sleep. We tend to think of sleep as "wasted time," and that may be the reason why studies show that the vast majority of Americans don't get enough sleep. Pressed as we are for time, we just assume that we can get by with less. Even doctors are largely unaware of the critical importance of sleep. They treat insomnia with drugs (many of which actually disturb sleep quality), but few physicians today bother to take a sleep history. Routine intake questionnaires rarely include a section on sleep habits.

But among researchers, sleep is an extremely hot topic. Entire journals are devoted to the subject, and sleep centers are opening in research facilities around the world. This explosion of interest has been fueled mainly by neurobiologists who are starting to unravel the complex way in which the brain directs the healing powers of the body. And one of the most startling discoveries has to do with what goes on while you sleep. When you begin to understand these mysteries, you'll never look at a cup of coffee in quite the same way. That's because sleep can be a youth-restoring, powerfully rejuvenating, deep healing experience—or, it can be merely a continuation of the day's tension, conflict, and frustration. For most of us, the difference is a drug called caffeine.

The World Health Organization (WHO) in Geneva reports that more than 30 percent of people in industrialized countries experience episodes of sleeplessness, and about 12 percent of adults have chronic insomnia.

Source: A. La Voie, "Sleepless in Seattle, and All Around the Globe," Medical Tribune News Service, June 27, 1997.

As you may know, a night's sleep is divided into roughly ninety-minute cycles in which brain activity changes dramatically. In Illustration 3, you can see that during each cycle, the brain goes through four stages, from S1 (shallow sleep) to S4 (deep sleep). Most people are familiar with S1 because that is when we dream and have rapid eye movement (REM). But in reality, each stage provides the body and brain with essential repair, rejuvenate, and rebuild benefits. Dreams, for example, are absolutely critical for maintaining mental and emotional health. We don't know why, but if you prevent a person from dreaming for just a few nights, that individual will start to experience clear signs of psychosis. It was once thought that caffeine enhanced dream sleep, or at least lengthened the S1 phase of the sleep cycle. But recent research shows that caffeine (and numerous other drugs) can disrupt this crucial function.[32]

As important as dreams are to the mind, deep sleep (S4) is essential for the health of the body. Interestingly, scientists have learned a great deal about deep sleep from studying coma patients. The purpose of coma, you see, is to deactivate all nonessential functions of the body and brain in order to devote every possible ounce of energy to the task of healing. Likewise, the body uses deep sleep to mobilize all available resources for healing and rejuvenation. During S4 sleep, there is a massive creation of new cells throughout the body. Every tissue benefits, but most activity is centered on building immunity and restoring the nervous system. We all know how wonderful we feel after a good night's sleep. That's because deep sleep provides a level of rest that cannot be obtained in any other way. In a very restful night, you may experience deep sleep at two and possibly three phases. But when there's caffeine (or its metabolites) in your bloodstream, you are unlikely to experience deep sleep at all.

ILLUSTRATION 3

A NORMAL SLEEP CYCLE

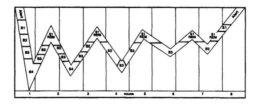

Caffeine has been found to shorten total sleep time, increase the duration of Stage 2, shorten Stage 3, and often eliminate Stage 4 (deep sleep).

Sources: S. H. Onen, F. Onen, D. Bailly et al., "Prevention and Treatment of Sleep Disorders through Regulation of Sleeping Habits," *Presse Médicale*, 1994;12;23(10):485–89; and M. H. Bonnet and D. L. Arand, "Metabolic Rate and Restorative Function of Sleep," *Physiology and Behavior*, April–May 1996;59(4–5):777–82.

Those who promote caffeine as a harmless drug like to cite research showing that coffee and soft drink users become tolerant to the stimulant effects and no longer experience insomnia. You must understand that insomnia is not the issue. Insomnia (the inability to fall asleep) deals only with the quantity of sleep. The real issue here is sleep quality. Caffeine tolerance may allow you to fall asleep, but if S4 sleep is disrupted, you will wake up feeling tired instead of renewed.

Research shows that people who consume more than 250 milligrams of caffeine per day tend to have poor sleep quality.[33, 34] What's more, they are generally unaware of this critical problem. In one study, habitual coffee drinkers were allowed to drink coffee until midday (in order to prevent withdrawal). Later in the day, they were given either caffeine or placebo, and on days when they received placebo, their sleep quality improved significantly.[35] As a result, they felt much better the following day. But for millions of Americans, caffeine-induced sleep disorders remain hidden and undiagnosed. These people drag themselves out of bed and remain tired through the day.

I don't think it is being overly cynical to suggest that this is precisely what the caffeine industry wants. After all, if you're groggy in the morning, you'll reach for their product. By midmorning, that first cup will wear off, so you'll reach for another. You'll have a caffeine beverage with lunch and most likely another in midafternoon—all because your body really didn't rest. You fell asleep but never got to experience the depth of sleep that you need most. Is the problem widespread? Recent surveys suggest that 25 percent of U.S. adults have trouble falling asleep, 23 percent awaken frequently, 25 percent wake up too early, nearly half of all Americans are dissatisfied with the quality of their sleep, and one out of every ten is taking some medication to help them sleep.

While this certainly qualifies as an epidemic, I believe those numbers don't come close to identifying the magnitude of the sleep problem. That's because we have limited information. In a sleep laboratory, we'd be hooked up to a monitor that would record every stage of sleep on a device called an electroencephalogram (EEG). The scientist conducting the study could tell us, "You never made it into S4 sleep last night. Better cut back on the caffeine." But in real life, most of us simply look at the clock, wonder why we feel exhausted, and then stumble into the kitchen to make a pot of coffee.

Take another look at Illustration 3. Did you notice that this normal sleep cycle takes place over a span of eight hours? Do you normally get a full eight hours of sleep? I didn't think so. In fact, few American adults devote enough time to this critical repair and rebuild cycle, and we suffer greatly for it.

CASE STUDY

Amy came to my office with a five-year history of fibromyalgia. During the interview, she was surprised at how interested I was to know her caffeine history. In fact, no one had ever explained to her the connection between caffeine and her painful disorder.

Now I believe that if you give a person enough time, he or she will usually tell you the cause of their illness. Amy's story was classic. She was a "one cup in the morning" woman with a low-stress job in Thousand Oaks, California, a town about twenty-five miles north of Los Angeles. Life changed dramatically for her when she landed the "job of her dreams" in LA. The commute was an hour and a half on a good day, and to assure that she would not be late, Amy started leaving the house at 6 A.M. That meant she had to get up at 5 A.M. sharp. Her usual bedtime (before the LA job) was 11:30 or midnight, which gave her about seven hours of sleep, "barely enough" as she described it.

But to get the same amount of sleep on her new schedule would mean going to bed at 10 P.M. and she was just not tired at ten. In fact, if she went to bed at ten, she just tossed and turned until midnight anyway, so she gave up and assumed that she could "catch up" on her sleep over the weekends.

Unfortunately, it doesn't work that way. It is possible to "make up" for one bad night's sleep, and maybe even two nights. But according to most sleep experts, after two consecutive nights of poor sleep, the damage starts to accumulate. You'll learn exactly how that damage contributes to fibromyalgia in Chapter 5, but right now I want to tell you why Amy couldn't fall asleep before midnight. Actually, you probably already know.

Getting two hours' less sleep made Amy tired, but she had to be "up" for her new job, so she started drinking coffee while driving to LA. She bought a special "commuter mug" and didn't notice that it held twenty ounces, about twice what she normally drank. What's more, she seldom had time for her usual breakfast, and so this coffee was invariably consumed on an empty stomach. As the weeks went by, she started having another mug of coffee at mid-morning and one or two cola beverages in the afternoon. It wasn't long before she started having shoulder and neck pain. Her friends at work were quick to suggest that she get a better chair and elevate her wrists when using the computer. She bought special back supports for the car seat and desk chair, and tried stretching exercises twice a day, but the pain only got worse. That's because none of these measures dealt with the cause of her problem.

The trap that Amy was caught in is extremely common.

You probably know someone with the same story, and right now, it's easy to see the elements of that cycle: reduced sleep led to increased caffeine consumption, caffeine disrupted what little sleep Amy was able to get, and the loss of sleep quantity and sleep quality contributed to her fibromyalgia, the primary symptoms of which are pain and fatigue.

ILLUSTRATION 4

THE CAFFEINE-SLEEP-DISEASE CYCLE

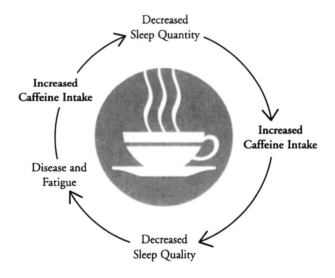

Decreased
Sleep Quantity

Increased
Caffeine Intake

Increased
Caffeine Intake

Disease and
Fatigue

Decreased
Sleep Quality

Coffee and Sleep: Debunking More Myths

Time of Day

There is a popular notion that coffee before 3 P.M. can't disturb your sleep. In fact, caffeine *at any time* of the day can cause sleep problems, especially if you are under stress. Researchers at the Institute of Pharmacology in Zurich,

Switzerland, gave a moderate amount of caffeine (200 milligrams) to healthy subjects at 7 A.M. By 11 P.M. blood levels of caffeine had fallen more than 80 percent and *still* the subjects experienced significant sleep disturbance, especially in the S4 stage.[36] This may be due to the stimulation of cortisol, or to some unidentified brain-body dysfunction created by caffeine earlier in the day.

WHO'S MOST AT RISK?

We also tend to think that caffeine-related problems are mostly experienced by people in the workforce. In reality, those hardest hit appear to be the elderly. Even though seniors tend to cut back on coffee, the caffeine they do ingest is detoxified much more slowly and their nervous systems are much more sensitive than those of younger people. Research is now showing that sleep disturbance among the elderly is a *major* factor not only in age-related physical degeneration but in mental degeneration as well.[37, 38] Investigators from the National Institute on Aging have identified another culprit: hidden caffeine. Their 1995 report showed that those taking any caffeine-containing medications were nearly twice as likely to have sleep problems compared to age-matched controls.[39] Avoiding these medications is not an easy task. Today, more than 2,000 OTC and prescription medications contain caffeine.

Critical Point #10: Your Fatigue Quotient

While the connection between poor sleep and fatigue is obvious, caffeine contributes to fatigue in at least three other ways. Adrenal exhaustion results in profound tiredness, as can blood sugar abnormalities associated with caffeine use. And we've already seen in Chapter 2 (Test #4) that the muscle tension resulting from stress can use up tremendous amounts of energy.

How ironic that the very substance people turn to for energy is a major cause of their fatigue. It gets worse, of course, when you understand that the cumulative effect of fatigue and poor sleep is more serious illness. In fact, fatigue is one of the top three reasons why Americans seek medical help.[40] In 1994, there were over 15 million doctor visits for this problem. The tragedy is that, for the most part, physicians are unaware of the caffeine connection. Surveys show that fewer than 10 percent of patients receive advice from their doctor to reduce caffeine. Even with heavy coffee drinkers, the percentage is less than 15 percent.[41]

The popular press, however, may be catching on. A while ago, *U.S. News & World Report* ran a feature article on the growing epidemic of fatigue in America.[42] Boxed out on page one of the article was a list of "the most common causes of prolonged fatigue." Caffeine addiction was number two on the list, and, overall, caffeine was a factor in five of the seven points listed.

THE BLOOD SUGAR ROLLER COASTER

Hypoglycemia results when blood sugar levels fall below normal. Since blood sugar (or glucose) is the fuel that runs our muscles and brain, hypoglycemia typically produces fatigue, depression, and anxiety. There is no single cause of hypoglycemia. It is an imbalance in the complex process of energy metabolism involving the liver, pancreas, and adrenal glands.

Caffeine plays a major role because it stimulates the fight-or-flight stress response described earlier. As part of this response, the liver rapidly raises blood sugar levels. This is felt as a "lift" by the person who drank the coffee (especially if the coffee contained added sugar) but the body must then deal with the metabolic emergency of hyperglycemia (elevated blood sugar). This is accomplished by the pancreas, which secrets insulin, driving the blood-sugar level down.

In some individuals, however, blood sugar may decrease to levels below normal, resulting in hypoglycemia and the all-too-familiar "letdown" feeling a few hours after the coffee lift. Of course, many people simply reach for another cup of coffee, which starts the roller-coaster cycle all over.

Although this model of "caffeinism" is well understood, it is not clear why some people are more sensitive than others. Experts believe this has to do with the individual's age, weight, body composition, overall health, and other factors.

CASE STUDY

Jeff had a promising career as an architect. He worked in a huge Los Angeles firm, and competition for advancement was fierce. When he came to see me, Jeff had been at the company for five years, but his position was anything but secure. At any moment, he knew he could be replaced by an ambitious and energetic intern. There were only two ways Jeff could demonstrate his value to the firm: work harder and work longer. I was not surprised when he told me that he drank about twelve cups of coffee a day.

At the age of thirty-four, Jeff was feeling old. He remembered a time, not so many years back, when he would bounce out of bed in the morning, work hard, and still have energy to play softball in the evening. As he sat talking to me, however, his manner was anything but bouncy. The dark circles under his eyes told me that he was sleeping poorly. And although he had been a collegiate All-American, I could tell that Jeff was out of shape and about twenty-five pounds overweight. At his last physical, his doctor listened to his complaints, announced, "You're depressed," and handed him a prescription for an antidepressant.

But Jeff was smart enough to know that his depression was not the cause of his fatigue. It was the other way around. He was even aware that caffeine was part of the problem, but he didn't think there was any alternative. Everyone at work was a caffeine addict. It was part of the culture.

The first thing I did with Jeff was to create an agreement. If he would follow my Off the Bean program step by step without fail, I would guarantee that in sixty days, he'd feel better and have more energy. It was a no-lose proposition for Jeff. After all, if I was wrong, he could always go back to the coffee. We measured his blood pressure, heart rate, and weight. He filled out a questionnaire like the one in Appendix C, and we took a photograph. That kind of documentation is extremely valuable in charting one's progress.

I have no doubt that if I had simply told Jeff to cut out coffee, he would have left my office and never come back. But the program made sense to him, and in just two weeks, he was able to reduce his caffeine intake by 50 percent with no headache or fatigue. He called a few days later to tell me that for the first time in years, he had awakened before the alarm clock went off. By the end of the month, he was down to one cup of coffee in the morning and a cup of tea in the afternoon.

During the next thirty days, Jeff experienced remarkable improvements in his energy level. Before, his days had been like a roller coaster, with peaks of creativity and alertness alternating with mental fog and profound fatigue. Now he was sailing through the day with consistent energy and clarity. Even the dreaded three-o'clock slump had disappeared. His appearance had improved and he'd lost weight, but the most important benefit for him was his attitude. Jeff felt like himself again: optimistic, energetic—and happy!

Now the Hollywood ending would be Jeff becoming a partner in the firm, but that's not what happened. The experience of near burnout convinced Jeff that the price of success in that arena was much too high. So he took his renewed energy and went to work for a smaller company. At his new job, he didn't have to watch his back constantly, so he was able to spend more time in creative pursuits. A year later, he was doing quite well and enjoying life immensely, along with a few cups of caffeine-free herbal tea every day.

Critical Point #11: Malnutrition

Malnutrition is one of the most well-defined effects of habitual caffeine intake. It contributes in a very logical way to a host of disorders that we will explore in Chapter 5. Caffeine, and possibly other ingredients in coffee and tea, causes an increased loss of thiamin and other B vitamins in the urine.[43–45] There is evidence that caffeic acid also decreases the bioavailability of thiamin so that less of this vital nutrient is absorbed from food.[46] Since the B vitamin status of many Americans is borderline to begin with, regular consumption of coffee and soft drinks can contribute to deficiency and a raft of symptoms, including neurological damage.[47]

Then there is the loss of calcium and other minerals. Researchers at Washington State University's Department of Food Science and Human Nutrition found that as little as 150 milligrams of caffeine caused increased loss of calcium, magnesium, sodium, and chloride in the urine.[48] The losses were far greater when the caffeine intake was raised to 300 milligrams. Research just published in the *Annals of Nutrition and Metabolism* found that caffeine increased potassium loss by nearly one-third.[49] To make matters worse, such mineral loss appears to be accelerated when caffeine is mixed with sugar.[50] Studies show that the mechanism behind this mineral-wasting phenomenon may have to do with the fact that caffeine impairs the kidneys' ability to hold on to calcium, magnesium, and other minerals.[51] Most recently, zinc was added to the list of nutrients depleted by caffeine.[52]

As you read this, you might be wondering how caffeine affects your bones. In fact, all that calcium loss cannot help but increase your risk for osteoporosis, and perhaps hypertension as well. As you will see in Chapters 6 and 8, caffeinated soft drinks create special problems for women. The caffeine causes increased urinary loss of calcium, while another ingredient, phosphoric acid, interferes with the absorption and metabolism of that important mineral. The result? Studies have shown that high caffeinated soft drink consumption is associated with increased fracture risk among women[53] and girls.[54]

ANEMIA ANYONE?

Perhaps an even greater nutritional problem has to do with the effect of caffeine on iron absorption. In the late 1970s, researchers stumbled upon an important discovery. Nutritionists were looking for ways to increase iron intake and came up with the idea of fortifying sugar with the mineral. (No comment!) However, they found that when iron-fortified sugar was added to coffee, very little iron was absorbed. This prompted further investigation, and in 1981, the *American Journal of Clinical Nutrition* reported research showing that caffeine may oxidize available iron, converting it to a form with dramatically reduced bio-availability.[55]

Other studies showed that a single cup of coffee can reduce iron absorption from a meal by as much as 75 percent. What's more, this dramatic inhibition of iron absorption occurred even when the coffee was consumed an hour after a meal. And if you think you can compensate for this handicap by taking vitamins or minerals, you're wrong. Coffee and tea both reduce the effectiveness of iron supplements.[56, 57]

The salient point here is that over 30 percent of American women spend their entire lives with suboptimal iron status. In many cases, that leads to iron deficiency and a disorder known as anemia (deficiency in the blood's oxygen-carrying ability), but low iron can seriously affect energy, immunity, and even brain function long before anemia develops (see Chapter 6).

Critical Point #12: Caffeine and Immunity

We have already explored the disastrous effects that excess stress hormones have on immunity (Critical Point #7).

But caffeine and other methylxanthines may also exert negative pressure directly on your body's defense system by reducing the activity of monocytes and natural killer (NK) cells.[58-61] When you understand that these immune cells are your best protection against viruses and cancer, you begin to see the seriousness of the problem.

Now here's some good news. Recent research has shown that the number and immune strength of monocytes and NK cells can be *enhanced* by the administration of DHEA.[62, 63] Remember, however, that excess stress hormones will decrease and/or deplete your body's own production of DHEA so that in order to benefit from DHEA, reduction of caffeine intake is imperative.

CAFFEINE VERSUS MELATONIN

Melatonin is another vital hormone, and it's an extremely hot topic in immunology these days. For decades melatonin was thought simply to regulate the sleep/wake cycle in humans and animals. Now research is showing that it has powerful and important immune functions, including anti-cancer activity and the antioxidant ability to "scavenge" dangerous molecules known as free radicals. You've probably heard a great deal about other antioxidants, such as vitamin C and vitamin E, but melatonin's role is only now coming to light. One group of researchers, after presenting stunning evidence of melatonin's ability to protect cellular DNA, concluded that this hormone "may prove to be the most important free radical scavenger discovered to date."[64]

Like DHEA, production of melatonin decreases with advancing years. Again, this was first thought to be one of those inevitable consequences of aging, but if you are smart, you'll start to question anything that is said to be inevitable. And when you look for the reason why melatonin levels fall with age, you come face-to-face with a familiar duo: caffeine and stress.

You'll remember that stress leads to decreased DHEA through a kind of metabolic "competition." The adrenals just can't produce large amounts of both DHEA *and* stress hormones. But melatonin is produced by the pineal gland in the brain as well as other cells in the intestinal tract, so the mechanism by which stress lowers melatonin is not fully understood.

We get a clue, however, from recent research showing that melatonin (in addition to its sleep and immune system duties) is also an anti-anxiety agent.[65] It may be that stress simply "uses up" or depletes this vitally important hormone. We also know that cortisol radically disrupts the normal secretion of melatonin,[66] and that stress and coffee (even decaf) can damage cells of the intestinal tract that secrete the hormone.[67]

The most recent (and most damning) piece of evidence illustrates that caffeine directly suppresses melatonin production. Researchers have long known that exposure to bright light decreases melatonin, while dim lighting promotes secretion of the hormone. A new study in the journal *Brain Research* showed that when normal human subjects were given caffeine or placebo, caffeine resulted in significantly lower levels of melatonin, even when lighting conditions were dim. As expected, bright light conditions lowered melatonin as well, but the combination of bright light and caffeine produced a striking decrease, far more than would result from either condition alone. In other words, bright light and caffeine had an additive effect in depressing the subjects' production of melatonin.[68]

Thus, whether through depletion or through impaired production, stress, anxiety, and caffeine combine to reduce the amount of melatonin available to our bodies. And that, according to leading experts, is a metabolic catastrophe that leads to crippled immunity, impaired sleep, and accelerated aging.[69, 70]

Imagine you lived in a country that was always under threat of attack. No matter where you went, there was a perpetual state of alert. Not only that, but your defenses were constantly being depleted and weakened. Does that sound stressful? Caffeine produces the same effect on your body, like fighting a war on multiple fronts at the same time. All organ systems are strained during times of stress, but most important are the adrenals, which must supply hormones to activate the body's emergency functions.

Remember, however, that the caffeine "emergency" is not a real threat to survival. While the adrenals are busy fighting a phantom enemy, real enemies may go unchecked. The adrenals are responsible for helping mount an immune attack against a wide range of pathogens. Studies show that adrenal hormone production may triple during acute infection.[71] If stress is prolonged, adaptive mechanisms may fail, leading to serious and chronic illness.[72]

Let's face it, remaining healthy and strong throughout life is a battle. Caffeine is the Trojan horse. It looks like a gift but instead delivers adrenal stress, low blood sugar, mood and energy swings, fatigue, depression, malnutrition, and disturbed sleep. By now, you are starting to see the full scope of how caffeine affects the quality of life. In Chapter 5 we're going to see how these twelve critical points contribute to specific disease states. I want to emphasize again how insidious this downward spiral is. Caffeinism is a gradual and at first imperceptible disorder. And because all your friends are also getting tired and becoming sick more often, it's natural to assume that these signs and symptoms are inevitable.

Of course, some of the effects are obvious. You can measure increases in blood pressure, and you can feel the coldness resulting from constriction of blood vessels in your fingers. But most of the stress is very subtle. There is no way to measure irritability, for example. People who have never known you off coffee just assume that is your personality.

Another gradual effect of caffeinism is that your concentration becomes one-dimensional. You tend to lose the big picture because you can't step back from what you're involved in. Coffee concentration is good for some tasks but terribly limiting when, for example, you have to deal with any kind of adversity or setback. Coffee cuts you off from the brain's higher centers of reason and evaluation because you are forcing your brain into defensive, emergency overdrive.

In yet another ironic example of wrong thinking, we often view such limitations as advantages. We talk about a "competitive edge" as if success depended only upon aggressiveness. In reality, this type of success often comes at the price of burnout and ruined health, and I have seen it scores of times in my clinical practice and in the first-class cabin of 747s.

I travel a great deal, and very often find myself sitting next to successful businesspeople. It is amazing to me how often they will maintain a frenzied work pace throughout the flight, tapping away at their laptops, talking on the phone, faxing letters. And all the while, the flight attendant keeps their coffee cups filled.

During a meal, when there's a lull in the action, it's natural to strike up a conversation and, as you can imagine, it often centers around what we do for a living. More times than not, the man or woman is in a high-pressure executive position. They're usually heavy coffee drinkers and almost always have significant health problems directly related to stress. I'm a good listener, and I often feel like a therapist as my neighbor describes his or her physical and emotional pain. In short, the vast majority of these successful people feel like they're trapped on a treadmill.

But there are the exceptions, people who live with no frenzy or turmoil. These people are generally healthier, more fit, and definitely happier than the treadmill crowd. And the most significant difference is not their income but their attitude. They tend to drink less (or no) caffeine, and they understand that true success is a balance. I have heard remarkable wisdom from these people, about how their lives changed when they realized that business does not have to be self-destructive. I've talked with award-winning salespeople who experienced dramatic gains after getting off caffeine. Many have described a completely different approach that opened doors that before had been slammed in their faces. What made the difference? One man told me, "I was less aggressive but far more effective. I was able to relate to the customer's needs more clearly, and once they realized that I was not trying to steamroll them, they were more open to what I had to say."

With sales, as in life, we make decisions every day that affect how we feel. The lessons for me has been clear, because I am convinced that what we get out of life depends on the kind of energy we put into it. The caffeine-driven go-getter may accomplish a great deal at first, but suffering is sure to follow. With the tools presented in this book, I believe that we now have a much more rewarding alternative.

CHAPTER 4

Caffeine and Your Mind

If you ask people what caffeine does for them, most will tell you that it sharpens their minds. However, this perception is only true in the sense that stress increases alertness. We know, for example, that we tend to remember traumatic events very clearly. Everyone remembers what they were doing the day Kennedy was shot. Eons ago, this survival mechanism helped us to remember (and thereby avoid) dangerous situations when such an ability meant the difference between life and death.

But today, millions of people create artificial stress by ingesting caffeine numerous times every day, and then they marvel at the way it "sharpens" their minds. In this chapter, we'll look at the mental and emotional downside of caffeine, what happens to your brain and nervous system when they are subjected to this constant stress. We'll look at three different aspects of caffeine: the physiological effects; how those affects alter mind, mood, and behavior; and finally the emotional consequences, including anxiety, depression, and other psychological disorders.

Studies show conclusively that caffeine contributes to anxiety, irritability, panic attacks, depression, and anger.

With high levels of caffeine in your blood, even the small annoyances of life can gain tragic proportions. The irony of it all, of course, is that when people are feeling stressed, they tend to drink more coffee. On the surface, that appears to make sense because much of the time we feel the need for a little more energy. But what you get from caffeine is really not energy; it's metabolic and neurologic stress.

Another part of the coffee illusion is created by advertisers who tell us that coffee is what you drink when you have to sort things out. Nothing could be farther from the truth. Even the term *coffee break* is absurd, as the net result of ingesting coffee is merely greater stress and decreased ability to cope.

Nuts and Bolts: Caffeine and Brain Function

In Chapter 3, we discussed how caffeine interferes with the normal control of neuron firing in the brain. Caffeine triggers a stress response that involves a surge in adrenal hormones and the classic fight-or-flight "emergency," affecting virtually every cell in the body.[1]

This stress response has an undeniable impact on the nervous system. We know that people living under threat of attack suffer greatly from the stress, even if the attack never comes. Likewise, caffeine creates background tension that ultimately reduces the quality of life, an effect that may go unnoticed because it is masked by other stressors.

However, unlike many other vicissitudes of life, we *can* do something about the levels of caffeine we consume. At some point, most people realize that peace of mind is a highly desirable experience. And the time to do something about your caffeine intake is before that peace is shattered.

The Stress/Distress Threshold

In Chapter 3, I presented the concept of a threshold point at which stress becomes damaging to the body. This is also true for the mind, and the undeniable fact is that caffeine lowers that threshold point by creating anxiety, irritability, anger, and hostility. In other words, events that we would normally cope with successfully send us flying off the handle. Our responses can take many forms, from outward expressions of frustration to silent rage.

THE STRESS/DISTRESS THRESHOLD

Managing Life's Challenges		Influence of Caffeine		Overwhelmed by Life's Challenges	
Margin of mental and emotional health	Coping Skills awareness, ability to relax, sound sleep, cooperation, compromise, patience, flexibility, faith, optimism	Total Life Stress finances, health, family, relationships, career, world events, environment, anxiety, irritability, poor sleep	Coping Skills awareness, faith, optimism	Total Life Stress finances, health, family, relationships, career, world events, environment, anxiety, depression, irritability, poor sleep	Coping Skills awareness, faith
Total Life Stress finances, health, family, relationships, career, world events, environment					

99

Emotional Resilience

Life is complex and unpredictable, and to negotiate its challenges requires flexibility, understanding, and a sense of harmony and inner balance. The previous illustration at the left represents what could be called emotional resilience: the ability to "roll with the punches," to cope successfully and maintain a sense of peace in one's life.

For people amped out on caffeine, however, the margin of emotional health is very small. When the first life stress comes along—be it illness, financial woes, public speaking, final exams, relationship problems, or just getting a parking ticket—the experience destroys their peace of mind and overwhelms them.

Caffeine promoters deny this problem, but their data is artificial if not purposely misleading. For example, in research designed to evaluate the effect of caffeine on behavior, people who are under significant stress are usually removed from the study group, presumably because they would exhibit an "overreaction" to caffeine. Does this make sense?

A more accurate and meaningful line of inquiry would include such people because they are the most likely to be harmed. The best approach would be to evaluate the cumulative effect of stress resulting from both environmental and caffeine sources. One landmark study measured the effect of caffeine on military recruits and found that caffeine was a significant contributing factor to the development of combat-stress syndrome. The researchers concluded that "the use of decaffeinated coffee in military settings might reduce the prevalence of the various anxiety reactions, including combat-stress reaction."[2]

Such research fits perfectly into the model of emotional resilience and points toward a better understanding of the role of caffeine in health and disease. Now follow this line of reasoning to the next step, which is to acknowledge that emotional health and physical health are absolutely inseparable. Every day, more and more research is published in support of the body-mind connection, including studies that show stress to be not just a contributing factor, but a major factor in a wide range of health disorders. Thus, the model of emotional resilience can be expanded to include physical as well as emotional health.

"Stress plays a significant role in more than half of the complaints that bring patients to the physician's office."

Source: *The Physician and Sportsmedicine*, 1994;22(7):66.

The role of stress is perfectly illustrated by a report in the *Journal of the American Medical Association* showing that stress can alter brain biochemistry in such a way that the effects of subsequent events are greatly magnified. Animals exposed to stress, for example, will exhibit heightened aggressiveness long after the stressful event is over. And it's not just for a few hours. Abnormal brain chemistry and 200 percent increases in aggressive behavior have been observed for up to a month.[3] In other words, stress can produce long-lasting alterations in neurotransmitter production in the brain, resulting in higher levels of norepinephrine and a subsequent increase in anxiety and hostility. The take-home message here is that there is a cumulative effect of stress in our lives, and caffeine is an important part of the increasing harm that we experience.

ROBERTA BREAKS THE CYCLE

Roberta was a light coffee drinker and worked in a moderately stressful job as an administrative assistant. When her boss was promoted to CEO, the demands on her were greatly increased. Suddenly, she found herself working overtime, coming in early, and traveling three or four times a month. What's more, the intensity level of every day was increased because of her new responsibilities. She faced the challenge with determination—and caffeine. Soon, she was drinking coffee before she left the house, another cup as soon as she arrived at the office, a cup at midmorning, and a soft drink with lunch. Then there was tea or another soft drink in the afternoon.

The increased work hours started to cause problems at home. She was late picking up her son at child care more often than she was on time, and family demands only added to her stress. When Roberta came to see me, she was near the breaking point. She was experiencing headaches and muscle pain, and she hadn't exercised in months.

"All I need is a rest," she said. "Can you help me get through these next few months till my vacation?" I explained that I didn't agree with her line of thinking, and pointed out that unless she handled the underlying stress, she would be in the same plight a few weeks after her vacation. She insisted that a vacation would fix everything, so I drew the following diagram to make my point. I call it "the vacation illusion."

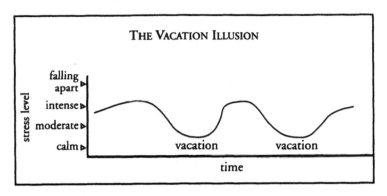

Roberta thought that she could push herself to the breaking point and that periodic vacations would prevent her from experiencing stress-induced disease and breakdown. Stress, however, has a cumulative effect, and this is compounded by caffeine. What she didn't take into consideration was that the damage being done to her nervous system would make her less and less able to cope with her job. For Roberta and millions of others, the vacation reality actually looks like this:

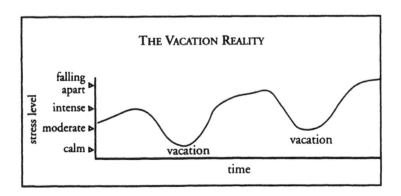

Note the upward slope of the stress curve. Each vacation provides less relaxation and rejuvenation, followed by greater stress, building to ultimate burnout. The question Robert asked, of course, was how to get off this upward spiral without quitting her job. And my answer was "Get off caffeine and give yourself a thirty-minute stress-management break every day."

Now you're probably thinking that without caffeine, you couldn't accomplish everything that needs to be done, so I will give you the same suggestion I gave Roberta: Follow my Off the Bean program, which includes a nutritional plan to enhance energy and mental acuity, and see how it makes life easier and more enjoyable. My program worked splendidly for Roberta. She was not only better able to cope with the various tasks of her job, but she found that she was working more efficiently with co-workers and spending less time "spinning her wheels." As she told me, "When I was running on caffeine, I thought I was doing a bang-up job, but I was really just banging around."

Don't Be Happy—Be Worried

To review, caffeine interferes with adenosine receptors, which normally control the rate of neuron firing in the brain. In addition, the drug interferes with the metabolism of GABA, an important biochemical that helps us filter information and plan sensible action strategies.[4] So the caffeine-stress combination, in effect, turns up the activity level in your brain while at the same time lowering your coping skills and decreasing your ability to relax. The result? Anxiety and irritability.

The amazing thing is that even without knowing how

this occurs, most people know that caffeine makes them nervous. Yet a common reaction is not to decrease intake of caffeine, but to reach for anti-anxiety drugs. Today, one out of every five American adults takes some form of tranquilizer or antidepressant. Since seven out of every ten American adults drink coffee, it's safe to assume that many individuals drink coffee *and* take tranquilizers. This behavior is equivalent to driving with one foot on the brake and one foot on the gas. No wonder so many people are falling apart.

Truth in Advertising

An ad recently ran in national magazines that asked, "Does your life have signs of persistent anxiety?" It went on to list symptoms such as sleep disturbance, irritability, muscle tension, restlessness, and fatigue. Is this a "quit coffee" ad? No, this was an advertisement for Buspar, a new anti-anxiety drug from Bristol-Myers Squibb. Nowhere did the ad mention that every one of these symptoms could result from the consumption of caffeine. Nor did the prescribing information (in the *Physicians' Desk Reference*) recommend that doctors query their patients regarding their caffeine intake before prescribing the drug.

Beyond Anxiety: Panic Disorder

For an estimated 5 million Americans, anxiety progresses to a condition known as panic disorder.[5] The onset of panic "attacks" usually occurs in the third decade of life, and it afflicts women three times more often than men. Panic disorder is characterized by unexpected, unprovoked and intense fear, usually including feelings of impending doom. The accompanying symptoms of rapid heartbeat, shortness of breath, palpitation, dizziness, sweating, and a feeling of helplessness make this condition truly and deeply frightening. A panic attack may last only minutes, or it may last hours.

Now I'm not saying that panic attacks are caused by caffeine, but look back at the model of emotional resilience and imagine a paper-thin margin of emotional health. Think of the possible triggers that could send someone's nervous system into a tailspin. One of the most significant is caffeine.

CHECKLIST #1: ANXIETY/PANIC DISORDER

Medical and scientific analysis of anxiety/panic disorder has revealed well-defined abnormalities in physiology and brain biochemistry in people who suffer from the condition.[6–10] These include:

1. Overproduction of adrenal stress hormones, including increased norepinephrine and cortisol.
   Is caffeine a factor? Yes ✓
2. Increased incidence of mitral valve prolapse (MVP).
   Is caffeine a factor? Yes ✓
3. Decreased nighttime melatonin production.
   Is caffeine a factor? Yes ✓
4. Dysfunction of GABA metabolism.
   Is caffeine a factor? Yes ✓

5. Increased neuron firing in the brain.
   Is caffeine a factor? Yes ✓
6. Decreased blood circulation to the brain.
   Is caffeine a factor? Yes ✓

What's more, in someone prone to this disorder, caffeine ingestion can trigger panic attacks.[11] Still, caffeine promoters dismiss this characterization of their product, claiming that if caffeine were so bad, nearly everyone would have an anxiety disorder. That response is reminiscent of the cigarette makers who (until recently) defended their product by stating, "If cigarettes are so bad, every smoker would get cancer." Of course not every smoker gets cancer and not every caffeine user has panic attacks. But it is important to understand that there is a continuum of effects. Everyone who smokes is destroying lung tissue, and in many cases that will progress to cancer. Likewise, everyone who abuses caffeine is harming his or her nervous system, and in many cases, that will progress to anxiety and perhaps panic attacks.

A Look at the Literature

Evidence of a connection between caffeine and anxiety/panic disorder is well established in the medical literature. Back in 1936, the *New England Journal of Medicine* reported that a woman became "confused, disoriented, excited, restless and violent" after ingesting a large number of caffeine pills. She was brought to the hospital, where the staff, ignorant of her caffeine binge, made the diagnosis of "psychoneurosis, anxiety type, with a hysterical episode."

Five weeks later, the same woman again took over 1,000 milligrams of caffeine tablets, and was returned to the hospital. When she did not improve, she was transferred to a psychiatric hospital, where she was strapped to her bed. After two months during which she made a slow recovery, she suddenly took a turn for the worse. Finally, someone noticed that she was drinking four cups of coffee per day. When the coffee was withdrawn, "she became entirely normal and was dismissed from the hospital."[12]

A more recent study published in the *Journal of Clinical Psychiatry* reported that caffeine is not only capable of triggering panic attacks, but can also increase their frequency and intensity.[13] Even moderate intake of caffeine has been found to worsen anxiety,[14] and in a typical vicious cycle, individuals with anxiety and depression have been found to exhibit increased sensitivity to caffeine.[15, 16] Finally, a report in the *Archives of General Psychiatry* found that caffeine produced significant increases in anxiety, nervousness, fear, nausea, palpitations, restlessness, and tremors in patients with agoraphobia and panic disorders. In fact, 71 percent of the patients reported that the behavioral effects of caffeine were similar to those experienced during panic attacks.[17]

Is the caffeine connection widely unrecognized? Surveys document that 70 percent of patients with panic disorder visited physicians ten or more times before they experienced relief of their symptoms.[18] The fact is that few physicians conduct a careful evaluation of caffeine intake, even though the medical literature is conclusive on the benefits of caffeine reduction in virtually all anxiety disorders.

Where Are You on the Caffeine/Anxiety Scale?

Emotional health is not an all-or-nothing state. There is a continuum of feelings and experiences that range all the way from deep serenity to panic. Where would you place yourself on this scale, and where would you like to be?

Deep Serenity	Mostly at Ease	Slightly Tense	Anxious	Panic
▲	▲	▲	▲	▲
You experience an extraordinary sense of peace in your life at all times.	You experience some stress but it is temporary and easy to relieve.	You experience tension or anxiety that is sometimes difficult to relieve.	You experience a level of tension or anxiety that is sometimes impossible to control.	You experience feelings of helplessness and are sometimes seized by intense fear.

The popular notion that habitual use diminishes this stress response has also been debunked. A landmark study published in *Psychosomatic Medicine* examined the effects of moderate caffeine intake on stress reactivity in both habitual and light consumers of caffeine. Psychosocial stress (e.g., giving subjects a demanding task and distracting them at the same time) caused an increase in the stress hormones epinephrine and cortisol, but the addition of a moderate amount of caffeine *more than doubled* the stress response.[19] Importantly, the researchers found that habitual and light caffeine consumers had basically the same increase in stress hormones, proving that people do not develop a tolerance to the anxiety-producing effects of caffeine. Rather, people simply become accustomed to the feelings of stress, irritability, and aggressiveness produced by the drug.

Damned If You Do . . .

The interesting thing about caffeine is that it potentiates or magnifies the stress in our lives. This effect occurs not only when one consumes it, but also when habitual drinkers are deprived of their "fix" for even a few hours.[20-22] Remember that caffeine is not a mood elevator except in the sense that metabolic stress tends to increase alertness. In other words, caffeine doesn't improve one's mood; it simply helps to avert the fatigue and depression associated with withdrawal. This fatigue and depression can come on quickly (within three hours of deprivation), and just about anyone can become dependent on caffeine, not only heavy or habitual users. Careful research conducted by the department of psychiatry and behavioral sciences at Johns Hopkins University School of Medicine shows that low to moderate caffeine intake (as little as one fourteen-ounce mug per day) can quickly produce withdrawal symptoms, including depression, anxiety, irritability, fatigue, and headache.[23]

The Depression Connection

Depression is the single most common psychiatric diagnosis in America. It is estimated that 23 percent of American women and 12 percent of American men will seek medical or psychiatric help for this problem at some point in their lives. These figures are staggering. We're not talking about transient blues or feeling a bit down, but rather clinical depression, which involves the inability to pull yourself out of the mood.[24, 25]

What's more, many experts believe these figures underestimate the true problem, since only one person in three suffering from depression seeks professional help. Medical research strongly suggests that the disorder is generally underdiagnosed, undertreated, and often inappropriately treated by health-care providers.[26]

Few people would say that caffeine makes them depressed, but that's only because the depressive effect is delayed. Studies show, for example, that most people given a group of substances over time will ascribe any changes in the way they feel to the last substance they took. Thus, feelings of tiredness and depression that come three hours after a cup of coffee are seldom associated with caffeine. We blame something else, like the weather or a boring job.

In reality, however, caffeine does contribute to depression in well-defined ways. The first is what I call the caffeine "rebound" effect. This has to do with the complex interactions between the stress response (adrenal stimulation) and brain biochemistry. We touched on this in Chapter 3 in the discussion of dopamine and addiction. There I presented evidence that caffeine raises dopamine levels in the brain in a way that is similar to amphetamines, albeit less dramatic.

The rebound depression is also similar, and to understand this, you don't have to be familiar with pharmacology. Have you ever felt a "letdown" after an exciting event—even something really good? The intense stimulation subsides and is then replaced by a creeping sense of depression or languor. This happens because your dopamine receptors, the brain cells associated with excitement, have all been fired. What follows is a metabolic rebound that you must experience until your stores of dopamine are replenished. Caffeine can trigger this stress/depression roller coaster, and it may involve more than dopamine, since caffeine also appears to stimulate serotonin release as well.[27]

The second way that caffeine contributes to depression is, of course, the withdrawal reaction, the most prevalent symptoms being headache, depression, and fatigue. Three facts are important to grasp in regard to withdrawal. First of all, each of the symptoms compounds or magnifies the depressive effect. Secondly, withdrawal can occur even in light caffeine users.[28] And third, withdrawal reactions can be evident even when caffeine is withheld for just a few hours.[29] Some people feel depressed or anxious if they're simply late for their morning or afternoon cup. That's not only a powerful motivation to consume the beverage, but it also creates an often-unidentified source of background stress.

CASE STUDY

A clinical report published in the *Journal of Affective Disorders* graphically illustrates the connection between caffeine and depression. A woman suffered for twenty years with recurrent depression. She was treated with a variety of drugs, including lithium, chlorpromazine, haloperidol, and Valium. After years of drug therapy, she decided to quit drinking coffee. Within one month, she was able to eliminate the Valium and all but one of her medications. At the time the clinical report was published, she had gone five years without a single episode of depression.[30]

Another Vicious Cycle

Depression can also occur as an adverse side effect of certain medications, and once again, caffeine is often a factor.

Consider the example of a fifty-year-old man with high blood pressure who is put on a popular class of drugs called beta-blockers (e.g., propranolol). Depression and fatigue are common side effects with these drugs.[31] Now the fellow is also drinking coffee, which contributes to his hypertension, and, faced with depression and fatigue, he then drinks even more coffee to break out of the depressed state. Thus, his blood pressure stays elevated and his doctor responds by increasing the medication dose, which causes the man to become more depressed.

A Word about Antidepressants

The pharmaceutical industry continues to spend billions to develop and market antidepressant drugs. Three main categories, including tricyclic antidepressants (TCAs), MAO inhibitors, and the new class of selective serotonin reuptake inhibitors (SSRIs) can all be very valuable, and all can have significant side effects. Of the three classes, MAO inhibitors have the longest list of serious side effects, mostly having to do with increased risk of heart disease. Common side effects include headache, dizziness, and insomnia. TCAs also have significant cardiovascular risks (elevated blood pressure, rapid heartbeat, palpitation, arrhythmias), and the new SSRIs, while having numerically fewer side effects, have as their primary disadvantage frequent reports of anxiety, insomnia, nervousness, and tremor.[32, 33] Believe it or not, with these common adverse side effects, none of these drugs list coffee as a beverage to avoid in their professional or patient literature.

CHECKLIST #2: DEPRESSION

Mental health professionals have observed that depression is often the other side of anxiety.[34, 35] In other words, a drug (like caffeine) that creates anxiety will ultimately contribute to depression. Depression is characterized by well-defined biochemical and behavioral abnormalities, all of which are aggravated by caffeine.[36-40] They include:

1. Overproduction of stress hormones, including increased ACTH and cortisol.
   Is caffeine a factor? Yes ✓
2. Strong association with insomnia and sleep disturbance.
   Is caffeine a factor? Yes ✓
3. Decreased nighttime melatonin production.
   Is caffeine a factor? Yes ✓
4. Dysfunction of GABA metabolism.
   Is caffeine a factor? Yes ✓
5. Alteration of serotonin levels in the brain.
   Is caffeine a factor? Yes ✓
6. Strong association with life stress.
   Is caffeine a factor? Yes ✓

But I'm Not Depressed!

If you're a coffee drinker, you may be thinking, "Well, I drink coffee and I'm not depressed." It's necessary to state again that everyone is different, and also that depression can be quite subtle. Throughout this book, I am suggesting that you will never know the full effect the drug is having on you until you experience what life is like caffeine free. Over the years, I have heard similar responses from hundreds of clients: "Wow, I never realized that caffeine made me so [select one: anxious, depressed, irritable]."

In addition, research shows that there are a number of variables affecting the depressive side of caffeine. A recent study measuring the stress hormone cortisol (raised by caffeine consumption) is revealing. Researchers found that in collegiate swimmers, there was a powerful correlation between cortisol levels and depression, but only during periods of intense training.[41] Thus, there appears to be a cumulative stress phenomenon, which may be present at certain times and absent at other times. Having this information and being sensitive to your moods will enable you to take the appropriate steps should you start to notice periods of depression.

Above all, I want you to avoid the common mistake of reaching for the coffeepot when you're feeling "blue." Coffee may help temporarily, but clinical and laboratory evidence suggests strongly that you will pay a steep price later on. Ironically, the group most likely to use caffeine in an attempt to change their state of mind are those suffering from clinical depression.[42]

DAVE KICKS CAFFEINE, SLEEPS BETTER, FEELS BRIGHTER

Dave was a typical, hardworking middle-management professional. And like so many, his intake of caffeine had slowly escalated to four cups a day, the last one coming around 3 P.M. to get him through the overtime hours. Always looking for the competitive edge, he read an article in a health magazine that recommended eight hours of sleep for peak mental performance. That was when he realized that he suffered from insomnia. He was having a hard time getting to sleep, and would often read in bed or watch TV until 1 A.M.

His doctor gave him Ambien, a sleep medication, and told Dave to cut back on coffee. So he dropped the 3 P.M. cup. He started falling asleep earlier, but then he noticed that he was getting "the blahs" almost every afternoon. Not realizing that it was related to caffeine withdrawal, Dave blamed his depression on the sleeping pills. When he came to my office, he said he was looking for a "natural sleeping pill that wouldn't make him depressed," but it didn't take me long to see the real problem.

"You don't have insomnia because of an Ambien deficiency," I told him. "Ambien may help, but I believe you will do much better by getting off caffeine altogether. Caffeine is keeping you awake at night and caffeine is making you depressed." Dave didn't like this suggestion, even though I assured him that he would have more energy, a better attitude, and a sharper mind with my Off the Bean program (see Chapter 10). Instead he went back to his doctor, who gave him a prescription for a popular antidepressant.

After a month on the two drugs, Dave felt worse than ever. He was falling asleep all right, but he awoke feeling tired. He felt that his motivation, the sharpness he needed in his competitive field, was gone. He wasn't depressed, but he also wasn't feeling great. By the time he got back to me, he'd stopped exercising, and he knew that was not a good sign.

"Look," I told him, repeating a rationale I had used a thousand times before. "If you try my program and don't feel a great deal better, you can always go back to your caffeine, sleeping pills, and antidepressants." So Dave agreed to give it a try, and over a period of three weeks, he got off coffee entirely. Shortly after that, he was able to discontinue both medications, and that's when his life really improved.

"At the end of a month," said Dave, "it was as if the sun broke through. I felt optimistic and powerful. And I was keenly aware that the energy and enthusiasm I was experiencing was coming from me, not a coffee mug. I got back into exercising, performed better at my job, and now look back on my caffeine addiction like a junkie who's finally kicked the habit."

Depression and Sleep

Dave's case illustrates another facet of the caffeine-depression connection. Sleep is disturbed in 90 percent of patients with depression. The conventional belief is that when people are depressed, they naturally have difficulty sleeping. New research, however, shows that this is not the case. A study published in the *Journal of Clinical Psychiatry* found that curing the depression does not necessarily eliminate the sleep problem.[43] The most likely explanation? Depressed individuals frequently use caffeine to give themselves a "lift." This habit perpetuates their sleep disorders and greatly increases the likelihood of recurrent depression.

What's more, sleep disturbance is a common side effect of antidepressant medications. New studies presented in Europe indicate that selective serotonin reuptake inhibitors (SSRIs)—which include the popular antidepressant Prozac—can seriously interrupt sleep patterns, making people feel drowsy during the day.[44]

The vicious cycle could not be more clear. Caffeine contributes to depression, but, not knowing this, people take antidepressant drugs. Both the drugs and the caffeine disturb their sleep, causing them to feel tired during the day, which causes them to drink more coffee. The only way to break this cycle is to get off the caffeine. Then you will be able to discern whether or not you truly need an antidepressant.

Depression or Fatigue: Which Comes First?

Fatigue is one of the most frequent reasons why Americans seek medical help.[45] It is also one of the most obvious causes of depression, and a source of some confusion among medical professionals. Mrs. Jones turns to her doctor for help with her fatigue and, after ruling out anemia and other disease factors, the doctor will often announce that she is "simply" depressed.

I find this response to be insensitive and unscientific. After all, it is entirely possible that the doctor was simply unable to find the cause of fatigue, and saying that she is depressed, while technically accurate, misses the point. In reality, anyone who becomes fatigued will ultimately become depressed.

The converse is also true. Depressed individuals will invariably experience fatigue. In fact, not all depressed people feel sad. Many just feel bone-weary. So we have another vicious cycle that requires a search for root causes, not a quick diagnosis and a prescription for antidepressants. The caffeine-depression connection is very clear, but caffeine's contribution to fatigue is often difficult to see. That's because we are so used to thinking of caffeine as an energizing substance.

It might be good to review the stress-fatigue cycle described in Chapter 3, remembering that caffeine does not provide energy at all, but only delivers a temporary shock to the nervous system that feels like a boost. Think of an exhausted fighter in his corner and the trainer slapping him in the face to get him ready for the next round.

The truth about caffeine and energy is finally getting out. Physicians are starting to warn their patients about caffeine "rebound," and an article in *U.S. News & World Report* listed caffeine addiction as a major cause of fatigue, including a "crash" that occurs after caffeine "buzz" wears off.[46] People who become aware of this powerful influence on energy and mood and take steps to improve their energy naturally (see Chapter 10) can experience remarkable improvements in their quality of life.

Mental and Emotional Effects of Caffeine

- Chronic caffeine ingestion may cause or exacerbate anxiety and may be associated with depression and increased use of anti-anxiety drugs.
- Caffeine may cause anxiety and panic in panic disorder patients.
- Caffeine may aggravate the symptoms of premenstrual syndrome.
- Chronic users who are caffeine-sensitive may have symptoms of caffeinism at relatively low doses.
- Individual who regularly consume moderate to heavy amounts of caffeine may develop caffeinism, or they may show signs of caffeine withdrawal syndrome after abstaining from the drug.

Source: G. L. Clementz and J. W. Dailey, "Psychotropic Effects of Caffeine," *American Family Physician*, May 1988;37(5):167–72.

Is Coffee the "Think Drink"? Think Again!

Students the world over use caffeine not only to stay awake, but also because they believe the drug will improve their performance on exams. Solid research, however, illustrates that as little as 100 milligrams of caffeine (a six-ounce serving) can cause a significant *decrease* in recall and reasoning.

One study compared scores on a memory test called the Auditory-Verbal Learning Test, or AVLT. College students who were given 100 milligrams of caffeine recalled significantly fewer words than those given a placebo beverage. These results were found in both single and multiple presentation trials. Interestingly, subjects given caffeine did fine at the beginning of the test, but were particularly weak in the middle to end portions of the study.[47] This illustrates that the "enhancement" of alertness provided by caffeine is both temporary and illusory.

Research has also found that caffeine ingestion is associated with *lower* academic performance and greater incidence of psychosomatic illness.[48] Ironically, when students are given a questionnaire to evaluate their expectation of benefits from caffeine, those with the highest expectations turn out to be those who consume the most caffeine and who experience greater levels of anxiety, depression, insomnia, headache, and fatigue.[49] I believe that heavy caffeine consumption is a significant factor in the epidemic of anxiety suffered by college students. One recent study found that 34 percent of students surveyed were experiencing anxiety sufficient to cause clinical symptoms of psychosomatic illness.[50]

Caffeine Boggles the Brain

How does caffeine decrease mental acuity and cause all these problems? There are a number of possible explanations, the first of course being stress. Nature did not design the stress response to enable us to engage in abstract or global reasoning, such as may be required for complex tasks or final exams. The stress response causes a shift of mental function to a very primitive survival-oriented part of the brain known as the limbic system.[51] Once again, this is great if you're engaged in a fight-or-flight situation, but not so great if you're trying to write an essay on the fall of the Roman Empire.

What's more, adenosine receptor antagonists (such as caffeine) have a depressive effect on other brain biochemicals, such as acetylcholine.[52, 53] Since acetylcholine is a neurotransmitter directly involved in memory and learning, this could account for some of the observed negative effects. In support of this theory, researchers generally have found that simple tasks such as assembly-line work are enhanced by caffeine consumption, while complex reasoning skills are diminished. Subjects asked to perform auditory recognition tasks, for example, where they had to process verbal information, did worse after ingesting caffeine.[54]

Other eye-opening research has found that caffeine causes a remarkable decrease in cerebral blood flow. You don't have to be a neurochemist to see that such an effect would not be good for memory, mood, and learning. Caffeine produces this effect, known as cerebral vasoconstriction, by interfering with the normal relaxation of blood vessels in the brain.

> "Caffeine, even in small doses, is a potent cerebral vasoconstrictor."
>
> Source: R. J. Matthew and W. H. Wilson, "Substance Abuse and Cerebral Blood Flow," *American Journal of Psychiatry*, March 1991;148(3):292–305.

Is the effect significant? One study illustrated that a dose of 250 milligrams (approximately fifteen ounces of coffee) produced approximately a 30 percent decrease in whole-brain cerebral blood flow.[55] This is not only unfortunate, it's dangerous, because at the same time, caffeine increases blood pressure in the brain, leading to an increased risk for stroke.[56] Researchers have also found that caffeine reduces the oxygen level of brain tissues.[57] With all of the attention on brain health today (concerning depression, Alzheimer's and Parkinson's disease, as well as stroke) don't you think it's a little odd that this data has not even made it to the evening news?

The Great Gaurana Hoax

Recently, manufacturers have been tripping over themselves to market products containing guarana, a South American herb. Guarana (botanical name, *Paulinia cupana*) is in chewing gum, "energy" drinks, a popular soft drink, and nutritional supplements purported to enhance sex drive, mental acuity, and stamina. It's hyped as an ancient Aztec secret, but the only secret is that guarana contains more caffeine by weight than coffee beans. Manufacturers usually fail to mention that salient fact.

It's also interesting to note that no manufacturer of guarana products has provided reliable evidence of their effectiveness. In fact, studies have been performed that soundly debunk the product claims. One group of researchers gave memory and learning tests to elderly volunteers. Those given guarana performed no better than those given placebo.[58] Another study found that guarana actually had negative effects on a variety of learning tasks.[59] The same is true for yerba maté, another herbal source of caffeine.

The DHEA Connection, Part II

In Chapter 3, we learned that DHEA is a hormone that contributes to youthful energy, vitality, and sex drive. Aside from the fact that it is converted by the body to testosterone and estrogen, DHEA also plays an important role in memory, mood, and learning. Recent studies have found that depressed individuals improve when DHEA levels are optimized, and this improvement includes enhanced memory and feelings of well-being.[60] But before you run to the health-food store to buy DHEA, you must realize it's not that simple. Stress and caffeine can abolish nearly all of the neurological benefits you might obtain from DHEA.[61]

If you want the improvements in brain function that optimal levels of DHEA can provide, you'll have to cut back on caffeine. That's because there is a tug-of-war going on in your body between DHEA and stress hormones. When stress hormones predominate, your immune system, emotional state, energy, vitality, and DHEA levels all suffer—and aging is accelerated as a result.

Can Caffeine Damage Your Brain?

Neurological damage from caffeine ingestion is far from proven, but consider the evidence. We know that elderly individuals with symptoms of memory loss and disorientation have degeneration of neurons in an area of the brain known as the hippocampus. In animal studies, raising stress hormone levels produces neuron damage in that precise location.

What's more, human studies support the concept of stress-induced hippocampal degeneration. Using magnetic resonance imaging (MRI), researchers have found reduced hippocampal activity in people under high stress conditions such as depression and post-traumatic stress disorder.

David Morgan of the University of South Florida's Institute on Aging explains, "We think that exposure to stress hormones, particularly high levels over a long period of time, may be responsible for the minor learning deficits we have as we get older."[62] He goes on to assert that stress hormones may be responsible for the chronic degenerative diseases that cause most deaths in older people. The message is clear: Keeping levels of stress hormones as low as possible may determine to a great extent the quality of life in your later years.

Caffeine and Mental Illness

If a person were injected with 500 milligrams of caffeine, within about an hour he or she would exhibit symptoms of severe mental illness, among them, hallucinations, paranoia, panic, mania, and depression. But the same amount of caffeine administered over the course of a day only pro-

duces the milder forms of insanity for which we take tranquilizers and antidepressants.

Mental and emotional health requires a sense of stability, and we have seen that caffeine creates a roller-coaster
effect throughout the nervous, endocrine, and cardiovascular systems. Thankfully, mental health professionals are
starting to take a close look at the caffeine connection.
Regarding the treatment of anxiety, recommendations are
now being published to *start* with avoidance of caffeine,[63]
and the latest edition of the *Diagnostic and Statistical Manual of Mental Disorders* (DSM) includes an entire section
on caffeinism.

However, research concerning caffeine and mental
health is mixed, in great part because of the way many
studies are designed. In Chapter 1, I presented a study
where hospitalized psychiatric patients were switched to
decaf coffee without their knowledge.[64] When these individuals did not improve, the conclusion was made that
caffeine is not harmful to mental health. Given what we
know about the severe emotional and physical symptoms
associated with caffeine withdrawal, would anyone wonder why these people did not improve?

To evaluate the matter fairly, we need research that takes
into account not only withdrawal, but the fact that it can
take three weeks or longer for stress hormones to return to
normal after discontinuing caffeine. In addition, it would
be useful to know whether psychiatric patients consume
higher amounts of caffeine than the general population.
One survey of psychiatric hospital admissions found that
patients consumed approximately five cups of coffee per
day.[65] Another put the total even higher and noted that
the heavy caffeine users were also most likely to suffer
from depression.[66]

In fact, a recent study revealed that about 40 percent of hospital inpatients consumed sufficient caffeine to produce multiple symptoms of caffeinism—including anxiety, depression, and paranoid delusion. Based upon these startling results, the authors recommend that all psychiatric patients be questioned regarding their caffeine intake, and suggested that caffeinism should be viewed as a primary contributing cause of anxiety-related emotional illness.[67]

Another facet of this important issue has to do with adverse reactions and long-term damage that may be caused by caffeine's interaction with commonly prescribed psychiatric drugs. Researchers are warning mental health professionals that caffeine can interfere with and even negate the therapeutic benefits of these medications.[68]

Does any of this information surprise you? The fact is that caffeine has powerful neurological effects, and it is unreasonable to expect that the drug would not cause harm to those whose nervous systems are already shattered and stressed.

As if more evidence were required, two revealing studies have recently been conducted with psychiatric patients. In the first, researchers gave schizophrenic patients a dose of caffeine equivalent to about four cups of coffee. The caffeine raised blood levels of stress hormones and produced significant behavior disturbances, as well as increased blood pressure.[69] The second study measured the effect of withdrawing caffeine from the diet of severely retarded adult patients. Two weeks without caffeine produced no real improvement in sleep pattern or behavior, but reintroduction of caffeine was accompanied by a highly significant increase in ward disturbance ratings.[70] These findings are consistent with the fact that it would take three weeks or longer for caffeine-free patients to exhibit positive behavior changes.

"Our data suggest that inquiry into caffeine consumption should be included routinely for psychiatric patients, e.g., at admission, because patients with a psychotic disorder undergo a higher risk for an excessive caffeine consumption."

Source: M. Rihs, C. Muller, and P. Baumann, "Caffeine Consumption in Hospitalized Psychiatric Patients," *European Archives of Psychiatry and Clinical Neuroscience*, 1996;246(2):83–92.

"[D]eleterious effects may result from the interaction of caffeine with commonly prescribed psychotropic drugs. . . . Increased public education about potential health problems related to caffeine consumption is suggested, and further controls of caffeine in psychiatric settings are recommended."

Source: A. Kruger, "Chronic Psychiatric Patients' Use of Caffeine: Pharmacological Effects and Mechanisms," *Psychology Reports*, June 1996;78(3 Pt 1):915–23.

Common Profiles of Caffeine Abusers

A great many people are addicted to caffeine and abuse it without being aware of the consequences. Depending on individual sensitivity, as little as two cups of coffee per day has been shown to produce anxiety, insomnia, irritability, and dizziness.[71]

Dr. Michael Liepman, a clinician who works in addiction psychiatry at Michigan State University/Kalamazoo Center for Medical Studies, has identified the following types of patients who commonly abuse caffeine. Are you among them?

1. Patients with insomnia who are unaware that caffeine can disturb sleep for up to eight hours. These individuals often obtain sleep medications (from physicians who do not take a caffeine history) and then become doubly addicted, often escalating dosages of both drugs over time.
2. Patients with anxiety disorder (panic disorder, generalized anxiety disorder [GAD]) whose symptoms are aggravated by caffeine.
3. Alcohol abusers who drink to counteract the anxiety and/or depression produced by excess caffeine intake.
4. Recovering alcoholics who switch to caffeinated beverages once sober from alcohol. They become anxious, experience an overwhelming craving for alcohol sedation, and then relapse.
5. Hyperactive-appearing children who start on caffeinated beverages and chocolate (a source of caffeine and theobromine). Such children often become wild and uncontrollable, either ending up on stronger stimulants or sedating themselves with alcohol, marijuana, or other drugs.
6. Patients on sedating drugs who increase their intake of caffeine to resist the sedation.
7. Patients who are taking drugs that include caffeine (e.g., painkillers) without knowing that they contain caffeine.
8. Fetuses, newborn infants, and nursing infants whose

mothers ingest caffeine from multiple sources. The babies have disturbed sleep, which causes the mothers to become sleep-deprived, whereupon the mothers increase their caffeine intake in order to function.

This last group is arguably the most serious because there are two "victims," both of whom are caught in a spiral of addiction and pain. We know, for example, that when pregnant women consume caffeine, their babies are often born with a caffeine dependency. If these babies are bottle-fed, they will experience withdrawal symptoms, and if you can imagine a newborn baby with insomnia and a splitting headache, you understand the tragic consequences. Even if they are breast-fed, breast milk does not contain as much caffeine as they were getting in the womb, and that may also trigger withdrawal symptoms.

Then there's the mother, who now has to deal with a child who cannot be consoled. Readers who have raised fussy children will understand the strain that this creates. Multiply fussy times ten, and you have the stress of a baby addicted to caffeine. As mentioned above, these mothers often turn to caffeine to get through the day, and thus fall farther into the abyss of stress, disturbed sleep, neurological damage, and emotional pain.

To Sleep, Perchance to Dream . . .

As described in Chapter 3, sleep is a critical factor in emotional and physical health. A perfectly healthy and optimistic person will start to exhibit clear symptoms of emotional illness after only three nights of disturbed sleep. In my clinical practice, I took a careful sleep inventory and found that fewer than 25 percent of my patients had satisfactory sleep habits, in terms of duration, consistency, and restfulness. The vast majority woke up feeling tired. And in most cases, significant improvements were achieved simply by reducing or eliminating caffeine.

There is no mystery to this. Medical research conclusively shows that as stress hormones increase, sleep duration and quality suffer greatly.[72, 73] In many cases, this produces a well-defined vicious cycle of caffeine intake → anxiety → depression → impaired sleep → increased caffeine use.[74]

Reducing or eliminating caffeine is obviously the way to interrupt this cycle and restore a sense of balance in one's life. Invariably what surprised my patients was the profound difference they felt. As sleep improves, you would expect an increase in energy, but the ripple effect of benefits also included decreased pain, better mood, decreased reliance on prescription and over-the-counter drugs, enhanced immune function, and improvements in memory and learning. Most important, patients reported "feeling themselves" again. In some cases, where caffeine consumption had been lifelong, they were literally discovering who they were for the first time.

Anger and Hostility

Getting off caffeine also tended to reduce feelings of irritability and hostility. This, of course, turns out to be extremely valuable both from an individual and a social perspective. In the section on heart disease (Chapter 5) I will present the connection between caffeine intake, stress hormones, and behaviors like anger and hostility. You'll learn that these behaviors are clearly linked to increased risk for stroke and heart attack.[75] Well, as you can imagine, cardiovascular disease is not the only condition affected by anger and hostility. Mind-body research (known as psychoneuroimmunology) tells us that the cycle of stress hormones and caffeine plays an important role in many if not most health disorders, even traffic accidents.

According to the National Highway Traffic Safety Administration, rage is a key factor in two-thirds of all fatal car crashes.[76] That's about 28,000 highway deaths each year. In addition, of course, are the untold numbers of nonfatal accidents caused by tailgating, speeding, weaving, exchanges of insults, honking, screaming, and actual gunfire.

Issues surrounding caffeine affect each and every one of us. We live, work, and play within a social framework that depends upon personal interaction. We know that the quality of this interaction depends to a great extent on the level of harmony, peace, cooperation, patience, and forgiveness we are able to maintain. We also know that caffeine often works to the detriment of these factors.

- A study of locomotive engineers showed that coffee consumption was linked with increased negative mood and decreased positive mood.[77]
- A sample of 144 inmates from a maximum-security penitentiary reported that those who consumed high levels of caffeine experienced poorer general mood levels than any other group. Caffeine consumption in this sample population *averaged* 800 milligrams per day—well above the amount considered damaging to health.[78]

- Importantly, there appears to be a time-dose factor in the development of caffeine and stress-related disorders. The body is able to compensate for increased stress hormone levels, but not forever. At some point (and this depends on myriad individual factors that are impossible to predict) the body's stress management system (known as the hypothalamic-pituitary-adrenal axis, or HPA) starts to malfunction. This results in a well-defined breakdown pattern with clear biochemical abnormalities and symptoms of physical and emotional illness.

Recently, a group of researchers wanted to test the hypothesis that people with borderline hypertension could be distinguished from those with normal blood pressure simply by looking at the health of their HPA axis. Sure enough, there was a high correlation between abnormal stress hormone levels and the incidence of borderline hypertension, proving that a failure of the stress management system is a factor early in the disease process. Importantly, this biochemical defect also produced a characteristic alteration of mood and behavior, marked by feelings of exhaustion and emotional distress. The researchers referred to this condition as "a defeat type of reaction to stress."[79]

The good news is that the converse is also true. There are steps you can take that will reliably lower your stress hormone levels and even restore balance to the HPA axis. As you well know, getting off caffeine is an important first step, but yoga, meditation, prayer, tai chi, and biofeedback can also help a great deal, and have been shown to produce often dramatic improvements in energy and mood, with decreased tension, decreased anger, and increased feelings of well-being.[80, 81]

Background Stress—The Saboteur of Health

At this point, you know that there are serious health risks associated with caffeine consumption, and we have explored many of these in detail. The arguments I present are carefully documented from the scientific and medical literature. Some health risks are easy to quantify. For example, you can have the level of cortisol in your blood checked, or you can compare the incidence of various diseases among coffee drinkers and nondrinkers. But there are more subtle factors at work as well, what I call disposition and outlook.

The image I get regarding life for most people today is one of pots on a stove. We're constantly putting on lids to prevent pots from boiling over, and switching pots to "back burners." Well, what if we were able simply to turn down the heat? Wouldn't that make a great deal of sense? In other words, life is complex. If you can simplify things (i.e., by taking pots off the stove), good for you. But sometimes that's not possible or even desirable, and life remains complex and busy. In that case, reducing the background level of stress and tension is critically important to maintaining the balance and quality of your life.

Getting off caffeine is like turning down the heat. Everything becomes more manageable. There may still be half a dozen pots on the stove, but they're simmering nicely instead of boiling over. Once again, the decision is up to you as to which experience of life you desire.

Another View

When I am challenged by representatives of the caffeine industry, their arguments are most often based upon the lack of scientific consensus regarding caffeine and mental health. I admit that this is so. There is no universal agreement concerning the effects that caffeine produces in the body or the mind. But I would like to make two points:

First, no one is arguing that caffeine is good for us. The only debate concerns the degree to which it is harmful. Second, I would like to suggest looking at the issue from a different angle. Take the association between caffeine and anxiety disorders. This chapter presents solid and convincing evidence that caffeine causes anxiety in great numbers of people. In many cases, anxiety affects the quality of life to the point of producing incapacitating emotional illness such as panic disorder. Still, there are those who will say the data is not strong enough. To them I put the following question: Do people suffering from anxiety improve when they reduce or eliminate caffeine?

The answer to this question is a resounding yes. Not only do I know it from clinical experience, but careful research has also proven the benefits of caffeine reduction. A landmark study published in the *British Journal of Clinical Psychology* found that patients suffering from anxiety tend to consume more caffeine than the general population. In fact, more than one-third of their study group was categorized as "heavy caffeine users." After a period of caffeine reduction, these patients saw their symptoms decrease by a mean of 42 percent and, importantly, the improvement was directly proportional to the caffeine intake. In other words, those who reduced caffeine a little improved a little, while those who made very significant reductions in caffeine intake showed the greatest improvement.[82]

Take the Challenge!

Most people have no idea what life would be like without the background of caffeine and stress hormones coursing through their veins. Even if you're only having a few cups a day, chances are your personality is affected in ways that may be too subtle for you to associate with caffeine. As you've seen in this chapter, caffeine's contribution to anxiety and depression alone are reasons enough to kick the habit.

I want to encourage you to conduct a trial period without caffeine. You owe it to yourself. Use the Off the Bean program in Chapter 10 to break the habit. Remember that you must go through the entire detoxifying process, which takes a minimum of three weeks, before you can begin to measure the results—and that it takes sixty days total before you can fully assess the benefits of being caffeine free.

Assure yourself that if you don't feel significantly better, you can always go back to caffeine. But at least you'll know that you explored the option, and are not simply a slave to the coffeepot. Not only your mood, but your entire outlook on life, stands to benefit as a result.

CHAPTER 5

Specific Health Disorders: The Caffeine Connection

Caffeine and Cardiovascular Disease

I know, you've heard it a thousand times: Cardiovascular disease is the nation's number one killer. But have you ever thought about what that actually means? If we translate the abstract numbers into concrete terms, the picture becomes much more real and immediate. Only then will we be motivated to do something about it—in our own lives and in the lives of those we love.

Cardiovascular disease (CVD) encompasses disorders of the heart and blood vessels, including heart attack, stroke, chest pain, hypertension, rheumatic heart disease, and atherosclerosis (hardening or blockage of the arteries). In 1997, more than 960,000 Americans died of cardiovascular disease. Remarkably, there are societies on earth where CVD is rather rare, so we know that it's not one of the inevitable consequences of aging. In fact, CVD is preventable. Nevertheless, unless people take action toward prevention, things will go on just as they have for decades.

In America today, nearly one-third of men between the ages of fifty and sixty will die within the next ten years from cardiovascular disease. And if that surprises you, consider that this disease now kills more women than men. More people die of cardiovascular disease than succumb to all cancers, all accidents, pneumonia, influenza, suicide, and AIDS combined: one life every thirty-three seconds.[1]

HEART DISEASE

Coronary heart disease (or heart disease) is by far the most common form of cardiovascular disease. According to the American Heart Association, every twenty seconds, an American suffers a heart attack, and every sixty seconds somebody dies from one. If you picked up your morning paper and read that three jumbo jets had crashed the day before, you would be greatly alarmed. What if this happened every morning, 365 days a year? That's the impact heart disease has on our nation, and yet the efforts at prevention are limited. Sure, there have been significant advances in hospital coronary care units, and more people are trained in CPR, but that's not prevention—that's simply rapid response.

The goal, after all, is to prevent heart attacks, and present efforts toward that end fall into two categories: drugs and dietary change to lower cholesterol, and drugs and dietary change to lower blood pressure. As valuable as these measures are, they are still not primary prevention. What about preventing cholesterol levels and blood pressure from rising in the first place, and what about all of the other risk factors in heart disease?

Given a complex issue, people (especially the media) naturally look for a simple explanation. Heart disease was thus reduced to a "cholesterol problem," which of course turned out to be untrue. Plenty of people have high cholesterol and never have heart attacks, and every day people with low cholesterol are rushed to the hospital in cardiac arrest.

Even adding the blood pressure factor does not produce an accurate picture of heart disease, but these two considerations are the only ones that receive much attention. And since coffee-induced increases in cholesterol and blood pressure appear to be relatively small, the professional and popular press have written off coffee as a risk factor. But nothing could be farther from the truth.

"The strong association between coffee consumption and coronary heart disease risk found in several different studies and the implications for the large population at risk are compelling arguments for concern about adverse cardiovascular effects of caffeine consumption."

Source: Neal L. Benowitz, M.D., "Clinical Pharmacology of Caffeine," *Annual Review of Medicine*, 1990;41:277–88.

CHECK YOUR PRESSURE

First of all, increases in blood pressure due to caffeine are often quite significant. Even in moderate doses, caffeine can raise blood pressure in healthy young men and women to the level of borderline hypertension.[2, 3] In those with existing hypertension, caffeine can be even more dangerous. The key factor, once again, is stress.

The first hint of this intriguing phenomenon came in 1969, when researchers tested caffeine's effect on blood pressure in rats. They found that caffeine produced only modest increases in blood pressure and were about to write it off; but they decided to repeat the experiment on stressed rats. Sure enough, when the rats were given caffeine and then placed in a crowded situation (i.e., under stress), their blood pressure increased dramatically.[4]

Since then, the same pattern has been identified in humans. When subjects are relaxed, caffeine does not appear to raise blood pressure significantly. These are the studies most often cited by the caffeine industry. But is this an accurate representation of most people's lives? Real life is stressful, and caffeine multiplies the increase in blood pressure and the subsequent damage.[5]

Throughout this book, I have emphasized the point that any evaluation of caffeine must look carefully at those who are most vulnerable. In this regard, recent research on men with borderline hypertension is quite revealing. It was found that in this group, the increase in blood pressure after ingestion of caffeine was greater than that found with healthy controls. What's more, this group also had an exaggerated response to caffeine combined with a stressful task.[6] In other words, caffeine intake is most dangerous for those who are most vulnerable (read: most stressed), a pattern that we will see numerous times in subsequent chapters.

HABITUAL COFFEE DRINKERS: ALSO AT RISK

It was long believed that habitual coffee drinkers did not suffer the increased blood pressure seen when caffeine is administered to non–coffee drinkers. Recent research, however, has revealed that caffeine can affect blood pressure in just about anyone.[7] One study with sixty "heavy" coffee drinkers found that caffeine continued to cause increases in blood pressure, and the authors emphasized in their conclusion that these effects "do not appear to habituate with regular use."[8]

As it turns out, the hypertensive effects of caffeine appear to be related to *changes* in blood caffeine levels. While habitual drinkers tend to maintain levels of caffeine through repeated doses throughout the day, these levels drop during sleep. In other words, the lower a person's caffeine level first thing in the morning, the greater the hypertensive effect of those first few cups of coffee. Experts estimate that at least 25 percent of the general population has early-morning blood levels of caffeine low enough for normal caffeine consumption to raise their blood pressure.[9]

Now, this brings up a very intriguing point. According to national health statistics, an individual is more than 50 percent more likely to have a heart attack on a Monday than on a Saturday. At first, everyone took this as simple evidence that Mondays are high-stress days and Saturdays are relaxed days. But researchers were surprised to find that the pattern held even among those with low-stress jobs. It turns out that caffeine is the critical factor. Since most people consume less coffee on the weekends, a coffee drinker's blood caffeine level will tend to be lowest on Monday morning, just when he or she is likely to slam down the most coffee. The resulting increase in blood pressure, while temporary and unlikely to show up in a scientific study, may well prove fatal.

"The cardiovascular effects of caffeine may persist throughout the day with repeated administration of moderate amounts of caffeine. Habitual caffeine use does not necessarily lead to complete tolerance, which suggests that caffeine's cardiovascular effects could contribute to an increased risk of cardiovascular disease."

Source: J. D. Lane and D. C. Manus, "Persistent Cardiovascular Effects with Repeated Caffeine Administration," *Psychosomatic Medicine,* July–August 1989;51(4):373–80.

RESEARCH CAPSULE
Diet Pills and Caffeine: A Deadly Duo

Prior to the Controlled Substances Act of 1970, most diet pills contained amphetamine drugs, which effectively suppress appetite but cause addiction and dangerous side effects. When the FDA banned amphetamines, manufacturers created similar effects (and side effects) with the combination of two central nervous system stimulants, caffeine and phenylpropanolamine (PPA). In the mid-1980s, the FDA moved against this dangerous mix because of a number of deaths associated with its use. Too late for some users, research found that while both drugs alone increase blood pressure, the combination of caffeine and PPA could result in massive increases, triggering stroke and heart attack.[10–13] That's why today the active ingredient in most diet pills available without a prescription is phenylpropanolamine alone.

However, while caffeine-PPA combinations may be banned, people using PPA diet pills still drink coffee, sometimes lots of coffee. What's more, PPA is frequently overused. The reasons for this become clear once you understand how PPA works. Again, it's related to stress hormones, this time norepinephrine.

As described in Chapter 2, norepinephrine (NE) is a powerful biochemical produced in the adrenals and nervous system that affects mind, mood, and behavior. PPA (like amphetamines) causes a rapid release of NE, which creates stress but feels like "energy." NE also suppresses appetite. The problem is that amphetamines and PPA do not increase the brain's synthesis of NE. If you're releasing more NE but you're not replacing NE stores in the brain, you will ultimately experience a rebound "letdown." As brain levels of NE fall, users must take more and more PPA to experience the same amount of appetite suppression. Such overuse may not only raise blood pressure, but also cause insomnia, irritability, headache, anxiety, and panic. When caffeine is added to the equation, the likelihood (and severity) of adverse effects is multiplied, due most likely to the fact that PPA can produce dramatic increases in blood caffeine levels.[14] Cases have been reported where individuals suffered manic psychosis after ingesting caffeine and PPA.[15]

"The effects of the widely consumed drugs caffeine and phenylpropanolamine are mediated through activation of the central and sympathetic nervous systems. Severe, life-threatening, and occasionally fatal hypertensive reactions have been reported after their combined use."

Source: C. R. Lake, D. B. Rosenberg, S. Gallant et al., "Phenylpropanolamine Increases Plasma Caffeine Levels," *Clinical Pharmacology and Therapeutics*, June 1990; 47(6):675–85.

THE WHOLE STORY

Most people assume that caffeine raises blood pressure because it makes your heart beat faster or harder. If this were the case, you would expect your blood pressure to return to normal fairly soon after a cup of coffee—and that doesn't happen. The fact is that caffeine causes vascular resistance, a condition in which the blood vessels (especially in the extremities) constrict and reduce blood flow.[16] This stress response was very useful a few thousand years ago in the face of imminent physical harm. Vascular resistance reduced blood loss from injuries. But today all it does is raise your blood pressure and make your fingers cold.

Actually, vascular resistance affects many areas of the body and mind. As discussed in the previous chapter, caffeine reduces circulation in certain areas of the brain. Once again, the fight-or-flight/survival part of the brain remains unaffected, but areas associated with long-term memory and learning can be impaired.

Put on your physiology hat. Can you think of another condition in which vascular resistance could cause a major problem? How about the increased circulation associated with exercise? Here the muscles are working hard and starved for oxygen and fuel. Under conditions of vascular resistance, the entire system can go into hyperdrive, elevating blood pressure much higher than it would be at rest. A study with healthy young men (none of whom had high blood pressure) published in the *American Journal of Cardiology* showed that a modest amount of caffeine taken before exercise produced dangerous elevations in blood pressure in 45 percent of subjects.[17] When a similar experiment was conducted with men at risk for hypertension, the results were even more alarming.[18]

THE CALCIUM CONNECTION

Research has identified an important connection between calcium metabolism and hypertension, accounting for the fact that calcium supplementation lowers blood pressure in about 25 percent of patients. Because caffeine is known to disturb calcium metabolism, a study was recently conducted to explore the effects of caffeine abstinence on blood pressure. The results? After two weeks off caffeine, two important measures of calcium status (serus ultrafiltrable calcium and parathyroid hormone) improved markedly in nearly all of the subjects.[19] These results illustrate clearly that caffeine stresses calcium metabolism, and that those desiring to control their blood pressure would do well to get "off the bean."

CHECK YOUR OIL

Scores of studies have been performed to evaluate the effects of coffee and caffeine on blood cholesterol levels. Most have found that coffee (including decaf) is associated with elevated cholesterol, and these increases are not always small.[20–22] In fact, blood cholesterol levels appear to rise in direct proportion to the number of cups of coffee consumed,[23–29] and we now know what causes this rise in blood cholesterol. It's not the caffeine, as once thought, but two other chemicals (diterpene alcohols) naturally found in coffee: cafestol and kahweol.[30, 31]

How does all this impact coronary artery disease? Most experts today agree that for every 5 percent increase in serum cholesterol over 200 milligrams per deciliter, there is a 10 percent increase in risk for heart attack or stroke. That means that stress and coffee can make a tremendous difference in your risk for these killer diseases. What's more, coffee intake is associated with elevations of the most dangerous fraction of cholesterol, known as apolipoprotein B, and this correlation has been found at moderate intake of two or more cups per day.[32]

BEYOND BLOOD PRESSURE AND CHOLESTEROL

As I mentioned, the caffeine/cardiovascular disease debate has, until recently, been limited mainly to a discussion of blood pressure and cholesterol. Since there is no universal agreement on how much these risk factors are raised by caffeine, it has been possible for the caffeine industry to duck the entire issue. But no more.

That's because six additional risk factors are coming to light, and caffeine is involved in each and every one.

"One point most authorities do agree on: Patients prone to cardiac arrhythmias should avoid caffeine. The amount in just a few cups of coffee can cause problems."

Source: Paul Cerrato, B.S., M.A., *Journal for the American Association of Office Nurses.*

---

1. ARRHYTHMIA AND BLUES

The proper function of the heart as a pump depends upon an intricate series of electrical impulses that contract chambers and open valves in perfect timing. This rhythm is the pace of life, sending blood continuously to more than 75 trillion cells in your body.

When the heart muscle is stimulated out of the proper

time sequence, pumping action becomes uncoordinated and blood flow becomes weak. If proper rhythm is not restored, these conduction and rhythm disturbances (collectively called arrhythmias) are usually fatal. Scientists do not understand exactly what causes arrhythmias, but they do agree that caffeine is associated with increased risk among those prone to the disorder.[33, 34] It is also important to note that the amount of caffeine required to disturb heart rhythm is not great. Intake of less than 300 milligrams per day has been associated with greater incidence of arrhythmias.[35, 36] Since a fourteen-ounce mug of coffee contains around 200 milligrams of caffeine, less than two mugs can easily put you into the increased risk category.

Even in healthy individuals, the combination of stress and fatigue has been shown to increase risk for arrhythmias.[37] Think about that. When you're feeling beat, haven't slept well, or you're just pushing too hard, how often do you resort to drinking coffee to get through the day? The resulting strain on your heart can be significant. Caffeine can also cause tachycardia (rapid heartbeat) and can exacerbate the symptoms of mitral valve prolapse (MVP), a common heart defect. In fact, MVP may be an important key in our understanding of the arrhythmia-caffeine connection.

Mitral Valve Prolapse (MVP)

The mitral valve lies within the heart, regulating the flow of blood from the left atrium to the left ventricle. When the valve is prolapsed (fallen or weakened), it malfunctions, and as the heart beats, blood may flow back into the atrium. MVP is rarely serious, but it does produce occasional or periodic symptoms, including shortness of breath, fatigue, light-headedness, and dizzy spells. The cause is unknown, but there is a significant genetic factor. Individuals with one affected parent have a 50 percent chance of inheriting MVP.

While MVP can cause heart murmur, palpitations, and chest pain, most individuals with the disorder have no noticeable symptoms and are unaware of the condition. Still, MVP significantly increases one's risk for arrhythmia,[38, 39] and the combination of caffeine and MVP can be dangerous. Interestingly, caffeine researchers often *remove* individuals with MVP from their investigations, presumably because such individuals would exhibit negative effects greater than the average person. But that's bad science. Conservative estimates are that 7 to 10 percent of the population has MVP. That's millions of Americans, and these are precisely the people who *should* be studied because they are among the most vulnerable to caffeine's adverse effects.

Aside from mitral valve prolapse, there are other arrhythmia risk factors that appear to operate in conjunction with caffeine intake. Caffeine can cause a sudden contraction of the aortic muscle, as well as dramatically increased stress hormone release in the heart itself. In an individual whose arteries are already partially blocked, such events can produce arrhythmia and heart attack.[40]

There are also reports that caffeine can increase the incidence of paroxysmal atrial tachycardia (PAT) and ventricular beats, other types of heart rhythm disturbance. These arrhythmias are often associated with exertion, and doctors have reported increased incidence of PAT with caffeine (coffee or tea) when taken as much as twelve hours prior to exercise.[41]

This brings up an important point concerning caffeine research: Long-term effects are often ignored. After all, you only see what you're looking for. But new research using continual heart monitoring technology enables us to look at the full spectrum of caffeine effects, including something known as heart rate variability (HRV). HRV has been shown to correlate very strongly with sudden death, and while moderate caffeine ingestion appears to produce no abnormal HRV in young adults, it has been shown to aggravate abnormal HRV in overweight, middle-aged subjects.[42]

"There is a two times (200 percent) greater likelihood of ventricular premature beats after coffee ingestion."

Source: T. K. Leonard, R. R. Watson, and M. E. Mohs, "The Effects of Caffeine on Various Body Systems: A Review," *Journal of the American Dietetic Association,* 1987;87(8):1048–53.

---

2. CORONARY VASOSPASM

When an artery is blocked, tissue beyond the block is deprived of oxygen and quickly dies. If this occurs in an artery leading to the heart, it causes a heart attack (medical term: myocardial infarct or MI). If the block is in an artery leading to the brain, it causes a stroke. In both cases, the major cause of blockage is the narrowing of an artery from the buildup of plaque, a process known as atherosclerosis. Often, the fatal combination is atherosclerosis and a blood clot that lodges in the narrowed artery.

But in approximately 20 percent of fatal heart attacks, an autopsy reveals that the victim had clear arteries. What caused the blockage of blood (and therefore oxygen) to the heart resulting in massive cell death and heart attack? Often it is a spasm of one or more arteries leading to the heart. Known as coronary vasospasm, this event can shut off blood supply as effectively as a clot or atherosclerosis.[43] You need to know that the risk for such a tragedy is related in part to your intake of caffeine.

In fact, caffeine contributes to coronary vasospasm in multiple ways. We know that caffeine, by stimulating the release of stress hormones, lowers the stress threshold (review Chapter 3) so that situations that would otherwise have been handled become distressful. With this caffeine-induced stress "magnifier," the risk of vasospasm is increased.[44]

Caffeine also contributes to magnesium deficiency, a condition that makes arteries more prone to spasm.[45] In typical vicious-cycle fashion, the combination of caffeine and stress exacerbates the low magnesium state.[46] What's more, if there is also a buildup of plaque within the artery, the tendency for arteries to spasm increases the overall risk for heart attack tremendously.

On the other hand, it is important to understand that the entire scenario of magnesium deficiency, elevated stress hormones, and hypersensitive arteries can be silent. You don't feel any of these dangerous developments like you would, for example, if your arteries were being occluded by plaque. In those cases, there are often clear warning signs such as breathlessness upon exertion or chest pain. But research shows that a person prone to vasospasm can have a completely normal electrocardiogram and be symptom-free[47]—that is, until they end up facedown on the sidewalk after their morning jog.

3. HOMOCYSTEINE

Early in 1997 the *American Journal of Clinical Nutrition* published research confirming a strong association between coffee consumption and elevated blood levels of a biochemical known as homocysteine.[48] Elevated homocysteine is a powerful contributor not only to heart disease, but also to stroke, miscarriage, birth defects, and possibly Alzheimer's disease. And the data is incontrovertible. A huge study group (over 16,000 people), almost equally divided between men and women, was evaluated, and the researchers were careful to factor out variables like smoking, vitamin intake, and history of cardiovascular disease. The study's conclusion is definitive and crystal clear: As coffee intake increases, so does the level of dangerous homocysteine in the blood.

But when I went on-line to see what my cardiologist colleagues were planning to do about this remarkable data, I found only stony silence. The consensus of opinion was to "wait for more information." In other words, no medical organization was even going to mention this report to their members, let alone recommend moderation of coffee intake.

More Information Comes In

A few months after the coffee and homocysteine report appeared the *Journal of the American Medical Association* (JAMA) published another landmark study, this one looking at homocysteine and heart disease.[49] Turns out the homocysteine factor is far more important than anyone thought. In fact, the JAMA study concluded that, in terms of risk for cardiovascular disease, elevated homocysteine is "equivalent to [high cholesterol] or smoking." People with the highest homocysteine levels had *more than three times the risk* for cardiovascular disease than those with low homocysteine.

There are now over fifty studies that illustrate precisely how homocysteine increases your risk of cardiovascular disease. While this is not the place for a detailed lesson in physiology, I'm not sure you'll be hearing anything about the matter soon from your doctor, and it's too important to ignore. This information could very well save your life (or at least a painful and expensive trip to the hospital).

You know that proteins are composed of amino acids. One of those amino acids, methionine, is commonly found in meat and dairy products, and when the body processes or metabolizes methionine, homocysteine is created as a by-product. Normally, the body breaks down the homocysteine into harmless metabolites, but there are a number of factors that either prevent this breakdown or overwhelm the body's ability to clear homocysteine from the blood.

Caffeine raises homocysteine levels in two ways. We know that the elimination of homocysteine from the blood requires optimal amounts of folic acid, vitamin B-12, and vitamin B-6. Caffeine depletes these vital nutrients. Secondly, caffeine appears to interfere with the normal breakdown of homocysteine. A diet high in meat and dairy products, on the other hand, tends to overload the system. Combine the two and you have real trouble. Add smoking to the mix and you're a walking time bomb.

What Exactly Does Homocysteine Do to the Body?

Research suggests that homocysteine damages blood vessel walls. These injury sites, known as lesions, start to collect the substances your body sends to repair the damage. This material builds up over time, accumulating protein, calcium, and cholesterol from the bloodstream and forming plaque, which ultimately blocks the artery.

Other researchers have found that homocysteine increases the stickiness of platelets, cells in the blood that are essential for clotting. As platelets become more sticky, the likelihood of abnormal clot formation (and subsequent stroke or heart attack) increases dramatically.

Elevated homocysteine also affects the blood vessels' ability to dilate. Remember that every time your heart beats, your arteries must expand (dilate) to accommodate the increased pressure. As homocysteine levels increase, however, the blood vessels lose this elastic ability and are damaged as a result.[50] Consider that as we age, most people's overall blood pressure increases.

Consider also the damage done to rigid blood vessels under conditions of strenuous exercise. Normally, blood pressure rises and arteries expand to meet the body's increased need for oxygen and fuel. But when homocysteine levels are high, blood pressure increases and the blood vessels don't expand. The result: accelerated damage, cardiovascular disease, and increased risk for heart attack and stroke.

Who's at Risk?

While all caffeine users are at increased risk for elevated homocysteine, the following groups have been identified as *very* high-risk populations.

1. People with other risk factors. If you have high blood pressure or high cholesterol, or if you smoke, even a

small increase in homocysteine will greatly increase your risk of cardiovascular disease.[51]

2. Diabetics. People with diabetes are at increased risk because homocysteine appears to be far more damaging to their blood vessels. What's more, they have reduced ability to clear homocysteine from their bodies. This greatly increases risk for heart disease, as well as degeneration of the eyes and peripheral circulation.[52, 53] In fact, there are a number of reasons why diabetics should not drink coffee (see list on pages 199–200).

3. People with rheumatoid arthritis. Recent research has shown that people with rheumatoid arthritis also have a defect in homocysteine metabolism that makes them particularly vulnerable to even slight elevations of this biochemical.[54] That may account for the observation that people with rheumatoid arthritis often improve on a vegan diet (no meat, eggs, or dairy), which is naturally low in methionine.

4. People with a family history of Alzheimer's disease. Alzheimer's disease is also characterized by abnormally high homocysteine levels.[55] While a cause-and-effect relationship has not been confirmed, the rationale for homocysteine-induced brain degeneration is not far-fetched. Homocysteine appears to accelerate free radical activity, a process known to damage nerve cells.

5. The elderly. Studies indicate that as many as 50 percent of individuals over age sixty-five have elevated levels of homocysteine.[56] Coffee drinkers in this group are therefore likely to have far more serious consequences than they might have experienced in their younger years.

What's Being Done?

As far as I can see (and I've looked extensively), nothing is being done. A review article on the health effects of coffee was published in the *Medical Tribune* on June 25, 1997.[57] This magazine is read by more physicians than any other medical publication. The word *homocysteine* did not appear in the article. Instead, the American Heart Association was quoted as saying, "[M]oderate coffee consumption does not appear to increase a person's risk of heart attack." In their current publication dealing with caffeine, the AHA statement is even worse: "Whether or not *high intakes* of caffeine increase the risk of coronary heart disease is still under study" (my italics).

In reality, the caffeine-homocysteine-heart disease connection has been thoroughly and exhaustively examined. Conclusive research has even been published in the AHA's own journals![58] It's just that no one appears to be willing to draw the obvious and important conclusions from the mountain of data already in hand.

RESEARCH CAPSULE

You've heard about HDL (high-density lipoprotein), the "good" cholesterol that lowers your risk of heart disease? Your doctor may have encouraged you to exercise regularly in order to raise the level of this protective factor. Well, if your homocysteine levels are high, all the HDL in the world won't protect you. Research just published in the *American Journal of Cardiology* shows that homocysteine is so damaging that it virtually eliminates any protective benefits obtained from high HDL.

Source: H. R. Superko, "Elevated High-density Lipoprotein Cholesterol Not Protective in the Presence of Homocysteinemia," *American Journal of Cardiology*, March 1, 1997;79(5):705–06.

Three Steps You Can Take

Research appearing in the pages of dozens of medical journals now supports a prudent and effective approach to reducing your blood levels of homocysteine. You're not likely to read about these steps in a magazine or hear about them on the evening news. You probably won't hear them from your doctor, and that's because these important measures do not involve the purchase of expensive, patented drugs. Instead, they involve three simple steps:

1. Decrease your intake of meat and dairy products, and increase fresh fruits and vegetables.
2. Decrease or eliminate your intake of coffee.
3. Take a daily vitamin supplement that provides 400 micrograms of folic acid, 20 micrograms of vitamin B-12, and at least 5 milligrams of vitamin B-6.

A+B = Huh?

A: "We conclude that an elevated homocysteine level is now established as a strong and independent factor associated with all categories of atherosclerotic disease in both men and women."

Source: I. M. Graham, L. Daly, Helga Refsum et al., "Plasma Homocysteine as a Risk Factor for Vascular Disease: The European Concerted Action Project," *Journal of the American Medical Association*, 1997;277:1775–81.

B: "In conclusion, we found a strong dose-response relation between coffee intake and plasma homocysteine concentration. . . . Given the widespread use

---

of coffee, even small adverse consequences will have important health implications."

Source: O. Nygard, H. Refsum et al., "Coffee Consumption and Plasma Total Homocysteine: The Hordaland Homocysteine Study," *American Journal of Clinical Nutrition*, 1997;65:136–43.

C: "[M]oderate coffee consumption does not appear to increase a person's risk of heart attack."

Source: American Heart Association

4. HOSTILITY AND ANGER

Numerous studies have shown that hostility and anger significantly increase risk for heart disease and stroke.[59] We now know that these emotions are tied to stress hormones in a vicious cycle: Anxiety and stress cause increased production of epinephrine and cortisol, which then affect mood, mind, and behavior in such a way as to create more stress, hostility, and anger. A common trigger? Caffeine.[60]

Importantly, the damage caused by the additive effects of caffeine and stress is often silent. Small arteries may spasm, cutting off blood supply to vital areas of the heart for short periods of time. The risk for rapid heartbeat (tachycardia), flutter, and arrhythmias all increase during periods of intense stress, but the victim, caught in the emotional spiral, is often completely unaware of the damage being done.

As you can imagine, one outburst of anger is not likely to give you a heart attack. The research is conclusive, however, regarding people in whom hostility and anger are common experience. At different points in life, we may find ourselves in jobs or situations that stimulate anger and aggressiveness. Ironically, those are also the times when we tend to drink the most coffee. Breaking this destructive cycle, therefore, involves changing our habits and awareness.

> "We have found that anger can cause a weakness in the pumping action of the heart."
>
> Source: G. Segall, M.D., of Stanford University, *Medical Tribune*, 1991;32(14):17.

5. THE MAGNESIUM CONNECTION

Adequate magnesium is essential for normal heart function and even a slight deficiency of this mineral can have adverse effects on the heart and blood vessels. Diet surveys and blood tests show that millions of people consuming a typical American diet are not obtaining sufficient magnesium from their food.[61, 62] Most of them are also drinking coffee, which has been shown to deplete magnesium from the body.[63, 64] You don't have to be a Ph.D. in public health to see that this is a major problem. Low magnesium increases the risk for arrhythmia, congestive heart failure, heart attack, coronary vasospasm, hypertension, and stroke.[65–67] One recent report in the *American Heart Journal* noted that "the intricate role of magnesium on a biochemical and cellular level in cardiac cells is crucial in maintaining stable cardiovascular function."[68]

> "It should be realized that preventing the patient from a magnesium deficit is the first, and the application of magnesium the second best strategy to keep the patient free from cardiac arrhythmias."
>
> Source: M. Zehender, "Magnesium as an Anti-arrhythmic Therapy Principle in Supraventricular and Ventricular Cardiac Arrhythmias," [German], *Zeitschrist for Kardiologie,* 1996;85 supplement 6:135–45.

Here is yet another vicious cycle. Research shows that Type A individuals (high-stress personalities) lose significant amounts of magnesium when faced with a stressful situation compared to Type B individuals (easygoing personalities.)[69] But we also know that Type A people tend to drink a great deal more coffee than Type B folks. And it doesn't really matter which factor comes first (stress or caffeine intake). The result is that the people who need magnesium the most are the ones whose stores are most depleted.

When was the last time your doctor measured your magnesium level? Chances are it never happened, even if you are at risk for heart disease. Once again, that's because nutrition, diet, and exercise are usually overlooked in favor of the "quick-fix," drug-oriented approach. Some blood panels measure serum magnesium, but that reflects only the amount of the mineral that was being transported in your blood at the time the test was taken. It does not indicate the amount of magnesium in your body. You can obtain that important information by measuring the magnesium in red blood cells. Known as RBC magnesium, this valuable test can be done by most laboratories, but you'll have to ask for it and pay for it yourself. Insurance companies, for the most part, do not yet understand the remarkable preventive benefit of maintaining optimal levels of magnesium, even though the data has been available for twenty years.

A special note for individuals with any form of heart disease: A new study has conclusively shown that oral supplementation with magnesium can significantly reduce the incidence of arrhythmia.[70] This does not mean, however, that you can drink all the coffee you want and simply take a magnesium pill. Coffee will deplete magnesium rapidly, even from a supplement, and increase your risk for heart disease in multiple ways. A sensible strategy for staying alive and healthy: Decrease or eliminate caffeine. Supplement with a high-potency multimineral providing at least 400 milligrams of magnesium and 100 milligrams of potassium per day.

6. ALTERED BLOOD CLOTTING

When a person is killed by a stroke or heart attack, there are always direct and indirect causes. We've been discussing the indirect causes, those factors that contribute to the blockage of an artery. But the direct cause (the blocked artery) is also fairly complex, insofar as arteries do not usually build up sufficient plaque to stop all blood flow. The killer factor is often a blood clot that travels to the narrowed artery and plugs it up.

Today, it is common for people with atherosclerosis to be given "blood thinners," drugs that decrease the clotting ability of the blood. The fact is, however, that millions of Americans are walking around with what is known as silent ischemia. Plaque has built up in their arteries, but not to the point of causing pain or abnormal heart activity. Health experts are concerned because the number of people with silent ischemia is increasing dramatically, and not just because the baby boomers are reaching their fifties. The most frightening thing is that this condition is being diagnosed in people who are in their thirties and forties.

Silent ischemia is "an accident waiting to happen." If a person should form an abnormal clot and if that clot finds its way into a narrowed artery leading to the heart or brain, he or she is finished. You need to remember that in a large percentage of cases, the first sign of cardiovascular disease is a fatal heart attack.

Anyone who has owned a house will tell you that plumbing requires regular maintenance, and even then, after thirty or forty years, large sections may have to be replaced. And that's steel and copper pipe. Your plumbing (over 1,000 miles of blood vessels) is delicate tissue, subject to the same forces of pressure, erosion, wear, and tear. And the way the body fixes leaks involves clotting. You might not know that in addition to the cuts, punctures, nicks, and scrapes that are visible signs of clotting, you spring internal, invisible "leaks" on a regular basis, and your body fixes itself remarkably—like having a self-repairing plumbing system in your house.

But this mechanism must be finely tuned. If your blood clots too slowly, you can hemorrhage. If your blood clots too fast, you'll tend to form unnecessary clots that can wreak havoc in the body. Interestingly, the clotting mechanism is very much affected by what we eat and drink. A diet high in meat and dairy products will tend to increase the "stickiness" of your platelets, thereby making your blood more likely to clot abnormally fast.

I started wondering about the effect of coffee on blood clotting when I was studying the stress response. We know that adrenaline accelerates blood clotting, and from an evolutionary point of view, this makes perfect sense. After all, throughout human history, the events that got our adrenaline up were threats to our survival, and those threats often resulted in injury. The stress response thus produces alterations in the blood to make it clot faster.

But today, as I have explained, stress is remarkably different. Instead of facing a saber-toothed tiger or a club-wielding foe, we're facing deadlines, crammed schedules, traffic jams, and mortgage payments. None of these involve physical injury, but we cannot change our genes. Stress still produces alterations in blood clotting, and on top of this, millions of people accelerate the clotting mechanism of their blood every morning when they slam down their first cup of coffee.

Caffeine actually appears to affect blood clotting in two ways: by magnifying the normal stress response (resulting in higher stress hormone levels), and by raising homocysteine levels (see "3. Homocysteine," this chapter). This may account for a large part of the increased risk for stroke associated with coffee drinking.

A group of investigators reporting in the *American Journal of Epidemiology* found a strong association between caffeine and heart disease. In fact, the increased risk for heart attack was seen starting at one to two cups of coffee per day.[71] At that modest level of consumption, the risk for heart attack increased 40 percent. In men who drank at least five cups per day, the increased risk was 200 percent or more.

The data regarding risk for women is even more serious. One recent study examining dietary factors and heart disease found that the association between caffeine intake and heart attack was stronger than that for meat, butter, and total fat. In fact, coffee drinkers had almost twice the risk of heart attack compared to women who did not drink coffee.[72] Research by other investigators has found that consuming more than thirty-six ounces of coffee per day caused a 250 percent increase in the risk of heart attack in women.[73]

By looking at individual risk factors for heart disease, the caffeine industry has been able to snow the public and even most of the medical community. But real people do not have single risk factors; they have *multiple* risk factors, and there is an additive or even a multiplying effect when they are all considered.[74] One important study, for example, found that women consuming more than twenty-four ounces of coffee per day had almost twice the risk of heart attack compared to non–coffee drinkers. That's fairly alarming, but when the researchers looked at the combination of caffeine consumption and elevated cholesterol, coffee drinkers faced astounding odds. Moderate coffee drinkers with high cholesterol had more than seven times the risk of heart attack, while heavy coffee drinkers had eighteen times the risk of non–coffee drinkers.[75]

Likewise, when measured at rest, caffeine raises blood pressure only a little. But when you add stress (either physical or mental), caffeine can raise blood pressure significantly.[76] Caffeine has also been shown to increase stress hormone release in the heart muscle. If this is viewed as a single risk factor, the data is not that alarming. But tens of millions of Americans have partial blockage of their coronary arteries, which produces decreased blood flow or ischemia. When this factor is included, a different picture emerges. One group of researchers has stated that a modest intake of caffeine in an individual with ischemia might product a *three- to six-fold increase* in cardiac stress hormones. They conclude, "We hypothesize that [this release of stress hormones] lies behind the reported connection between cardiac events and methylxanthines, for instance sudden cardiac death following coffee consumption." [77]

THE ADDITIVE EFFECT OF CORONARY RISK FACTORS

Complete this checklist to see if caffeine is likely to increase your risk for cardiovascular disease:

	YES	NO
1. Has anyone in your family suffered from heart disease?	___	___
2. Are you a woman?	___	___
3. Do you have mitral valve prolapse?	___	___
4. Is one of your birth parents a diabetic?	___	___
5. Do you smoke?	___	___
6. Are you overweight?	___	___
7. Are you under a significant amount of stress at home or work?	___	___
8. Have you ever noticed that your heart beats faster after consuming coffee?	___	___
9. Have you ever noticed any irregularity in your heartbeat, such as the sensation that it "skipped a beat"?	___	___
10. Do you have high blood pressure?	___	___

	YES	NO
11. Does (did) either of your parents have high blood pressure?	____	____
12. Is your cholesterol level greater than 180 milligrams per deciliter?	____	____
13. Have you ever experienced ringing in the ears for any length of time?	____	____
14. Have you ever been diagnosed with transient ischemic attacks (TIAs)?	____	____
15. Have you ever found that you were out of breath just climbing a flight of stairs?	____	____

Key:

2–4 "yes" answers: Caffeine will increase your risk for cardiovascular disease.

5–7 "yes" answers: Caffeine will seriously increase your risk for cardiovascular disease.

8 or more "yes" answers: Research suggests that caffeine could be the precipitating factor in your premature death.

Here is a typical situation in which blood levels of homocysteine (and nutrition in general) are all but ignored. A fifty-two-year-old man goes to his doctor for a physical. He's slightly overweight, and his cholesterol and blood pressure are too high. (By the way, this describes about 30 million American men.) The doctor writes a prescription for drugs to lower the patient's cholesterol and blood pressure, and sends him home.

The problem is that these drugs have significant side effects, not the least of which is decreased sex drive and fatigue (just what a fifty-two-year-old man does not need). In fact, there is good evidence that aggressive use of drugs to lower cholesterol and blood pressure actually *increases* overall mortality, but that's another (sad) story. The point I want to make is that prescribing drugs is not the same thing as health care. In this case, significant factors related to this man's condition were completely ignored.

This man needed diet and lifestyle counseling and follow-up. Research shows conclusively that a low-fat diet combined with stress reduction can dramatically reduce the risk of cardiovascular disease, and may even reverse CHD damage.[78]

For someone with high cholesterol and high blood pressure, knowing his homocysteine and magnesium levels is also critically important. Studies show that supplemental vitamins B-6, B-12, and folic acid can lower homocysteine.[79, 80] Obviously, a magnesium supplement can improve tissue levels of that vital mineral. We know that coffee raises homocysteine and lowers magnesium. Real health care would include recommendations for this patient to reduce or eliminate coffee and supplement his diet with a good high-potency multivitamin. Since that multivitamin would also include important antioxidant vitamins such as vitamins C and E, the patient's risk for heart disease would be further reduced.[81, 82]

What's more, the reduction or elimination of caffeine would also lower the patient's risk for coronary vasospasm and arrhythmia. And reducing coffee intake is an essential step in any program to lower blood pressure and cholesterol. In fact, when nutrition, lifestyle, and caffeine reduction are the treatment focus, research strongly suggests that medications are unnecessary.[83, 84]

Imagine the two choices before you. On the one hand, you modify your diet, learn (and practice) a stress management technique, and add some nutritional supplements. You experience increased feelings of well-being, greater stamina, some weight loss, a better sex life, and an improved health report from your doctor on your next visit. Compare this to making no lifestyle or dietary changes but taking prescription drugs every day. You keep the same habits to which you may be attached but that compromised your health in the first place. You experience a variety of drug side effects such as loss of libido and decreased energy, but that's not the bad news. The bad news is the realization that you're going to have to take these drugs for the rest of your life, because without them, your blood pressure and cholesterol will quickly rise to dangerous levels. Now, the question is, What kind of health care do you want?

Caffeine and Gastrointestinal Health

WHAT'S YOUR GUT FEELING?

I was going to title this section "Gastrointestinal Disease" and discuss the various pathologies connected with caffeine, such as ulcers and irritable bowel syndrome, but I realized that such an approach would be far too narrow. It is critically important to remember that health is not simply the absence of a specific, named disease. People whose gastrointestinal tracts (stomachs and intestines) are inflamed and irritated are certainly not healthy, even though they may not be experiencing enough pain and discomfort to send them to the doctor. People who self-medicate with antacids every day are certainly not healthy, even though they may never be diagnosed with gastro-esophageal reflux disease (GERD).

The wider and more accurate view of gastrointestinal health is one that looks at optimal function and what compromises optimal function, not what destroys this remarkable tissue or necessitates the use of drugs and surgery. In this context, you need to know more about the GI tract. I promise this will not be boring or useless information. Rather, this "interior view" of your body might make you think twice about the things you eat and drink, and have a dramatic effect on your health and wellness.

THE HOLE IN THE DOUGHNUT

It's important to understand that food, once swallowed, is still technically "outside" the body (much like the hole is outside the doughnut) until it is digested and absorbed through the intestinal tract into the bloodstream. The misconception is that this occurs easily, that by some automatic process everything we eat is broken down and absorbed, and the remaining undigested fiber is simply eliminated as waste.

In reality, the digestive process is neither easy nor automatic. It is an intricate and continuous process, with numerous mechanical and chemical reactions taking place simultaneously. Furthermore, each step of the process is dependent on previous steps, so a defect in one phase will almost certainly hinder the entire process to some degree.

This critical function, by which we are nourished and thrive, deserves close attention. For the health-conscious individual, that means learning what can be done to optimize digestion and what habits and practices to avoid.

PERSPECTIVE

As I have mentioned previously, the genes that control every cell in your body haven't changed even a fraction of a percent in the last 25,000 years. That means your digestive tract is identical to that of early *Homo sapiens,* designed, quite simply, for hunting and gathering. The idea that we should postpone hunger satisfaction until a preset time called lunch or dinner is, from a scientific point of view, extremely bizarre, not to mention the fact that our meals today contain a mix of highly refined, chemicalized foods, for which we are entirely unprepared, consumed in gargantuan quantities.

Medical anthropologists today are starting to understand that the changes in eating habits brought about by the agricultural and industrial revolutions have placed an enormous burden on our digestive systems. In short, our technology has outstripped our biology. Our genes have stayed the same, while virtually everything about what and how we eat has changed completely. I believe this is the principal reason why each year, over 30 million Americans suffer from acute or chronic digestive dysfunction.[85]

Caffeine is one of those substances (along with refined sugar, "fake fats," and hydrogenated oils) that is completely foreign to the human gastrointestinal tract. Which is not to say that we can't detoxify the compound. Chapter 3 describes how your body accomplishes this arduous task. Rather, it is the effects of caffeine that we need to explore and, believe it or not, we're just beginning to get a clear picture. One leading researcher has noted, "Despite more than a century of effort to elucidate the actions of methylxanthines [primarily caffeine] in man, one of the major conclusions to be drawn is that there is a need for further studies." [86] Here is what we know:

FUNCTIONS OF THE GASTROINTESTINAL TRACT

The GI tract has five major functions:

1. *Microbial Defense:* Throughout human history, most of the foods and beverages we consumed were contaminated with bacteria and mold. The GI tract therefore contains a highly specialized germicidal system comprised of hydrochloric acid (HCL) and a variety of immune defenses, including secretory IgA (sIgA).
2. *Digestion:* The complex starches, fats, and proteins we consume must be broken down into simple units that can be absorbed into the bloodstream.
3. *Essential Barrier:* The GI tract has the formidable task of keeping out any substance that should not enter your bloodstream, including bacteria, food contaminants, allergy-causing agents, and a variety of toxins produced during the process of digestion.
4. *Absorption:* Balanced against this barrier function, the GI tract must at the same time facilitate the absorption of the substances you need. This requires precise conditions of acid balance, enzyme activity, and timing.
5. *Elimination:* As an organ of elimination, the intestinal tract rids the body not only of unusable food components, but also of a wide array of toxins and metabolic waste.

Each of these functions is critical to overall health and wellness, and caffeine alters or interferes with all of them.

Caffeine Reduces Microbial Defense

There is evidence that caffeine interferes with the secretion and immune activity of secretory IgA, and stress is once again the principal factor. As the stress hormone cortisol rises, sIgA tends to fall. This has been demonstrated even in mother's milk.[87] What's more, the inverse relationship between cortisol and sIgA becomes more apparent when subjects are given a deep relaxation technique. As stress hormone levels fall, sIgA increases significantly.[88] This gives us both new insight into the value of relaxation and yet another reason to reduce caffeine intake. Optimal health cannot be achieved with compromised immunity.

Coffee may also reduce the germicidal ability of the stomach, in what first appears to be a paradoxical effect on HCL secretion. It has long been known that coffee (even decaf) is a strong stimulator of HCL secretion.[89] But that may not be the case when the beverage is taken with a meal. Research shows, in fact, that caffeine consumed with food can actually decrease the normal and necessary acid response to a meal.[90] This reduces both the digestive and the decontamination activity of your stomach.

Caffeine Impairs Digestion

Depending on when it is consumed in relation to food, coffee can either raise or lower production of HCL by the stomach. If acid levels rise too far or too fast, one group of problems is created, including increased risk for ulcer. If HCL secretion is reduced, food will tend to ferment and putrefy, leading to the production of toxic by-products. Coffee has been found to produce a chain reaction of maldigestion throughout the entire GI tract[91]—an especially important issue among the elderly, as digestive efficiency tends to decrease with age.

What's more, coffee may also speed gastric emptying, meaning that the contents of the stomach are passed prematurely into the small intestine, cutting short the important gastric phase of the digestive process.[92]

Caffeine Impairs the Barrier Mechanism of the GI Tract

If material from the stomach is released too early, it tends to be excessively acidic, and this may injure sensitive intestinal tissue. Thermal or acid-related injury to this tissue is known to compromise the barrier function of the gut, leading to the absorption of materials that you really don't want in your bloodstream.[93]

As you can imagine, this may set up a vicious cycle where reduced microbial defense combines with impaired barrier production, leading to the absorption of toxins, bacteria, and allergy-causing molecules. Colitis, for example, has been characterized as an intestinal "barrier dysfunction" syndrome,[94] and food allergy is directly related to the breakdown of the intestinal wall's barrier mechanism.[95]

Caffeine Impairs Nutrient Absorption

When you think about your GI tract, it is easy to understand the importance of absorption. After all, that's how the baked potato, broccoli, and filet of sole that you ate for dinner ultimately becomes you.

I have presented ample evidence in Chapter 3 that caffeine reduces the absorption of a number of vital nutrients. You may want to review that material, but let me simply list here the vitamins and minerals that are known to be affected.

Thiamin and other B vitamins
Calcium
Magnesium
Potassium
Iron
Zinc

Of course it is entirely possible that caffeine and coffee impair the absorption of other (or even most) nutrients. It's just that tests have not been conducted with the others. In animal experiments, coffee and tea were both found to decrease the bioavailability of protein.[96]

Caffeine Disturbs Normal Elimination

Coffee is a frequent cause of both constipation and diarrhea, the effect differing from individual to individual and also depending on when it is consumed. Coffee on an empty stomach causes diarrhea, and this is a common experience.[97]

But caffeine can also cause constipation due to its diuretic action. In other words, caffeine tends to pull water out of the digestive tract, leading to hard stools that are difficult to pass.[98, 99]

Now, of course, many people claim that caffeine helps them maintain normal bowel regularity, but that is the same as relying on laxatives. Either way, you're using a drug to induce bowel movements, and ultimately many coffee drinkers become dependent on this laxative action.[100] Without the caffeine stimulation, they experience what is known as "rebound constipation."[101]

HEARTBURN

Of course it's not the heart that's burning, but the sensitive tissue of the esophagus. It's burned by acid regurgitated (refluxed) from the stomach, thus the medical term *gastroesophageal reflux disease,* or GERD. The undeniable coffee connection has to do with the effect that coffee (even decaf) has on the valve between the esophagus and the stomach.

For some reason, coffee reduces the pressure on this valve so that the highly acidic contents of the stomach are allowed to pass up into the esophagus.[102] Obviously, there are cofactors. Overeating increases one's risk to GERD, as does obesity, maldigestion, and lying down after eating. But the coffee factor is quite significant, as demonstrated by the fact that you can stimulate heartburn in a sizeable percent of perfectly healthy people just by giving them coffee.[103]

It was once thought that coffee-induced heartburn resulted from a hypersecretion of stomach acid, but it appears that the coffee-induced valve defect is the primary cause. Heartburn sufferers, in fact, have been found to produce *less* stomach acid when given coffee.[104] I mention this in order to point out the folly of treating coffee-induced heartburn with antacids. Notwithstanding drug company hype, people don't get heartburn due to an antacid deficiency. The prudent approach to eliminating the problem (and not just masking the symptom) is to quit drinking coffee.

Of course, the coffee industry does its best to downplay the heartburn issue, and once again, the reasoning is along the lines of, "If coffee caused heartburn, everybody would be suffering." But the truth is that, for unknown reasons, some people are just more sensitive than others. In addition, certain types of coffee appear to create more severe symptoms.[105]

IRRITABLE BOWEL SYNDROME (IBS)

IBS is a common condition affecting approximately 20 percent of Americans.[106] The complaints are constipation (perhaps alternating with diarrhea), abdominal pain (dull or crampy), bloating, abdominal rumbling, and flatulence. Now you might think with symptoms this common, researchers would have discovered the cause, but, once again, the picture is only now coming into focus. Brand-new evidence suggests strongly that there is a coffee connection involving two factors.

First is a group of rather caustic acids found in coffee. These acids, actually present at a higher level in decaf coffee, can irritate the GI tract directly, causing cramps, discomfort, and diarrhea. Second, there is GABA. Our last discussion of GABA (gamma amino butyric acid) focused on this biochemical's role in mind, mood, and behavior, and how it acts as a natural stress reducer in the brain. We now know that GABA is also produced in the gastrointestinal tract, for much the same purpose.

The GI tract is essentially a tubular muscle with a variety of bulges, twists, and turns. Material is moved from the stomach to the small intestine and on to the large intestine through a series of rhythmic contractions known as peristalsis. Laxatives work by irritating the sensitive intestinal tissue, which triggers accelerated contractions. Actually, anything that irritates the GI tract will tend to have a laxative effect, and that includes anxiety. We all know the "gut-wrenching" feeling of stress.

So nature placed in this system a large number of cells to manufacture GABA, as well as receptors for GABA that would calm the GI tract.[107–109] From Chapter 4, we know that caffeine interferes with GABA metabolism,[110] and this explains why people with IBS experience a worsening of symptoms when they drink coffee, as well as the widely variable effects of coffee from person to person.

Scientists are now referring to the complex network of immune and nervous system cells within the intestinal tract as the "brain of the gut."[111] Stress is perceived differently by different people, and its effects throughout the body reflect this difference. What you must know is that coffee lowers the stress threshold in your GI tract just as it does elsewhere in your body and mind. GABA is the neurochemical that is supposed to keep your GI tract functioning at "normal," and the combination of stress and caffeine overrides that GABA message, creating the symptoms of IBS and possibly much worse. Colitis has been positively linked to anxiety and stress,[112] and animal research has found that the GABA receptors are a first-line defense against colon cancer.[113]

THE ULCER STORY

You've probably heard that caffeine and stress don't really cause ulcers, that the real cause is a bacteria known as *Helicobacter pylori* (*H. pylori*). Here's an intriguing fact: *H. pylori* is an extremely common bacteria. Millions of Americans test positive for this organism, and by age seventy, 80 percent of the population has been infected, yet only 10 percent develop ulcers.[114]

Obviously, there must be other risk factors, and any investigation will quickly identify stress, caffeine, and coffee. Coffee contributes to ulcer formation in a number of ways. The harsh acids are a direct factor and, as mentioned, these acids are higher in decaf coffee. But caffeine itself is a problem because it stimulates acid secretion in the stomach and interferes with the protective action of GABA. In fact, coffee, tea, and soft drinks have all been shown to stimulate acid secretion, especially when consumed on an empty stomach.[115, 116]

We also know that caffeine and chronic stress elevate blood levels of cortisol, which suppresses a number of immune functions, including production of secretory IgA. As we have learned, sIgA is a powerful antimicrobial agent, especially effective against guess what? *H. pylori!*[117] That means that when IgA levels are low, *H. pylori* is allowed to proliferate and cause ulcers. When IgA levels are high, *H. pylori* and other pathogens in the mouth, throat, and gastrointestinal tract are quickly destroyed. When viewed in this way, *H. pylori* is actually a secondary risk factor. Stress, caffeine, elevated cortisol, and suppressed IgA production are the primary factors contributing to ulcer risk.

Unfortunately, the modern drug-oriented approach to ulcers is simply a course of antibiotics and acid inhibitors. They may help in the short run, but if nothing is done to reduce cortisol and restore IgA production, the condition will recur. This is just one more example of "Band-Aid" health care ignoring the underlying cause of disease. Consider that in research predicting the incidence of ulcers in a large population, stress is the most significant factor.[118] And in research evaluating the drug-oriented approach to ulcer healing, the single most predictive factor for successful healing is the patient's anxiety level. In one study, those experiencing high levels of anxiety had a 400 percent increased risk for incomplete healing compared to those with low stress.[119]

It's an amazing but all-too-familiar scenario: Joe Executive goes to his doctor for his yearly physical. Joe's blood pressure is increasing, he's not sleeping well, and he has lots of discomfort after meals, and he uses antacids almost daily for the resulting heartburn. Caffeine is a known factor in all of these conditions, but his doctor doesn't even ask how much coffee Joe is drinking. There are two reasons for this: (1) It would involve a discussion, and today the average office visit with a primary care physician is twelve minutes and (2) the doctor is drinking four cups of coffee a day himself. He or she hasn't read the medical literature regarding caffeine and doesn't believe it's really doing anyone harm.

Six months later, Joe returns. His intestinal pain has increased, and he reports sharp stomach pain that gets slightly better when he eats. The doctor springs into action, writing prescriptions for a drug that will prevent Joe's stomach from producing digestive acid, and an antibiotic to kill *H. pylori.* Joe leaves the office thinking that he has received health care. But the fact is that Joe's suffering was not caused by a deficiency of ranitidine, sucralfate, amoxicillin, omeprazole, tetracycline, azithromycin, metronidazole, or any of the other drugs currently in use. All of these medications have side effects, and there is even evidence that chronic suppression of acid secretion can increase one's risk for gastric cancer. (Remember that stomach acid is an important part of gastrointestinal immunity.)

Please understand that I am not suggesting that one ignore an *H. pylori* infection. But evidence clearly indicates that drug treatment alone is frequently ineffective, precisely because it does not deal with the root problem. In fact, if dietary and lifestyle issues are not addressed, research shows that reinfection can be as high as 73 percent.[120] To get an idea of how shortsighted the drug-only approach is, imagine that Joe went to a fortune-teller before his first physical:

Fortune-teller: "You are suffering from severe indigestion and heartburn."

Joe: "That's right, I am."

Fortune-teller: "This is caused by stress, poor eating habits, and excessive coffee consumption. But your doctor will overlook these factors. Instead he will wait for your symptoms to become worse. In the meantime, a pathogenic bacteria will grow within your body and begin to eat away at your insides. This will cause open wounds in the extremely sensitive tissue of your intestinal tract, resulting in internal bleeding and acute pain. You will try to dull that pain with antacids, but it will become so bad you will return to the doctor, who will give you drugs. The therapy will include anywhere from two to four different drugs and the rate of success with this approach can be as low as fifty-three percent."[121]

Joe: "Wait a minute. That means I have nearly a fifty percent chance of not killing this bacteria?"

Fortune-teller: "That's right, and if the first course of drugs does not work, your doctor will try a second treatment plan using more powerful drugs at a higher dose. Of course, it is almost a certainty that the bacteria will have developed antibiotic resistance after the first course, so your chance of success grows smaller with each additional trial."

Joe: "Isn't there anything I can do?"

Fortune-teller: "Sure there is. Stop drinking coffee, tea, and soft drinks. Eat slowly and chew well. Eat smaller, more frequent meals, start an exercise program and make it a regular habit, learn a stress management technique and take some time off, sign up for a yoga class and learn the breathing exercises. Make sure to get at least eight hours of sleep a night, and slow down! Life's too short to suffer with internal bleeding from a perforated intestinal tract."

A FINAL NOTE CONCERNING ULCERS

Coffee promoters have done a good job of whitewashing the ulcer issue, often relying on the argument, "If coffee caused ulcers, everyone who drinks coffee would get one." The fact of the matter is that coffee doesn't "cause" ulcers, but once again, there is a continuum of gastrointestinal health with optimal function on one end, all the way to heartburn, irritable bowel, colitis, ulcers, and colon and rectal cancer at the other extreme. Where are you now and where do you want to be? Do you experience stomach or digestive problems more than a few times a month? If so, and if you are a coffee drinker, you may be heading for trouble. Keep in mind also that when coffee is administered to laboratory animals, in moderate but repeated doses similar to what humans consume, it produces "pathological changes in the gastrointestinal tract and ultimately ulcer formation."[122]

OTHER GASTROINTESTINAL RISK FACTORS

Temperature

Most people drink their coffee piping hot, and the resulting increase in gastrointestinal temperature has been shown to contribute to upper GI tract disorders.[123]

Food Allergy or Intolerance

Some individuals appear to be allergic to coffee (or possibly the chemicals it is treated with), and this can increase the adverse effects associated with the beverage.[124]

The Melatonin Connection: Intriguing New Research

In Chapter 3, I described the critical role played by melatonin in regulating immunity and sleep. I presented evidence that caffeine and coffee, especially when combined with other stressors, significantly reduce melatonin levels.[125]

In addition to being a primary neurohormone produced by the brain, melatonin is manufactured by a large number of cells in the gastrointestinal tract—another facet of the "brain of the gut." And melatonin's effect on the GI tract is more than calming. Researchers believe that melatonin's principal role in the GI tract is to promote healing and boost immune defense. New studies show that melatonin is particularly effect against stress-induced injury to the sensitive lining of the intestinal tract and stomach.[126] Not only is melatonin essential for the protection of this tissue, but it has also been shown to enhance tissue DNA synthesis, indicating that it is also an agent for repair and cancer prevention.[127]

• • •

We are finally understanding that the gastrointestinal tract is an incredibly complex and sensitive environment. So much of our health depends upon maintaining the right balance of acids, enzymes, and hormones. Moreover, this biochemical balance must be matched by the proper mechanical function of valves, muscles, and organs.

When we eat natural foods (the foods this system was designed for) and consume these foods in reasonable quantity at a reasonable pace, things tend to go quite well. But today's diet presents a level of digestive challenge unknown in human history. For eons, the only beverage humans consumed was water. Today, Americans consume more soft drinks than any other liquid, and most of that is caffeinated. What's more, we consume coffee and tea in prodigious amounts, and then wonder why we don't feel well.

Of course, I'm not saying that everyone who drinks coffee is going to suffer with gastrointestinal problems, but many people do, and they usually don't make the connection. In clinical practice, I saw hundreds of patients whose irritable bowel syndrome, colitis, food allergy, gastritis, heartburn, bloating, and abdominal pain improved or healed completely once they got off coffee. I concur with the advice given by Dr. Henry D. Janowitz, author of *Good Food for Bad Stomachs*: "People with stomach ailments should avoid coffee and other caffeinated products."[128]

Oh My Aching Back (and Wrist and Shoulders and . . .)

For years I had a practice in a comprehensive medical group that included physicians, chiropractors, psychotherapists, and massage therapists. Usually I could tell by looking at a patient's chart if he or she needed to be referred to massage therapy. Experience told me that habitual caffeine users were very likely to be holding enough tension in their muscles to cause a significant amount of discomfort and pain. And I was right 95 percent of the time, even when pain was not one of the patient's listed complaints.

I am still amazed at the amount of pain that people become accustomed to living with. After a while, we just sort of get used to it, assuming that it is an inevitable part of growing older. Therapeutic massage, of course, brings pain and tension to the "surface" of our awareness, and often prompts us finally to take steps to alleviate this suffering. Many, however, simply keep returning to the massage table instead of eliminating the underlying cause.

The first step I recommend for someone experiencing chronic muscular tension is to get off caffeine. Massage therapists, chiropractors, and physical therapists—anyone who works physically with a patient's body—can always tell a difference when the patient gets off caffeine. For many, that step alone will reduce pain to a remarkable degree. Others need bodywork or yoga to release the deep level of tension that we all tend to accumulate as we go through the trials and challenges of life.

It helps to understand that tension is simply part of the stress response left over from Paleolithic days when stress meant imminent peril. When faced with a fight-or-flight situation, tension helped to steel the body against injury. But it's no longer a survival asset. Tension today destroys our sense of ease. It creates a level of pain that may flare up or smolder, but either way, it diminishes the quality of life.

If you suffer from chronic pain and your physician has not recommended you stop drinking caffeine, it's probably because he or she has been told caffeine is a muscle relaxant. That is partly true, in that certain muscles in the body do relax in response to caffeine, but these are only the smooth muscles, such as those lining the airways. The vast majority of skeletal muscles contract in response to caffeine, and those are the ones that ultimately produce tension-derived pain.

Very often, muscle tension combines with other factors, such as inflammation, to cause pain. Such is the case with a common condition known as carpal tunnel syndrome (CTS) in which pain is produced by a narrowing of the nerve channel in the wrist. CTS sufferers wear wrist splints, take painkillers, often resort to surgery, and frequently none of those treatments is effective. That's because the underlying muscular tension must be reduced, and that won't happen as long as the individual is drinking caffeine.

In a study of nearly 1,500 office workers, caffeine use was found to be a primary risk factor for CTS. In fact the correlation of caffeine use and this affliction held in both directions. In other words, people who did not use caffeine had very low risk for CTS and those who used caffeine had the highest risk. Since cigarette smoking is associated with caffeine use (and could confuse the issue), the researchers removed from the data anyone who smoked. Even then, caffeine remained a primary risk factor.[129]

Other research with chronic back pain illustrates the same association. In one study, individuals with chronic back pain were found to be consuming an average of nearly 400 milligrams of caffeine per day, while matched controls (people the same age and occupation without back pain) averaged less than half that amount.[130] Of course, this does not prove that caffeine causes the pain. It is possible that pain sufferers turn to caffeine to help manage pain.

To clear up that possibility, researchers administered caffeine to volunteers and found that in fact, caffeine produced head and neck pain in a significant percent of volunteers.[131] This would tend to confirm that caffeine is a contributing cause of pain syndromes from carpal tunnel to neck, shoulder, and back pain.

THE CALCIUM CONNECTION

To understand just how caffeine produces muscle tension, you need to know that the drug disrupts calcium ion flow through what are known as calcium-release channels. Smooth muscle lacks these caffeine-sensitive calcium-release channels, so there is no contraction.[132] Skeletal muscle, however, is rich in calcium-release channels, and thus caffeine can cause contraction or spasm.[133] In fact, the sensitivity of muscle tissue to caffeine has been used by veterinarians to predict muscle damage from strenuous running.

A procedure called the caffeine contracture test measures the degree to which a muscle contracts in response to caffeine. Horses whose muscles contract severely in response to caffeine will be very likely to incur damage from strenuous running.[134] A syndrome of muscle pain after exertion has also been identified in humans, and once again, the marker appears to be increased sensitivity to caffeine.[135]

THE ULTIMATE TEST

Of course, the best way to evaluate the relationship of caffeine to your muscle pain is to get off the drug and see how you feel. Many people have been amazed when an unlooked-for benefit from quitting caffeine was relief from pain caused by neck, back, and shoulder tension. But remember, if you're suffering from chronic pain, going cold turkey off caffeine is likely to make your condition worse before it gets better. Therefore I urge you to employ the Off the Bean strategy presented in Chapter 10. That will minimize withdrawal symptoms and ease you into a different life—one in which you are free of the background stress and tension created by caffeine.

Headache

Forty-five million Americans suffer from chronic headache. Seventeen million are migraine sufferers. The relationship of caffeine to headache is confusing, not because the data is inconclusive, but because for half a century, a major cause of headache has been promoted as the cure. Caffeine is a common trigger for migraine and other types of headache.[136] There is no mystery here. As we've seen, caffeine increases tension in the jaw, shoulders, back, and neck. It has a powerful vasoconstrictive effect in the brain. As little as 250 milligrams of caffeine has been shown to decrease total brain cerebral blood flow by 30 percent.[137] New research also shows that headache sufferers commonly have low magnesium levels (measured as serum ionized magnesium),[138] and we have already learned that caffeine depletes the body of this essential mineral. Now consider the following common scenario.

The person with a headache doesn't know that it was caused or triggered by caffeine, so he or she looks for a painkiller (analgesic). Studies show that in 95 percent of cases, the analgesic drug contains caffeine.[139] Such painkillers work, especially if the headache was caused by caffeine withdrawal, but the caffeine ultimately triggers another headache. Ultimately, the hapless sufferer becomes dependent on the painkiller for even a modicum of relief, but the headaches increase in frequency and intensity. This may go on for many years, creating a cycle of pain and depression that destroys the quality of life.[140]

And the cycle is not uncommon. Very often the patient's doctor is the one to recommend a caffeine analgesic. And often it is the same doctor who must ultimately admit the patient to a hospital for analgesic abuse detox. The standard analgesic detox program looks like this:[141]

1. Withdrawal of caffeine-containing analgesics
2. Treatment of the withdrawal headache (which may last one to two weeks)
3. Therapy to reduce migraine triggers, including avoidance of caffeine

What's wrong with this picture? Is it not crystal clear that if someone had told the headache sufferer to avoid caffeine in the first place, a decade or more of pain and suffering, addiction, and depression could have been avoided?

WITHDRAWAL AND BEYOND

A caffeine deprivation (withdrawal) headache results from the normal opening (dilation) of blood vessels that are constricted by caffeine. In other words, habitual caffeine intake keeps blood vessels in the brain constricted. When caffeine is not consumed, these blood vessels return to their normal blood-flow potential, and it is this increased circulation in the brain that causes the throbbing agony of a caffeine withdrawal headache. In studies where caffeine is withheld or simply delayed, headaches result from habitual ingestion of as little as 100 milligrams (one cup of coffee or two cola beverages) per day.[142, 143]

Ultimately, of course, the brain becomes accustomed to normal blood flow and the headache subsides. In Chapter 10, I will explain how to decrease or eliminate caffeine without suffering so much as a single headache. But the point to keep in mind is that habitual caffeine users are disrupting normal and essential blood flow to the brain. This is not a good thing, even if the body does get used to such abuse.

And the caffeine-headache connection goes well beyond withdrawal. Caffeine itself contributes to headache even when it is consumed moderately and consistently.[144, 145] One landmark study demonstrated significantly increased risk for headache at caffeine intakes of 250 milligrams per day.[146] Yet I continue to come across reports in the medical literature and popular press that caffeine is a cure for headache. Perhaps the most bizarre is a recent article in the *Medical Tribune* advising people who wake up with headaches to have a cup of coffee before they go to bed.[147]

Today, the most popular herb sold in America is *Ginkgo biloba*. Ginkgo has been shown to enhance peripheral blood flow, especially in the brain, and thus may be helpful in the prevention and treatment of Alzheimer's disease and some types of vascular disorders.[148, 149] But clinicians are starting to report that some people taking ginkgo are experiencing headaches. Do you see why? Ginkgo dilates the same peripheral blood vessels in the brain that caffeine constricts. Thus habitual caffeine users are taking ginkgo and giving themselves withdrawal headaches: the worst of both worlds.

STUMBLING INTO ADDICTION

Here's a classic example of how caffeine addiction and the commensurate headache can insidiously sneak into a person's life. At sixteen years of age, Caroline was attending a boarding school and came down with mononucleosis. Sent home for a month to recover, she began drinking coffee for the first time in her life simply as a way to cope with the profound fatigue.

Upon returning to school, where students were not allowed to drink coffee, Caroline began to experience blinding, almost incapacitating headaches in the midafternoon. She was given Excedrin, two of which delivered a whopping 130 milligrams of caffeine to her 100-pound body. The analgesic relieved her headache but also kept her awake until 3 A.M. As a result of disturbed sleep and endocrine stress, full recovery from her illness, which is normally accomplished in four to six weeks, took Caroline more than three years. What's more, she became addicted to painkillers and was not free of headaches until, as an adult, she eliminated all sources of caffeine in her diet.

THE OPERATION WAS A SUCCESS, BUT THE PATIENT IS ADDICTED

Post-surgery headache has been noted in the medical literature for decades, and was until recently attributed to a side effect of anesthesia. Then, a few years ago, someone made the observation that people who abstain from caffeine do not experience such headaches. Ultimately, it was found that the "postoperative headache" was in fact a caffeine withdrawal headache, since surgical patients are not allowed to drink before their operation.[150]

Sensible solution: Get off caffeine. Preposterous solution: Put caffeine in the patient's intravenous drip. Action taken: The preposterous solution, of course!

I'm not making this up. It's called prophylactic (preventive) intravenous administration of caffeine, and it's currently being recommended for habitual coffee drinkers who are undergoing surgery.[151]

A New View on Caffeine Withdrawal

"Although the phenomenon of caffeine withdrawal has been described previously, the present report documents that the incidence of caffeine withdrawal is higher (100 percent of subjects), the daily dose level at which withdrawal occurs is lower (roughly equivalent to the amount of caffeine in a single cup of strong brewed coffee or three cans of caffeinated soft drink), and the range of symptoms experienced is broader (including headache, fatigue and other dysphoric mood changes, muscle pain/stiffness, flu-like feelings, nausea/vomiting and craving for caffeine) than heretofore recognized."

Source: R. R. Griffiths, S. M. Evans, S. J. Heishman et al., "Low-dose Caffeine Physical Dependence in Humans," *Journal of Pharmacology and Experimental Therapeutics* December 1990;255(3):1123–32.

OXYGEN, THE ESSENCE OF LIFE

Whether or not you suffer from tension or migraine headaches, you have to ask yourself if you want to consume a drug (caffeine) that clamps down the blood vessels of your brain and restricts oxygen delivery to billions of cells. In one more highly ironic twist of modern life, we now have oxygen bars springing up around the country, supposedly to rejuvenate patrons with a superoxygen hit. But many of these same people have just visited the espresso bar, where they loaded up on caffeine, thus making the oxygen unavailable to their cells. Better to forget the oxygen bar, stay off the caffeine, and enjoy the natural vitality that exercise, adequate rest, and good diet can provide. I predict you'll have fewer headaches and more brain power to meet any challenge the day may bring.

Aging

You're probably surprised to find aging in a section on health disorders. After all, every time the earth circles the sun, we're all one year older. But while that fact is inexorable, the consequences of aging are neither inevitable nor immutable. We are learning that aging does not have to include degeneration and decrepitude. It is possible, for example, to place two sixty-year-old women side by side and have most people believe that one is the other's daughter. Now mainstream medicine tends to focus on the older-looking individual because mainstream medicine is concerned primarily with the treatment of disease. On the other hand, I study the younger-looking one to see what can be learned regarding prevention and anti-aging strategies.

Over the years, this line of inquiry has paid rich dividends as research uncovers significant differences in the biochemical makeup of young- and old-looking individuals. We have discovered differences in hormone levels and radically different levels of other important repair and rebuild biochemicals such as insulin-like growth factor-1 (IGF-1). Much of that data was reported in my book *The DHEA Breakthrough* (Ballantine, 1996), and while this is not the place for an exhaustive review, there are critical points that need to be addressed in relation to coffee and caffeine. In addition, new and extremely exciting data is being published every month that reveals the importance of hormone production to longevity.

WHAT IS AGING ANYWAY?

There are a variety of theories that seek to explain the breakdown of human systems leading to death. Over the years, they are either refined or disproved as more information becomes available. When I was in graduate school, the genetic theory prevailed, that being the concept that "death genes" (or perhaps, a single death gene) programmed tissues to self-destruct. But in more than twenty-five years, such a gene has not been found. On the contrary, researchers have been able to create conditions in which tissues live far longer than expected. The critical factors in aging appear to be the efficiency by which nutrients are delivered, toxins are removed, and repair processes are maintained.

Indispensable to all these life functions is water. Water is not only the environment within which nutrient delivery, detox, and repair take place, it is an active and critically important participant in every chemical reaction that takes place in your body. One of the primary markers of aging, of course, is dehydration, and the loss of water from our tissues is accelerated by caffeine.[152] That means more lines and wrinkles on the outside, and a loss of metabolic efficiency on the inside.

Caffeine has significant diuretic effects even in habitual users. Even though considerable attention has been placed on the nutrients that are lost in the urine, hardly anyone has looked at the effects of the water loss itself. This is particularly ironic because coffee, tea, and soft drinks are today more widely consumed than water, thus creating a vicious cycle of dehydration and diuresis. What's more, rehydration after exercise is actually impaired by drinking caffeinated beverages,[153] and in yet another vicious cycle, dehydration appears to increase the toxicity of caffeine.[154,155] Therefore, the net effect of high caffeine use is accelerated aging, especially of the skin and kidneys.

CAFFEINE AND DETOXIFICATION

Detoxification, or the ability of the body to break down and eliminate toxins and waste, is a biomarker of the aging process. We are used to thinking of the liver, kidneys, and skin as the major organs responsible for this essential function, but each is entirely dependent upon water to get the job done. Thus, any degree of dehydration can seriously impair the detox process, accelerate aging, and increase risk to illness and disease.

While caffeine contributes to dehydration, perhaps the most important point to remember (from Chapter 3) is that caffeine itself must be detoxified by the liver, and that is not an easy process. In fact, high doses of caffeine may impair liver function, creating yet another metabolic stress. After all, the liver is responsible for detoxifying not only caffeine, but the vast majority of foreign materials that we are exposed to through water, air, food, and the environment. Most of these substances, collectively termed xenobiotics, are broken down by a group of enzymes known as the cytochrome P450 system (CP-450).

For years, scientists have used caffeine to evaluate stress on the CP-450 system. If a drug or therapy is toxic to the liver, that organ will take longer to detoxify a given quantity of caffeine.[156] The converse may well be true. Consider the liver function of an individual consuming large amounts of caffeine. It stands to reason that the liver's detoxification of other xenobiotics will be impaired. Evidence in support of this theory comes from research with anticancer (chemotherapy) drugs.

Remember that chemotherapy drugs are basically selective poisons that act chiefly upon rapidly dividing cells, such as those in a tumor. One of the problems encountered by oncologists is that these drugs become less effective over time. The body actually develops a tolerance or resistance to the drugs because the liver gets really good at detoxifying them.

Caffeine, however, has been shown to reduce the development of such tolerance, presumably by impairing the detox ability of the liver and inhibiting DNA repair.[157] Now, lest you think this is a good thing, consider the big picture. Caffeine is a drug that is consumed by millions of people, often in amounts of 500 to 1,000 milligrams per day. If it is impairing the ability of the body to detoxify xenobiotics, it is actually promoting disease (including certain types of cancer). The fact that it may have some benefit in enhancing the effectiveness of chemotherapy drugs is hardly cause for celebration.

HEREDITARY FACTORS IN DETOXIFICATION

In looking carefully at the CP-450 system, researchers have uncovered an extremely interesting phenomenon. Some people, termed "slow acetylators," have rather sluggish detox activity, and this appears to be purely genetic. Slow acetylators will have impaired caffeine clearance, and their detoxification of other drugs will also be impaired. Studies show that slow acetylators experience more toxic effects after caffeine ingestion, and often have serious allergic-type reactions to a class of antibiotic drugs known as sulfonamides.[158, 159]

It's important to understand that you have no way of knowing if you are a slow acetylator, because such testing is not done on a routine basis. Research suggests, however, that the condition may be extremely common. In one study, slow acetylator status was identified in 55 percent of the control group population.[160] Once again, this underscores the folly of blanket statements concerning the safety of caffeine. Safe for whom? At what dose?

REPAIR

The ascending theory of aging at the moment is one of accumulated error. Scientists marvel at the astounding ability of cells to repair and clone themselves, noting that our bodies are involved in a massive twenty-four-hour-a-day regeneration process. But as cells continue to copy themselves, the chance of error increases. Error, of course, results in the production of an abnormal cell, and when a critical mass of abnormal cells is reached, the tissue malfunctions or dies, thus contributing to the degeneration of aging.

The question, of course, is, What causes the error? Theoretically, every cell's DNA is a perfect blueprint for the entire life, repair, and replication of that cell, and as long as the blueprint is faithfully followed, error should not occur. But in biology, as in construction, mistakes happen. For example, what if the blueprint is damaged?

Imagine a construction office where someone spills coffee on the blueprint. It's quickly wiped off, but a part of the document is smudged. Construction must continue, so the general contractor guesses where the support beams are to be placed. As a result, eventually the building collapses.

Likewise, DNA can be damaged by an array of chemical and biological toxins. Collectively, these are called mutagens because they cause mutation. Fortunately, your body also produces cells that fix DNA. As you might have guessed, however, this DNA repair becomes less efficient as we grow older, and caffeine appears to play a role in the decline. There are three aspects to this:

1. Caffeine is a known mutagen. That is, it can cause replication error, either by damaging the DNA blueprint or disrupting communication of that information to other "builder" molecules like RNA.
2. Caffeine has been shown to inhibit DNA repairs.[161, 162]
3. Caffeine magnifies the DNA-damaging effects of other mutagens.[163, 164]

FREE RADICALS

Our bodies are also under assault by a group of metabolic and environmental toxins known as free radicals. These dangerous biochemical "thugs" are unstable molecules or atoms that are produced as a normal part of living. And under normal (or natural) circumstances, the body is able to control any damage they do by the stabilizing activity of antioxidants. Vitamin C, vitamin E, and beta-carotene are antioxidants that we obtain from food. Melatonin, glutathione, and superoxide dismutase are antioxidants that are produced by the body.

But today, very little is natural. Most people's consumption of antioxidant-rich fruits and vegetables is woefully inadequate, and at the same time, free-radical exposure has skyrocketed. Today, the pollution from industry and automobiles spans the globe and threatens the health and welfare of everyone, primarily by free-radical damage. This vastly increased exposure can overwhelm the body's ability to stem the tide of cellular destruction. Massive levels of free radicals are generated by cigarette smoke, auto exhaust, heavy metal and chemical pollution, electromagnetic fields, ultraviolet radiation, injury, illness, and stress. The accelerated aging seen in the deeply lined face of smokers is clear testimony to the damaging effects of free radicals.

GIVE ME A (COFFEE) BREAK

Recently, news that coffee contains antioxidants swept the nation.[165] But in fact, it only illustrated how desperate we are for good news about coffee. As it turns out, it is the vapors of brewing coffee that contain antioxidant elements, not the beverage itself. Even if you stick your nose next to your coffeemaker and inhale deeply, you will not receive much antioxidant benefit from coffee. The caffeine industry has also publicized studies that identify antioxidant properties of coffee, but these are invariably conducted in test tubes, not the human body.[166, 167]

In fact, caffeine may very well potentiate free-radical damage in a number of ways:

1. Caffeine directly reduces tissue levels of melatonin, an antioxidant critical to the protection of DNA.[168, 169]
2. In animal experiments, caffeine magnifies the free-radical damage produced by radiation exposure.[170]
3. Caffeine raises stress hormone levels, which are known to accelerate free-radical damage.[171]

AGE SLOWLY, NOT STRESSFULLY

The last point is probably the most important: Caffeine = Stress, and that clearly leads to degeneration and aging, not vitality and youthfulness. Researchers have identified what is called the stress-age syndrome, in which brain, endocrine, immune, and bioenergetic systems all start to fail due to changes brought about by the ravages of stress.[172–174]

Remember that caffeine and stress hormones also drive down levels of DHEA. As DHEA declines, so does the production of important repair biochemicals such as growth hormone and insulin-like growth factor-1 (IGF-1). In time, stress and caffeine contribute to adrenal exhaustion, whereupon a raft of important hormones are depleted. This destruction is not silent. You'll feel it every day in many ways as you simply can no longer command the vitality necessary for what were once everyday tasks.

Finally, it is important to consider the role of disease in the aging process. It is obvious that increased incidence of illness is both a cause and effect of aging. Thus, caffeine accelerates aging by impairing immunity, something that has been shown to occur through the elevation of stress hormones,[175, 176] nutrient depletion,[177, 178] and depression of DHEA.[179] Look at common infectious causes of death in the elderly such as influenza and pneumonia. It brings home the reality that we are only as strong as our immune systems.

Caffeine and Diabetes
(With a Note on Hypoglycemia)

A recent headline in the *Medical Tribune* announced DIABETES AT ALL-TIME HIGH IN U.S.[180] The story unfolded nightmare-like, with experts expressing alarm and bewilderment as to the cause or prevention of this epidemic. Since 1958, the number of Americans diagnosed with diabetes has increased 600 percent, from 1.6 million to more than 10 million. What's more, the Centers for Disease Control estimates that another 6 million Americans currently have diabetes but are unaware they have the disease.

These astronomical numbers do not begin to tell the story of suffering that diabetes brings. It is a major cause of cardiovascular disease and commonly leads to kidney disease, blindness, chronic infection, and foot and leg amputations. Nearly 20 percent of Americans over the age of sixty-five have the disease.

> "Diabetes is a common disease and becoming more common, and it is associated with some horrible consequences."
>
> Source: Linda Geiss, Center for Disease Control and Prevention, Atlanta.

Like other health professionals and public health experts, I have watched this national tragedy with growing concern. But here again, I part company with the mainstream medical community regarding the appropriate response. Conventional medicine turns for help to the pharmaceutical industry, which creates an ever-increasing number of drugs to manage diabetes. But this approach seldom eliminates the destructive and often fatal consequences of diabetes. What's more, these drugs have a laundry list of potentially serious side effects that may create additional problems for diabetics.

If diabetes were incurable, I would support drug treatment as a first-line approach, but the vast majority of patients have Type II diabetes, which in most cases can be virtually eliminated with nutrition and lifestyle modification. And one of those nutritional steps is the elimination of caffeine. Here's why:

1. *Caffeine raises blood sugar levels* and disrupts the blood sugar-regulating effect of insulin.[181] In fact, high-dose caffeine administration (the equivalent of six cups of coffee) has been shown to produce transient insulin resistance that is very similar to Type II diabetes.[182]
2. *Caffeine raises fatty acid levels* in the blood. Diabetics already have high blood-fat levels, and the addition

of caffeine can significantly increase their already high risk for heart disease.[183]

3. *Caffeine raises homocysteine levels,* which greatly increases the diabetic's risk for cardiovascular disease and degeneration of blood vessels in the eyes.[184, 185]

4. *Caffeine causes vascular resistance,* in which blood vessels constrict and circulation is reduced. Peripheral circulation is already impaired in diabetes, and the added effect of caffeine can prove disastrous.

5. *Caffeine raises stress hormone levels,* a primary risk factor for diabetes. Exposure to repeated stress increases the incidence of diabetes in rats.[186] Chronic stress, including feelings of irritability and hostility, has been linked to the development of insulin resistance, leading to the diabetic state.[187]

DRAMATIC IMPROVEMENT AFTER QUITTING CAFFEINE

Shirley was one of those "hard to manage" diabetics. Wide swings in blood sugar made it almost impossible to determine an effective dose of medication, and she suffered frequent bouts of hypoglycemia, causing her to be hospitalized twice. At one point, her doctor suggested that she quit drinking caffeine-containing beverages, but he mentioned it almost in passing and never explained why he thought it was a good idea. Consequently, she made an effort to reduce her coffee consumption, but she continued to have a large cup in the morning and another with lunch.

Then, at a support group meeting, a friend told her that quitting coffee altogether had helped him tremendously. Figuring it was worth a try, Shirley started drinking a caffeine-free herbal coffee. Within days, she noticed a leveling out of her blood sugar readings, and in two weeks, her blood sugar dropped to the high-normal range. Encouraged by this breakthrough, she started an exercise program and began watching her diet more carefully. Three months later, she was off medication and had "cured" her diabetes.

AN OUNCE OF PREVENTION

For those with a tendency toward diabetes (and that includes anyone who is obese as well as lean individuals with one or more diabetic parent), heavy coffee drinking can significantly increase risk. The reduction or elimination of caffeine is an important preventive measure. Still, to this day, the diabetes organizations have no recommendation regarding caffeine. Physicians are thus unaware of the benefits of caffeine reduction, and patients are kept in the dark.

CAFFEINE AND JUVENILE ONSET DIABETES

Without going into technical genetic descriptions, let me simply say that juvenile onset diabetes is similar to other hereditary diseases, in that the child inherits a susceptibility to the condition, not the disease itself. For the past century, scientists have puzzled over exactly what triggers the overt disease. Researchers in Finland and at the University of Pittsburgh believe they have found the answer.

In a landmark paper published in the prestigious *British Medical Journal*, they provide solid evidence that caffeine's known toxic effects on fetal development include damage to the pancreatic cells that produce insulin.[188] By charting the incidence of insulin dependent diabetes against the per person consumption of coffee in thirteen nations, these researchers illustrate a close correlation.

Critics, of course, will try to pass this off as mere coincidence, but the credibility of this type of analysis improves according to the number of corresponding points. In this case, there is a tight linear relationship for *every* country studied. Countries with the lowest coffee consumption have the lowest incidence of diabetes mellitus, and countries with the highest coffee consumption have the highest incidence of the disease.

HYPOGLYCEMIA

Hypoglycemia is often considered to be the "opposite" of diabetes. In reality, it simply refers to the state of insufficient (hypo) blood sugar (glycemia) that may be part of or a prelude to diabetes.

In nondiabetic individuals, hypoglycemia may be caused by consumption of simple carbohydrates, producing in an insulin surge that drives blood sugar levels below normal. Symptoms include disorientation, depression, fatigue, confusion, and poor concentration; all resulting from a shortage of glucose (fuel) to the brain.

Research has also confirmed that the hypoglycemic state can be induced and/or exacerbated by caffeine. Investigators at the Yale School of Medicine Clinical Research Center documented the following effects in human volunteers after ingestion of caffeine:

1. An immediate and sustained decrease of 23 percent in cerebral blood flow. This by itself can produce feelings of confusion and disorientation.
2. Increased blood levels of stress hormones, epinephrine, norepinephrine, and cortisol compared with placebo.

3. Marked symptoms of hypoglycemia even though the subject's blood sugar was considered low-normal.

The researchers concluded, "Our data suggest that individuals who ingest moderate amounts of caffeine may develop hypoglycemic symptoms if plasma glucose levels fall into the 'low-normal' range, as might occur . . . after ingestion of a large carbohydrate load."[189]

Commenting on the study, Dr. Richard Bernstein of Mamaroneck, New York, said, "Such an effect could be dangerous. For example, if a person has low blood sugar and also drinks caffeine, that person is more likely to be impaired."[190] And the lead researcher, Dr. David Kerr, noted that "these symptoms may be greatest for children who drink caffeinated beverages."[191]

The Adrenal Dysfunction Disorders: Allergy, Asthma, Fibromyalgia, Chronic Fatigue Syndrome, and Autoimmune Disease

Your adrenals produce or contribute to the production of about 150 hormones, every one of which is vitally important to health and wellness. Some of these hormones manage blood pressure; others manage stress. And all this activity is accomplished by two glands smaller than your thumbs, sitting on top of your kidneys.

In Chapters 3 and 4, I presented the scenario of adrenal stress resulting from the strains, burdens, and anxieties of modern life combined with the biochemical stress of caffeine. I described a "downward spiral" where the adrenals become exhausted and everyday problems then seem magnified out of proportion. That's because the adrenals are responsible for maintaining homeostasis (metabolic and emotional balance) during times of stress. Once the adrenal buffer is gone, you are constantly living on the edge of a breakdown. Your emotional resilience is reduced to a continual effort to cope—plus you become a prime candidate for asthma, allergy, fibromyalgia, chronic fatigue syndrome, and the autoimmune disorders discussed in this chapter.

Imagine if you had to live in a constant state of "emergency alert." It would be exhausting. In the same way, the adrenal glands, designed for episodes of stress (emergencies) in which tremendous energy is needed to fight or run away, find themselves in a situation where heightened activity is required *all the time*. And it's not just job stress. It's metabolic stress from poor food choices, pollution, and electromagnetic radiation. It's the pace of twentieth-century living and the breakdown of family (tribal) support groups and community. And on top of that, most people add caffeine, a drug that elevates stress hormones and can keep them elevated eighteen hours a day. For the poor adrenals, there's just no rest.

DELVING INTO ADRENAL FUNCTION

Until recently, no one bothered to look much at the adrenals. Even today, most doctors are only aware of two tests to evaluate adrenal function. One test (for Addison's disease) tells you if your adrenals are completely shot. The other (for Cushing's syndrome) tells you if your adrenals are in hyperdrive, most often from an adrenal tumor. Between these two extremes, there is nothing your doctor can tell you, other than that you appear "normal."

All that is starting to change as researchers discover adrenal factors in a wide range of health disorders. It turns out that the hormone balance maintained by the adrenal glands is much more fragile than we thought. This section will discuss what I call the adrenal dysfunction disorders. As you will see, adrenal weakness or adrenal insufficiency is the common factor that contributes to a number of serious health disorders.

And now the effect of caffeine on the adrenals is finally coming to light. The caffeine connection has been hidden by the fact that treatment for adrenal dysfunction disorders tends to be shortsighted and one-dimensional. As I have explained before, understanding the health effects of caffeine requires a long view, perhaps encompassing most of one's lifetime. And from that long-term view, a two-phase phenomenon is revealed.

PHASE 1: THE JOY RIDE

Phase 1 is what I call the honeymoon phase of caffeine consumption. This phase lays the groundwork for long-term, caffeine-related damage to your mind and body. Ever-increasing levels of stress hormones course through your veins, stressing your adrenals to the max. But for the present, you actually experience some beneficial effects from caffeine consumption. Caffeine can even seem like the answer to one or more of your health problems.

Here's a good illustration. In the current caffeine mania that is sweeping America, even health-food manufacturers and retailers have jumped on the bandwagon. Recently, articles have appeared in health-food magazines talking about the benefits of organic coffee. Some articles have discussed its mood-elevating effects, others imply that it is an aid to weight management, and a few even extol the drink as a natural treatment for asthma.

Now all of these "benefits" are real, to some extent, *but only in Phase 1.* We have already discussed how caffeine ultimately leads to depression. It's weight-loss "value" is similar to that of amphetamines, both in terms of temporary appetite suppression and ultimate side effects. And asthma? Caffeine can indeed reduce the symptoms of asthma—temporarily. And then in Phase 2, it makes them worse. That's why the long view is so important.

First of all, you must remember why caffeine has these temporary beneficial effects. It's all part of the stress response, the ancient survival mechanism that enabled us to survive in times of imminent danger. The increased respiratory efficiency that caffeine provides is purely a Phase 1 phenomenon; adrenal hormones are poured out to dilate the bronchial airways in order to send more oxygen to the muscles. But does that make caffeine a sensible treatment for asthma? Read the next section before you decide.

PHASE 2: PAYING THE PIPER

Habitual caffeine use ultimately leads to Phase 2, what has been called adrenal insufficiency or adrenal exhaustion. This condition bears more than a casual resemblance to the post-traumatic stress syndrome experienced by soldiers returning from combat. In effect, the adrenal glands simply wear out from chronic stimulation.

Throughout this book, I've talked about the myriad effects of caffeine-induced excess stress hormone production, from constricted arteries and elevated blood pressure to immune suppression and stomach ulcers. But this is only half of the story. As caffeine intake continues and the adrenals get weaker and weaker, a new set of problems arise that are related to stress hormone insufficiency. That's right—after a certain point, your adrenals are so exhausted that the pendulum swings the other way. And that's when you become most vulnerable to a whole new group of problems associated with adrenal exhaustion: namely, disorders related to inflammation and autoimmunity, among them allergy, asthma (inflammation of the bronchial airways), and even rheumatoid arthritis.

Consider this: We all know that adrenal hormones play a major role in the management of inflammation. (For example, prednisone is a synthetic adrenal hormone that is used to reduce inflammation in a wide variety of illnesses.) Adrenal hormones also help regulate the immune system, preventing immune cells from attacking healthy tissues. Rheumatoid arthritis has both an inflammatory and an immune system component. Recent research has shown that laboratory rats bred to have insufficient adrenal hormone production develop rheumatoid arthritis far more frequently than normal rats. It is also known that people with an adrenal disorder known as Cushing's disease are at high risk for depression, fatigue, and rheumatoid arthritis.

Recent research has found that abnormal adrenal hormone production in animals commonly leads to mood disorders. Clinicians have long noted that patients with rheumatoid arthritis frequently exhibit a type of depression characterized by fatigue, excessive sleep, and irritability. But it was always thought that this condition was the result of chronic arthritis pain. Now researchers are starting to think that the mood disorder and the inflammation may both be related to adrenal insufficiency.[192]

The adrenal insufficiency model of autoimmune disease makes sense when you learn that the onset of these disorders in humans is frequently associated with severe or chronic stress. Myasthenia gravis, for example, is an autoimmune disorder characterized by progressive loss of muscle strength and coordination. Current research suggests a strong adrenal stress component.[193]

THE DHEA CONNECTION

In Chapter 3, we learned that there is an inverse relationship in the body between stress hormones (primarily cortisol) and the "vitality hormone," DHEA, which is also produced by the adrenal glands. In Phase 1 of the caffeine/adrenal relationship, stress hormones are pumped out in excessive amounts. This action suppresses immunity and increases risk for a number of health disorders, especially cardiovascular disease. It also lowers production of DHEA, a hormone critical to the optimum functioning of your immune, cardiovascular, reproductive, and nervous systems.

Ultimately, the resulting stress leads to Phase 2 and adrenal exhaustion. The decrease in stress hormone production characteristic of Phase 2, however, does not result in increased DHEA. On the contrary, the exhausted adrenals are unable to produce either sufficient DHEA or cortisol, and this double whammy sets the stage for autoimmune disease. Men have a secondary supply of DHEA from testicular production, while women do not, which may help explain why women report more cases of autoimmune disease.

It is also interesting to note that a number of adrenal dysfunction disorders involve low levels of insulin-like growth factor-1.[194] IGF-1 is one of the body's chief repair and rebuild biochemicals, and its maintenance at optimal levels appears to be dependent on DHEA.

Until recently, however, very little attention was paid to the therapeutic benefits of DHEA. Asthma, allergy, and autoimmune disorders were treated with synthetic adrenal (glucocorticoid) hormones such as prednisone. And while these drugs certainly play an important role in the acute stage of inflammation, the adverse side effects make long-term use extremely unwise. Chronic use of glucocorticoid drugs can cause weight gain, hypertension, seriously reduced immunity, emotional disturbances, and bone mineral loss leading to osteoporosis.

DHEA may provide an alternative treatment. Researchers today are finding that, in at least one autoimmune disorder known as lupus, treatment with DHEA produces significant improvement.[195, 196] Most importantly, DHEA appears actually to help restore adrenal function.[197]

THE ALLERGY AND ASTHMA PARADOX

The relationship between asthma and allergy is well known. In most asthma patients, allergy is an important trigger. But few understand the connection between stress, caffeine, and these conditions. I believe that is because both allergy and asthma are commonly treated with adrenal hormones. For example, when a person has a serious allergy attack (anaphylaxis), the throat may swell, breathing may become difficult, and often the patient is rushed to the emergency room, where epinephrine (a synthetic adrenal hormone) is administered. Within minutes the swelling begins to subside and the patient improves. This is no mystery. It simply demonstrates that adrenal hormones are very effective in dampening the inflammatory response, no matter what the initiating cause might be.

Asthma is typically treated with adrenal hormones and a caffeine metabolite known as theophylline. So the short view would naturally be, "Well, I guess caffeine is good for my asthma." To get the truth, however, you need to take the long view. Chemically, theophylline is a dimethylxanthine, differing from caffeine only by the absence of one methyl group. (Caffeine is a trimethylxanthine.) When you consume caffeine, theophylline is one of the intermediate products that your liver makes as it breaks down and detoxifies the drug. Thus both the short-term and long-term problems associated with theophylline are very similar to caffeine.

Now, what would you think if you went to the doctor for your asthma and were told to take theophylline for the rest of your life? Your first question might be, "Is that safe?" To which a well-informed doctor might reply, "Well, actually, the drug is likely to upset your stomach, make you nervous, disturb your sleep, and suppress your immune system.[198–202] If you take too much, it might trigger an epileptic seizure.[203] Oh, and by the way, the immune suppression will primarily affect the immune cells you need to fight viruses and cancer.[204] But hey, for now, you'll breathe easier."

Obviously, in real life doctors don't give (and patients usually don't ask for) the long view. We want instant relief, even if there's a steep payback later on—and that's the hallmark of caffeine. In clinical practice, I saw hundreds of patients with allergy and asthma, and with uncanny frequency, they would relate to me the following scenario:

When they drank three or four cups of coffee during the day, they would be pretty much asthma-free for the whole day, but their condition would then be much worse at night when they could not suppress the symptoms with caffeine or theophylline. I would explain that they did not have asthma due to a caffeine or theophylline deficiency, and that their long-term chances of success in eliminating the problem depended to a great extent on how well they treated their adrenals.

Those who were willing to follow my Off the Bean program invariably experienced significant improvements. Of course the program was combined with a sensible diet and lifestyle approach that included reduced exposure to inhalant and food allergens as well as stress management and nutritional supplementation to reduce the hypersensitivity of their airways. Remember also that some people are allergic to caffeine itself, and avoiding the substance in any form leads to almost immediate improvement.[205]

THE HYPERSENSITIVITY CONTINUUM

Once again, allergy is not an all-or-nothing phenomenon. The best way to visualize allergy-related disease is on a continuum, from nonreactive all the way to a condition known as multiple chemical sensitivity (MCS) (see figure below). MCS patients are sometimes unable to leave their homes because even minimal exposure to outside air or pollution of any kind can trigger an allergic reaction.

Your position on this continuum is very much related to the ability of your adrenal glands to maintain adequate (but not excessive) levels of cortisol and epinephrine. Because caffeine and stress weaken the adrenal response, they exert a pressure that, over time, pushes us farther and farther to the right.

THE ALLERGY/SENSITIVITY CONTINUUM

Strong adrenal function	Compromised adrenal function			Adrenal exhaustion
△	△	△	△	△
Normal reactivity (Healthy)	Mild seasonal allergy	Chronic allergy/ asthma	Allergy/asthma requiring frequent medication	MCS syndrome

FIBROMYALGIA

Fibromyalgia is a chronic syndrome of pain that can range (and change) from tolerable to incapacitating. While the pain is arthritis-like, fibromyalgia is not a type of arthritis. The pain, rather than centering on the joints, is experienced more in muscles, tendons, and ligaments, and can shift unpredictably. For the moment, fibromyalgia remains a mysterious disorder, diagnosed from a symptom review and the existence of specific "tender points" on the body where even mild pressure causes undue soreness.

Current research suggest multiple causative factors, and there is a very significant caffeine-stress connection. New research has shown conclusively that patients with fibromyalgia suffer from an adrenal weakness that includes insufficient cortisol secretion.[206, 207] The pituitary hormone signal that stimulates adrenal production of cortisol (ACTH) may be more than adequate, but the adrenal response is still weak. Exercise, a positive stress that in a healthy person stimulates a rise in cortisol, produces only a modest response in the fibromyalgia patient.[208, 209] In effect, the syndrome fits perfectly into the Phase 2 model described above.

The simple solution is to give fibromyalgia patients synthetic adrenal hormones, but as we have already noted, the adverse side effects of these steroid medications are far too dangerous over the long term. We are left, therefore, wondering how to restore adrenal function naturally. That topic will be covered in Chapter 10. As you might have guessed, step one is to stop harming your adrenals with caffeine.

In fact, there are four good reasons why anyone with fibromyalgia should avoid all sources of caffeine.

1. *Recovery is unlikely as long as your adrenals are stressed.* Avoiding caffeine will greatly increase your

chance of recovery, a process that may take ten years or more.

2. *The restoration of deep sleep is critical to the healing process.* Sleep disturbance (specifically reduced S-4 sleep) is one of the most common and long-lasting symptoms of fibromyalgia.[210] The medical term for this disturbance is "alpha intrusion of Stage 4 sleep."

As we discussed in Chapter 3, deep (S-4) sleep is essential for repairing tissue damage. Anyone with disturbed Stage 4 sleep will have aches and pains from unrepaired microtrauma that occurs in the muscles and connective tissue. Whether from overexercise of a particular muscle group, a new activity that involves use of different muscles, or simply an activity that you haven't done in a while (gardening in the spring), minor muscular injuries are common and are normally repaired in deep sleep. In patients with fibromyalgia, these injuries appear to accumulate[211]—and any caffeine intake only worsens S-4 sleep disturbance.

3. *Caffeine causes anxiety,* which is part of the vicious cycle of stress and fatigue. The net result is that inflammation and pain are intensified.

4. *Caffeine exacerbates other symptoms of fibromyalgia, including:*
   - Decreased circulation to the fingers and toes (known as Raynaud's phenomenon)
   - Tension headaches and migraine
   - Irritable bowel

CHRONIC FATIGUE SYNDROME (CFS)

CFS is another multifactorial disorder with marked similarities to fibromyalgia. Many medical texts group the two conditions together for diagnosis and treatment. In CFS, however, the most striking feature is debilitating physical and mental fatigue.

What caught the attention of early researchers was the similarity of CFS symptoms to another condition known as post-viral fatigue syndrome. But the search for a viral cause (such as Epstein-Barr virus or EBV) turned out to be a dead end. EBV infection may play a role in chronic fatigue, but the vast majority of American adults test positive for EBV and only a small percent have chronic fatigue. There must be another factor that causes some individuals to fall apart in the face of viral or other infection, and that factor may very well be adrenal dysfunction.

As in fibromyalgia, recent research confirms that chronic fatigue patients have low adrenal function[212] and low levels of cortisol, both at morning and evening time points.[213, 214] The tie-in with fibromyalgia is obvious, but researchers are now beginning to see that CFS may be part of the wider picture of adrenal dysfunction[215]—in which caffeine intake is a major contributing factor.

I'm not saying that caffeine causes CFS or the other disorders we've discussed in this chapter. However, one should not ignore the proven and well-understood damage that caffeine inflicts on the adrenal glands and nervous system. It's important to take the long view, and CFS patients should be advised that using caffeine to get through the day will only prolong and deepen their debilitating illness.

There's yet another factor to consider. CFS patients have been found to have impaired clearance of metabolic toxins, in itself a significant biochemical stress. These metabolic toxins result from the normal metabolism of food, and they include bacteria, volatile fatty acids, amines, and bile acids. Additional bowel toxins are produced by parasites and yeast organisms. It is the job of the intestinal wall to prevent these substances from entering the bloodstream and surrounding tissues. In "Caffeine and Gastrointestinal Health," this chapter, I presented evidence that caffeine and coffee both tend to impair the barrier function of the intestinal tract, leading to increased absorption of toxic material into the body.

THE BOTTOM LINE

Anyone with allergy, asthma, fibromyalgia, chronic fatigue, or any other autoimmune disease will tell you that their symptoms worsen or flare up when they're under stress. In many cases, these people can pinpoint exactly when their condition first appeared and relate it to a specific trauma or stress in their life. If there is one essential lesson to be learned from this book, it is that stress is the invisible saboteur of health and wellness. Conversely, anything that you can do to enhance your experience of ease and peace will improve your life in myriad ways. The first step, as you know by now, is to get off the bean.

Men's Health

Earlier in this chapter, I presented a discussion of cardiovascular disease, by far the most significant health risk for men related to caffeine. But as male baby boomers reach their fifth decade of life, prostate health becomes a more and more pressing issue.

The most common symptom of prostate dysfunction is abnormal growth of the prostate, which then presses upon the urethra and causes problems with urination. Men with enlarged prostates (known as benign prostate hypertrophy or BPH) have trouble voiding their bladder, so pressure builds up and is difficult to release. Adding to the discomfort, this pressure also causes frequent awakenings to urinate during the night. Most importantly, BPH is a risk factor for prostate cancer, the second leading cause of cancer death in men.

As men age, the incidence of prostate infection and inflammation (prostatitis) also increases. All of these maladies are treated with drugs. Some work by inhibiting the metabolism of testosterone, some actually reduce testosterone production, and others fight underlying infection. Still, drug treatments of BPH, prostatitis, and prostate cancer are not what you would call remarkably successful. Surgery is being used more and more, and even the newest antibiotics often fail to eradicate prostate infections. Moreover, surgery and drug therapies often have adverse side effects, including decreased libido and impotence.

Thus, any man over forty is like to have a very uneasy feeling about his future health and sexuality. By age seventy, more than 50 percent will have enlarged prostates, and by age eighty, the number goes up to 80 percent. Here's the good news: Men can significantly reduce their risk for urinary and prostate problems by getting off coffee and caffeine. Milton Krisiloff, M.D., a urologist in Santa Monica, California, was one of the first to notice that dietary modification, including the elimination of all sources of caffeine, actually resolved prostatitis in the large majority of his patients.[216] In addition, he has clinical evidence that his simple program (the Krisiloff Diet) results in decreased PSA scores for many men. High PSA (prostate specific antigen) is an indication of increased risk for prostate cancer.[217]

Work by other investigators identifying an association between caffeine and urinary problems in men supports these clinical observations,[218, 219] and recently prostate cancer risk was found to be directly linked to intake of theobromine, a methylxanthine related to caffeine. In that study, men who consumed high levels of theobromine (commonly found in chocolate) had more than twice the risk of prostate cancer compared to men who consumed very little of that substance.[220]

ISSUES OF MALE REPRODUCTIVE HEALTH

By now most everyone knows that sperm counts among men in Western nations are declining, and the rate of decline is fairly alarming. A likely explanation for this is the increasing exposure to pesticides and environmental pollutants, many of which are powerfully toxic to the reproductive organs of men and women.[221]

As I have mentioned, coffee is the most heavily sprayed of all consumable commodities, but residues in the final roasted product are reported to be quite low.[222] Still, coffee and caffeine have to be considered in any discussion of reproductive health for three reasons.

1. Beyond the directly toxic effects, pesticides, fungicides, and herbicides can have cumulative effects on human health by altering hormone levels and hormone receptor sites in the body. These endocrine modulating effects can be virtually invisible for decades, producing symptoms only after many years of exposure. Thus, short-term research will miss important long-term causative factors.

2. Clearly negative health consequences to animals are produced when they are fed caffeine, and the ill effects are almost always centered on the nervous and reproductive systems. Rats fed caffeine suffer testicular atro-

phy and low sperm counts as a result. Studies show, in fact, that of all methylxanthines, caffeine has the highest reproductive toxicity.[223] What's more, the amount of caffeine required to produce these adverse effects is not massive. One study with rabbits found marked suppression of sperm formation at roughly the equivalent of three mugs of coffee for a 150-pound man.[224]

Now, I know that you cannot equate rabbits and rats to human beings, but animal studies do have relevance, especially when you consider that human beings with agricultural exposure to pesticides exhibit precisely the same constellation of symptoms.[225] And here's one more extremely intriguing observation: Men with agricultural exposure to pesticides who father children have an astronomical prevalence of female offspring (83.4 percent versus the normal of 48 percent).[226] The same thing happens when male rodents are fed caffeine.[227]

3. A wide range of human subjects has been studied to evaluate sperm counts and sperm motility. And whether you're looking at men facing final exams, running a race, or simply experiencing the stress of fertility testing, anxiety has a profound effect on sperm quality.[228–233] Motility (normal movement), sperm counts, and sperm morphology (size and shape) all suffer when men are stressed, and, as we have well established, one of the most reliable anxiety-producing influences in a man's life is caffeine.

PERHAPS MEN ARE NOT SO DIFFERENT AFTER ALL

We all want a healthy sex life for as long as possible. Men are often seen as being less willing than women to alter dietary habits and incorporate new healthy lifestyle habits. But if something simple like reducing caffeine consumption can keep us sexually vital and healthy, most men would choose to alter their diet any day over the pain of disease and the possible adverse effects of medical intervention.

The problem is that men often fail to recognize approaching danger until obvious symptoms send them to their doctor. And doctors are more likely to write prescriptions than provide dietary advice. So the issue becomes one of developing an increased sensitivity to the changes that occur in our bodies as we age, including the urinary pressure and delay that signals early prostate problems.

Clearly, caffeine affects women's reproductive capabilities, and we know that caffeine produces stress that can affect male sperm quality. If you are a prospective father, it certainly seems prudent to err on the side of caution and join your wife in eliminating caffeine from your diet.

GOUT: OH, MY ACHING FEET

Gout is a painful condition (considered a type of arthritis) that results from the deposition of uric acid crystals in cartilage, the bones of the foot, and kidneys. For unknown reasons, gout is primarily a male disorder, with only about 5 percent of patients being women.

There are a number of causes, mostly related to defects in uric acid metabolism, and these defects appear to be primarily genetic. As is almost always the case, however, heredity only predisposes one to the condition. Dietary and environmental factors play an important role. Diets high in sugar and protein have been shown to elevate uric acid levels,[234] as can caffeine.

The caffeine connection is demonstrated by a recent

case in which the patient, a forty-eight-year-old man, was "doing all the right things" to reduce his uric acid levels. He stopped drinking all alcoholic beverages, adopted a vegetarian diet, avoided sugar, and maintained ideal body weight. According to current medical knowledge, that was everything he could do. If he continued to experience gouty pain, he would have to take drugs to lower his uric acid levels.

At his wife's prompting, he stopped drinking coffee, and in a matter of weeks, his pain was completely gone. That's because one of the breakdown products of caffeine is methyluric acid, and that can add to the body's uric acid burden.[235] In fact, allopurinol, the drug that is used to treat gout, works by inhibiting the enzyme that converts methylxanthine (a caffeine metabolite) to methyl-uric acid.[236]

Now, besides an inherited tendency to accumulate uric acid, liver disease significantly increases the likelihood that caffeine will contribute to gout.[237] If you remember that the liver is responsible for the entire chain of breakdown steps in the detoxification of caffeine, this is not surprising. What is surprising is that the elimination of caffeine is not (yet) a standard recommendation for individuals with gout.

Caffeine and Your Eyes

Consider the astonishingly complex series of events that is taking place right now as you read this book. The miracle of sight is an amazing process involving highly specialized cells held perfectly within a fluid-filled sphere. Sight is the richest of our senses, accounting for about 75 percent of all of our perceptions.

Often likened to a camera, the human eye is far more impressive. The "film," for example, can be used over and over again as long as the conditions are right for repair and regeneration. In fact, the retina can capture more than ten images a second throughout life, sending information through the optic nerve directly to the brain.

In fact, every structure of the eye is under constant repair, nourished by extremely fine blood vessels and a fluid known as aqueous humor. The flow of aqueous humor maintains the internal or intraocular pressure, and if this flow is impaired, pressure may increase, damaging the eye and leading to a condition known as glaucoma. Glaucoma is a major cause of blindness, affecting approximately 3 million Americans, and fully one-third of them don't know they have the disease.

Caffeine significantly increases intraocular pressure in most people, especially when consumed in amounts of four or more cups a day.[238] If you have glaucoma, this pressure increase can occur at half that amount.[239] Experts believe that this results from changes in aqueous humor flow, and studies have shown a remarkable difference in the fluid dynamics of the eye between volunteers given caffeine and those given placebo.[240]

Perhaps even more serious (because it affects a greater number of people) is the decrease in microcirculation in the eye caused by caffeine. Here again, as in the brain and peripheral blood vessels, caffeine causes a marked constriction that limits the delivery of oxygen and vital nutrients to these tissues. Animal experiments show that this can inhibit the growth and repair of the lens of the eye.[241] Studies with human volunteers illustrate that caffeine's vasoconstrictive effect markedly reduces circulation to the macula, the central portion of the retina.[242] Macular degeneration is the leading cause of vision loss and blindness in people over sixty-five, with more than 16,000 new cases reported annually in the United States.[243] What's more, evidence suggests that the incidence of this condition is increasing rapidly.[244]

I find it remarkable that so little attention has been paid to the role of caffeine in eye health. Caffeine's diuretic effect can make your eyes so dry that wearing contact lenses is uncomfortable or impossible. Caffeine contributes directly to the two leading causes of vision loss and blindness. Today, health-food stores are filled with herbs, vitamins, and specialty products intended to decrease risk for macular degeneration, cataracts, and glaucoma, and yet no one is sounding the alarm regarding caffeine.

Antioxidants can help avert these common eye disorders by preventing free-radical damage to the lens, retina, and macula. *Ginkgo biloba* and bilberry herb also help by improving microcirculation. But none of these measures will have the best results if you continue to counter their salutary effects with caffeine.

CHAPTER 6

Caffeine and Women's Health

The hardest years in a woman's life are those between ten and seventy.
—HELEN HAYES (at eighty-three)

You've Come a Long Way

Women today are under a tremendous amount of pressure to balance the demands of family and career. Not that past generations of women had it easy—it's simply that the pace of life, and therefore the stress of life, has accelerated to the breaking point. What's more, women are facing these pressures alone, simply because the support systems of agrarian or tribal communities that were common centuries ago have largely disappeared.

In this book, I have tried to get across the equation that Caffeine = Stress. This is a critically important message, but it is opposed by powerful propaganda from the caffeine industry. Caffeine products are advertised as a "pick-me-up," with no mention of the fact that just a short time later they become a "drag-me-down."

It's always a surprise to me when I suggest that a patient cut back on caffeine and she reacts as though I'd asked her to betray her best friend. Even when I show her documented proof that caffeine is contributing to many (if not most) of her health disorders, she finds it hard to believe that her beloved coffee would do her harm.

With Friends Like These, Who Needs Enemies?

Let's face it. We all grew up with the idea that coffee was something you shared in special moments with a friend. This warm, fuzzy picture was conjured up by Madison Avenue ad men to get you hooked on caffeine products. The advertisers know that if they can just get you to consume a few cups of coffee or a few soft drinks a day, you will turn into a lifelong addict.

To illustrate how well this campaign has worked, one need only look at women's health literature. With very few exceptions, *nothing* is mentioned about eliminating caffeine, even though the connection between caffeine and women's health is undeniable and extremely important. In Chapters 3, 4, and 5 we looked at caffeine's contribution to a number of health disorders, including heart disease, digestive problems, diabetes, fibromyalgia, panic attacks, depression, and anxiety. This chapter will cover caffeine's impact on issues specifically related to women, such as premenstrual syndrome (PMS), menopause, fibrocystic breast disease, iron absorption, calcium deficiency, osteoporosis, fertility and conception disorders, and complications of pregnancy and childbirth.

The Gender Gap

When it comes to evaluating the potential dangers of caffeine, gender is the most important consideration. Yet the entire issue is usually overlooked or ignored. Compared to men, research shows that caffeine is much more damaging to women, producing adverse effects at lower intake. The effects are even more far-reaching when you consider the harm caffeine does to fetuses and nursing babies.

Given these facts, you may be surprised (and dismayed) to learn that roughly 75 percent of the human research on caffeine has been conducted on men. Hopefully, this chapter will serve to offset this astounding imbalance by describing exactly how caffeine affects women and what can be done to minimize the health risks associated with caffeine intake.

First of all, women detoxify coffee much more slowly than men. What's more, the half-life of caffeine (the time it takes the body to eliminate one-half of a given dose) changes according to a woman's menstrual cycle. In the luteal phase (roughly the last two weeks leading to menstruation), the half-life of a cup of coffee can be 7 hours, as compared to 5.5 hours in the follicular phase (the first two weeks of a woman's cycle).[1] Moreover, a number of factors specific to women, such as the use of birth control pills, reduce caffeine clearance even further. In fact, women on birth control pills require about twice the normal time to detoxify caffeine.[2]

All of this means that the cumulative effect of daily caffeine intake is very significant for women. A woman's second (and even third) caffeine-containing beverage will hit her glands, organs, and nervous system long before her body recovers from the first cup.

Caffeine just plain affects women differently than men, and it has to do with much more than the decreased clearance rate. In one study, for example, men and women were given the same 150-milligram dose of caffeine at the same time of day. The body temperature of the female subjects increased, while the male subjects experienced a decrease in temperature. In addition, an hour after caffeine administration, female subjects rated themselves as more sleepy, tired, and "disorganized" than the male subjects did, and on standard cognitive tasks, the female subjects found that caffeine made performance more difficult.[3]

Stress in general affects women more severely than men. Faced with threat or conflict, research shows that women tend to have a much greater stress response compared to men, resulting in higher blood levels of stress hormones.[4] This response does not mean that women are "weaker." On the contrary, I believe it indicates that women tend to respond to conflict more seriously than their male counterparts.

And they suffer for it. In one three-year study evaluating the effects of stress, elevated cortisol not only increased risk for cardiovascular and other diseases, as it did in men, but in women the stress response also predicted a decline in memory as well as cognitive and physical functioning.[5]

The Stress Chain Reaction

When the level of stress hormones (especially cortisol) is elevated, many of the body's maintenance and repair functions cease. How could it be otherwise? After all, this stress response was originally intended to get us out of imminent danger. To mobilize all available energy for survival, Mother Nature devised a way to shut down all noncritical functions in order to send blood, nutrients, and oxygen to the heart and skeletal muscles.

As I mentioned in Chapter 4, few of us today ever face the kind of danger that requires explosive action. Our stresses are the smoldering, chronic stress of twentieth-century living and twentieth-century caffeine consumption. But even though the stresses are different, our bodies' response is the same, and the shutdown of repair functions can weaken our bones, delay healing, and create lines and wrinkles in our skin. In short, caffeine and stress accelerate the aging process.

Phillip Gold, a researcher at the National Institutes of Mental Health in Bethesda, Maryland, compared the bone density of women with elevated cortisol to that of women with normal cortisol. Although all the women were age forty, those with elevated stress hormones had the bone density of seventy-year-olds.[6]

New Research Clarifies Heart Disease Risk

Remember how heart disease was once considered a "man's disease"? For years, the vast majority of research was conducted on men. Then someone noticed that just as many women die of heart disease—however, for different reasons. Apparently, women are more likely to have fatal heart attacks caused by coronary vasospasm, a constriction of the artery wall that shuts off blood flow to the heart.

The likelihood of coronary vasospasm is related to both stress and caffeine. A study examining the relationship between specific foods and the risk of heart attack in women found that *the women who consumed the most coffee had nearly three times the risk of heart attack compared to women who drank the least amount of coffee.* The association of caffeine and increased risk for heart attack was stronger than the risk factor for total fat added to food![7]

In the United States, breast cancer claims the lives of approximately 44,000 women each year. At the same time, more than 235,000 are killed by heart disease.

Job Stress and Caffeine Linked to Depression and Hostility

Faced with overwhelming workloads from their families and their employers, women today are falling apart in record numbers. Instead of being part of the solution, caffeine is very much part of the problem. North Carolina researchers found that women who were overworked and experiencing high levels of stress scored significantly higher on standard tests measuring depression, anxiety, and hostility.[8] In addition to the fact that such conditions are painful and reduce one's quality of life, all of these factors increase the risk for cardiovascular disease.

Other researchers from the University of California found that highly stressed female attorneys who worked more than forty-five hours a week were three times more likely to have a miscarriage during their first trimester of pregnancy, compared with those who worked less than thirty-five hours a week.[9] Again, caffeine, is a co-factor for two reasons: (1) People who work long hours have been shown to drink more caffeine; and (2) conclusive research has found a significant association between caffeine intake and miscarriage (see page 247).

Perhaps the new definition of "coffee break" should be "a break from coffee." I encourage all of my female clients (actually, I implore them) to replace the caffeine with herbal coffee, herb tea, or another noncaffeinated beverage (see Appendix A, "Resources").

Stress and Your Gastrointestinal Tract

It is well known that caffeine contributes significantly to anxiety, hostility, and depression. In turn, these are powerful risk factors for irritable bowel syndrome and ulcers (see Chapter 5). "Women with these characteristics [anxiety and hostility] were more than twice as likely to develop an ulcer," reports Dr. Susan Levenstein, who headed an eight-year study regarding psychosocial influences on health.[10] Women who were depressed at the start of the study were three times more likely to develop an ulcer over the study period.

A Little Dose'll Do Ya

Keep in mind that the damage done to the body and mind by caffeine is very much dose-related. A little caffeine will do a little harm, while lots of caffeine will do lots of harm. Determining factors include:

1. Your age, weight, overall health, and current medications. Remember that birth control pills greatly reduce the liver's ability to detoxify caffeine.

2. Your sensitivity to caffeine. For unknown reasons, some people are simply more sensitive to caffeine than others. This may be related to allergy, body type, adrenal health, or other factors.

3. Your activity level after consuming caffeine. What do you do after you consume caffeine? If you exercise, you can to some extent "work off" the stress hormones, glucose, and fatty acids that were released into your bloodstream. But if you sit at a desk, the biochemical events resulting from caffeine consumption will result in well-understood and documented damage.

Caffeine Causes Serious Nutritional Deficiencies

Calcium deficiency, osteoporosis, and iron deficiency are three of the most common nutritional problems in America today—especially among women. At the same time, coffee, tea, and soft drinks are the beverages most often consumed with meals. It turns out that the relationship between these nutritional problems and caffeine consumption is very well established.

Caffeine Facts for Women

FACT: Iron deficiency, inadequate calcium intake, osteoporosis, and depression are devastating problems for women.

Fact: Caffeine dramatically reduces iron absorption.

Fact: Caffeine increases calcium loss and risk of osteoporosis.

Fact: Caffeine produces short-term mood elevation, but contributes to rebound depression.

Reduced Calcium Absorption

Over 65 percent of American women have low calcium intake, a condition that is aggravated by caffeine's ability to accelerate the loss of calcium through the urinary and intestinal tracts.

One recent study provides a smoking gun to implicate caffeine in calcium deficiency. Researchers at Central Washington University investigated consumption levels of calcium and caffeine in women thirty-one to seventy-eight years old. All women consumed approximately 200 milligrams of caffeine daily, "the equivalent of one to two cups of coffee." This study showed that total urine output of water, calcium, magnesium, sodium, and potassium increased significantly for more than two hours following caffeine ingestion.[11]

Osteoporosis

Even with this conclusive evidence of caffeine-related mineral loss, health authorities hesitate to affirm that caffeine is a risk factor for osteoporosis. That's because the caffeine industry has created a smokescreen around the issue, using studies that supposedly show that no danger exists. Let's take a closer look.

One study commonly cited by caffeine proponents is titled "Caffeine Does Not Affect the Rate of Gain in Spine Bone in Young Women." But if you read the study itself (and not just the title) you will find that the subjects were college-aged women who consumed one cup of coffee per day. To say the least, this level of caffeine intake is representative neither of college students nor of most other American adults. Even the authors admit that the study does not in any way vindicate caffeine. They state only that "one cup of coffee per day, or 103 mg, appears to be safe with respect to bone health in this age group."[12] Surveys suggest that most American women consume that much caffeine before noon.

Besides, if you're trying to evaluate risk of osteoporosis, wouldn't it be important to look at postmenopausal women? Researchers at the University of California in San Francisco who did just that found a significant association between caffeine consumption and reduced bone mass. In fact, the caffeine–low bone density connection was found even in those women who took calcium supplements.[13]

Another way to explore the issue is to study middle-aged but still premenopausal women. In this category, leading researchers found that caffeine intake produced a double whammy on calcium levels. The drug increased calcium lost in the urine *and* increased calcium loss through the intestinal tract. Again, the amount of calcium lost was directly proportional to the amount of caffeine consumed.[14]

For the skeptic who wants to see proof that such calcium loss results in greater risk for osteoporosis, a very recent study conducted with women aged forty to fifty found that caffeine intake was conclusively associated with decreased bone density,[15] and research by the United

States Department of Agriculture confirms the findings. Results from the USDA study indicate that women who consume less than the RDA for calcium (65 percent of all women in the United States) face dramatic reductions of bone strength, especially when they consume more than two or three servings of coffee per day.[16]

Another research strategy is to take habitual caffeine users and see what happens when they stop. As expected, after only two weeks off caffeine, women showed significant improvements in calcium status even while consuming a low-calcium diet.[17]

Still another perspective (if you need one) may be gained by looking at the association of caffeine intake and hip fracture. Sure enough, data from studies covering nearly 90,000 U.S. women show a positive correlation between caffeine intake and hip fracture. The largest of the studies found that the risk for hip fracture for those who consumed the most caffeine was three times (300 percent) greater than it was for the group that consumed little or no caffeine.[18, 19]

There are actually two contributing factors that weaken a caffeine user's bones. We've discussed the direct factor of increased calcium loss, but there are also indirect factors associated with the increase in stress hormones. Caffeine raises cortisol levels, and with daily intake, that stress hormone may remain elevated for long periods of time. We also know that caffeine contributes to depression, and the combination of these two factors has telling effects. Women with a history of depression, for example, have weaker bones compared to age-matched women without depression.[20] Again, this is due simply to the chronic elevation of stress hormones that is part of the caffeine/depression scenario.

The goods news is that medical review articles are finally listing caffeine as a risk factor for osteoporosis.[21–27] The bad news is that no one seems to be paying attention. Material from the National Women's Health Network states that the negative effect on bones from a cup of caffeine is "more than adequately offset by a tablespoon or two of milk," and the position statement by the National Osteoporosis Foundation in Washington, D.C., states, "If calcium intakes meet NOF standards, NOF considers caffeine intake in the range of 2–4 cups of coffee per day to be without harmful effect on the skeleton." I do not mean to denigrate these organizations, both of which provide an extremely valuable service. It's just that in regard to caffeine, they are, like almost everyone else, unwilling to examine the evidence.

Caffeine, the Iron Robber

Not only does caffeine contribute to the loss of calcium, magnesium, zinc, and other valuable minerals, but it also contributes to serious iron loss. The data is incontrovertible. A 1983 study showed that one cup of coffee "reduced iron absorption from a hamburger meal by 39%." The study went on to state:

> When a cup of drip coffee or instant coffee was ingested with a meal . . . absorption was reduced from 5.88% to 1.64% and 0.97% respectively, and when the strength of the instant coffee was doubled, percentage iron absorption fell to 0.53% . . . The same degree

of inhibition as with simultaneous ingestion was seen when coffee was taken 1 hour later.[28]

I must explain the consequences of this astounding finding. Most women spend their entire lives malnourished in iron, and nearly 30 percent will be frankly anemic until they stop menstruating. This is because it is very difficult to absorb iron from food, and unless a woman has a great diet and perfect digestion, her monthly blood loss will tend to exceed her absorption of this essential mineral.[29] Add caffeine to that equation and the likelihood of insufficient iron approaches certainty. *Depending on the composition of a meal, a caffeinated beverage can reduce iron availability by a whopping 50 percent.*

What's more, caffeine impairs the absorption of any iron supplement taken to correct the deficiency. Documented cases have appeared in the medical literature showing that anemia was *incurable* until the patient stopped consuming caffeine.[30]

"Considering the high incidence of iron deficiency anemia worldwide and its likely association with immune function and mental development, these findings indicate that dietary habits such as coffee and tea consumption deserve more attention as potential causative factors."

Source: *American Journal of Clinical Nutrition,* 1988;vol. 48:645–51.

As you might know, the statistics on iron deficiency are alarming. Research shows that iron deficiency is the most common nutritional deficiency in the United States, Canada, Australia, and western Europe.[31] But what exactly does that mean? We're used to hearing about "iron-poor blood" causing a certain lack of zip and energy, but iron deficiency is much more than that. In fact, there are three distinct levels of iron deficiency, and I'll bet you've heard only about one. Don't feel bad. Your doctor may not know any more about this important issue than you do.

Anemia as a Measure of Iron Sufficiency . . . and Other Myths

Imagine that you had a financial adviser to manage your estate. One day, he calls you and announces that you will have to file bankruptcy because you are broke. "What?" you exclaim. "How is that possible? When you started managing my account, I had two million dollars!" "Well," he says, "about three years ago, I put all of your money in a gold-mining operation. Over the years, it has done quite poorly." "Why didn't you tell me I was losing enormous sums of money for three years?" you ask. To which he replies, "Well, technically speaking, you weren't completely broke, so as long as you had *some* money, I didn't think of bringing it up."

If this scenario sounds absurd and unbelievable, you have to understand that most doctors have followed this approach for decades with their female patients in regard to the precious commodity known as iron. That's because doctors have been looking only at the woman's complete blood count (CBC). If she's anemic (bankrupt), they tell her. If she's not anemic, they let it slide. The fact of the matter is that a woman will typically be iron deficient for *two to three years* before she becomes anemic.[32] At that point, anemia is difficult to cure. But if iron deficiency is identified in its early stages, it can easily be treated and anemia avoided.

Shocked reader: "It must be that there is no reliable way of determining the early stages of iron deficiency." Ah, but there is. It's a simple and inexpensive blood test that measures body stores of iron, called serum ferritin.

Shocked reader: "But my doctor does measure serum iron, and he always told me it was normal." Serum iron is a meaningless test. It only tells you how much iron is traveling through your blood. You can be frankly anemic—hardly able to get out of bed—and have normal serum iron.

Shocked reader: "Gosh, this serum ferritin must be a new test." Actually, the test has been available for nearly thirty years. Studies confirming its value as the definitive test for iron status were published in 1979, and verified repeatedly for the past two decades.[33–37] By now, the consensus among experts is that the only accurate way to determine iron nutriture is by evaluating ferritin and other iron parameters. What's more, serum ferritin is also the only iron indicator that is able to differentiate between true iron deficiency and anemia due to infection.[38]

Shocked reader: "If this is such a critical issue, why in the world has it not been diligently pursued?" Well, iron deficiency is primarily a problem for women, and most physicians and researchers are men. Additionally, the cure for the problem is a nutritional supplement and not a prescription drug, so the issue doesn't get much attention. There is, however, a growing body of research showing that ferritin is a critically important factor in evaluating (and even preventing) atherosclerosis,[39] so we may yet see the test performed routinely.

The take-home message here is that there is a *progression* of iron deficiency. You're not optimally nourished in iron one day and anemic the next. It's important to have a sensitive marker for iron status because there are clear symptoms way before the anemic state. Most symptoms are related to energy and mental alertness, so the connection with caffeine is more than casual.

For example, a woman with low iron stores is likely to have low energy and a hard time concentrating. Chances are she will also be depressed. And since she doesn't know these conditions are related to malnutrition, she will most likely chalk it up to growing older or her personality. What's more, she will probably resort to using caffeine in order to cope with these feelings, and that brings us to the next vicious cycle:

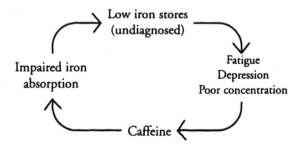

Iron Alert Action Plan

1. Monitor your serum ferritin level starting at menarch (the onset of menstruation). Make it a part of your yearly physical, or test at least every two years. Use the following guidelines derived from the latest biomedical information:

Ferritin Level	Iron Status
0–10	Severe iron deficiency
10–18	Marginal iron deficiency
18–40	Adequate
40–100	Optimal iron nutriture

2. If your ferritin is less than 10, I suggest that you work with your physician to correct the problem. You will need an effective iron supplement and follow-up. The most bioavailable form of iron I have found is a chelated iron, known as iron glycinate (see Appendix A). But be careful. Too much iron can cause constipation and abdominal cramping. This can be avoided by staying in the 30-to-90-milligrams-per-day range.

3. If your ferritin is between 18 and 40, premenopausal women should still consider iron glycinate at 30 milligrams per day.

4. In all cases, it is imperative that you maximize iron absorption from the food you eat, and that means reducing caffeine intake. If you continue drinking coffee, tea, or soft drinks with meals, the caffeine will reduce absorption of iron from any tablet you take as well as the meal. The only sensible approach is to get off the caffeine and soft drinks. If you're drinking tea, have it at "teatime" (midmorning or midafternoon), not with meals. Caffeine-free herbal coffee and herb tea, of course, will not interfere with iron absorption.

5. Vitamin C has been shown to enhance iron absorption. If your supplement does not already contain vitamin C, take a 200-milligram tablet of vitamin C with your iron.

6. Avoid other iron robbers: sugar, high doses of calcium supplements (especially calcium carbonate),

phytic acid (wheat bran), and oxalic acid (spinach, beet tops).

Suboptimal Iron Affects Mind, Mood, and Learning

Researchers at the Johns Hopkins School of Medicine recently highlighted an important defect associated with suboptimal iron status. In their study, seventy-three anemic girls who were "merely" iron insufficient were selected from four Baltimore high schools. They took either an iron supplement or a placebo for eight weeks. In just eight weeks, there were remarkable differences between the treatment group and the placebo group in memory, attention, and learning skills.[40] It turns out that iron is essential for the activation of enzymes that turn on key brain functions, including the secretion and activity of serotonin and dopamine, two neurotransmitters that affect mind, mood, and behavior. We now know that even marginal iron deficiency—what I call iron insufficiency—can contribute to mood, memory, and learning disorders long before anemia ever develops.

Premenstrual Syndrome (PMS)

Almost one-third of premenopausal women suffer from some degree of PMS—and recent research has confirmed that caffeine intake is related to both its presence and its severity.[41] Basically, the more caffeine you ingest, the worse your PMS will be.

One study, based on 841 responses to a questionnaire sent to female university students in Oregon, showed that caffeine consumption—whether coffee, tea, or soft drinks—was strongly related to PMS. The association started at one cup per day, and those consuming eight cups per day were *seven times* more likely to suffer with PMS as compared to abstainers.[42]

Ironically, women often try to deal with that worn-out feeling and other symptoms of PMS by increasing their caffeine consumption, which only makes the problem worse. One study confirmed that women with moderate or severe PMS have markedly different patterns of caffeine consumption than women with few or no symptoms.[43] And what about that depressed feeling that so often accompanies PMS? You guessed it: Episodes of depression during the luteal phase of the menstrual cycle have been linked with elevated cortisol and caffeine consumption.[44]

I urge women who suffer from PMS to prove or disprove these findings in the laboratory of their own bodies. Try eliminating all caffeine from your diet for a few months (it will take at least two months for a fair test). Then drop me a card, E-mail, or fax with your findings so I can tabulate the results.

RESEARCH CAPSULE
Tea Drinking Linked to PMS

A team of Chinese physicians and Annette MacKay Rossignol, an epidemiologist from Oregon State University, measured tea consumption of 188 women nursing students and tea factory workers in China. Over 90 percent of these women rode bicycles every day, and none used alcohol, tobacco, or oral contraceptives.

Their diets were virtually identical: vegetables, rice, pork, no beef, and very little refined sugar. Approximately 40 percent of the nursing students reported PMS, but in the tea factory, where much more tea was consumed, nearly 80 percent reported PMS. Women who consumed more than 4.5 cups of tea per day were almost 10 times as likely to suffer from PMS as women who drank none.[45]

Menopause

If you are suffering from (or trying to avoid) the negative side effects of menopause, you'll be very interested to know that caffeine is associated with decreases in levels of estradiol.[46] In other words, the more caffeine you consume, the lower your estradiol—and the more likely you are to experience the concomitant changes associated with low estrogen production.

In addition, caffeine ingestion also tends to lower blood levels of bioavailable testosterone in women, and raises levels of sex hormone binding globulin.[47] Since testosterone contributes significantly to a woman's libido and sense of strength and power, the result of these hormone changes at menopause may include androgen (testosterone/DHEA) deficiency and a decreased zest for life.

For women just entering menopause, caffeine is a significant factor in determining whether the experience will be easy or difficult. Research shows that during this period (known as perimenopause) a woman becomes more sensitive to the stimulant action of caffeine. Blood pressure, heart rate, and stress response (together known as cardiovascular reactivity) are all greater compared to premenopausal women.[48] In addition, caffeine appears to be a factor in the incidence of hot flashes. Research shows that eliminating caffeine can help reduce both the number of hot flashes and their intensity.[49]

Clinical Depression, Anxiety, and Panic Attacks

While depression is certainly not a female disorder, women account for 76 percent of all doctor visits for this malady. Depression is the single most common psychiatric diagnosis, and it is estimated that nearly 20 percent of American adults will seek medical or psychiatric help for this problem at some point in their lives.

One study demonstrated that chronic, heavy caffeine ingestion can be associated with depression and may also cause anxiety and panic in panic disorder patients—not to mention aggravating the symptoms of PMS. This same study showed that caffeine-sensitive users can have symptoms of caffeinism at relatively low doses, and individuals who consume moderate to heavy amounts of caffeine can have their woes compounded by withdrawal symptoms if they try to quit.[50]

In a study of agoraphobia and panic attacks, caffeine consumption exacerbated anxiety in 54 percent of the patients and triggered panic attacks in 17 percent. Fifty-one percent of female agoraphobics experienced worsening anxiety symptoms in the premenstrual phase.[51] When you remember that women with PMS tend to self-medicate by ingesting more caffeine and that the leading pain reliever for menstrual cramps contains caffeine, you can see why this is such a devastating scenario.

Fibrocystic Breast Disease

Millions of women suffer from monthly or chronic pain associated with benign breast lumps. The cause of this condition, known as fibrocystic (or cystic) breast disease, is not known, but research has identified contributing factors, among them caffeine.

The association between caffeine and fibrocystic breast disease was postulated as early as 1945, and since then it has been confirmed by numerous investigators.[52-55] In 1979, Dr. John Minton of Ohio State University College of Medicine discovered that women with this condition have abnormally high levels of a chemical messenger known as cyclic adenosine monophosphate (cAMP) in their breast tissue. Since caffeine is known to increase cAMP, Minton conducted an experiment to see if avoidance of caffeine would help.

It did. In fact, 82 percent of the women who strictly avoided caffeine experienced complete disappearance of breast lumps.[56] Similar results have been obtained by other researchers,[57, 58] and in 1997, the American College of Obstetricians and Gynecologists in Washington, D.C., observed that women who eliminate coffee and other caffeinated products tend to see improvement in this painful condition within four to six weeks.[59]

Breast Cancer

It is well known that fibrocystic breast disease is a risk factor for breast cancer,[60] so you would imagine that caffeine would be a risk factor too. But here the research is inconclusive. While animal research has identified a number of worrisome caffeine-related changes in breast tissue and growth,[61] most human studies have found no correlation between breast cancer and caffeine intake. Even in studies where there is an apparent connection, researchers question whether there is a true cause-effect relationship.[62] At this point, I believe the connection between caffeine and breast cancer is similar to that for other cancers—which, as we have discussed in Chapter 5, is unclear.

Fecundity and Delayed Conception

Fecundity is the likelihood that a sexually active woman using no birth control will conceive. Studies show that consumption of 300 milligrams or more (the equivalent of two mugs of coffee, or one mug and a few cola beverages) has a negative effect on fecundity. In fact, women consuming this common level of caffeine were more than twice as likely to suffer delayed conception of more than a year compared to women who consumed no caffeine.[63]

In a study reported in *Lancet*, 104 healthy women who had been attempting to become pregnant for three months were interviewed about their use of caffeinated beverages, alcohol, and cigarettes. In their subsequent cycles, women who consumed more than the equivalent of one cup of coffee per day were *half* as likely to become pregnant, per cycle, as women who drank less. What's more, researchers are confident that caffeine was the problem because there was a clear dose-response effect. In other words, the more caffeine the woman consumed, the less likely it was that she would conceive in a given month.[64]

To explore the issue further, researchers recently pooled data from five European nations over a two-year period and came up with similar results: Caffeine reduces fecundity.[65] The intriguing question is, How and why?

Consider the perspective that I've used throughout this book: the big picture of evolutionary biology. If Mother Nature's game plan is survival of the species, why would caffeine reduce fecundity? Could it be that elevated stress hormones send a message to the woman's body that it might not be the best time to conceive a child? More research is required to confirm this theory, as well as the multitude of additional issues that have come up regarding caffeine and childbirth. Perhaps the most serious is what happens *after* conception.

Complications and "Adverse Outcomes" of Pregnancy and Childbirth

My entire perspective on "adverse outcomes" changed radically the moment my wife became pregnant. Until that moment, I was able to look very scientifically at risk ratios and all the assorted statistics surrounding childbirth. But suddenly, when it was a real child ("my" child) inside the womb of the woman I love, these numbers became meaningless. It didn't matter how small the risk was. I didn't care if it was one miscarriage out of 10,000 pregnancies. If that one miscarriage or stillbirth or birth defect or any other "adverse outcome" could be prevented, I wanted to know about it. I became incensed when reading scientific reports that downplayed the risk associated with caffeine simply because the number of affected babies was small. I wondered how these researchers would explain that statistical concept to the distraught parents.

My wife and I now have two beautiful boys, and as I'm

writing this chapter, we're expecting a third child. I am extremely happy that Deborah never drank a lot of coffee. In fact, she dislikes the taste, doesn't drink much tea, and rarely touches soft drinks. All this is good news to me, because the more caffeine research I review, the more I am convinced that these beverages should be avoided by anyone who is pregnant.

Actually, that should include women who are even thinking of becoming pregnant, because intake of caffeine prior to conception is also a risk factor.[66] It is well established by now that women who consume caffeine-containing beverages have increased risk for spontaneous abortions (fetal loss), premature deliveries, and delivering infants with low birth weights.[67]

Miscarriage/Spontaneous Abortion/Fetal Loss

Whatever term you use, this event is a terrible tragedy. And while no one is going to say that caffeine "causes" miscarriage, the drug is a clear and well-understood risk factor. One landmark study found that when intake of caffeine from coffee, tea, and soft drinks was combined, the risk of miscarriage related to caffeine was more significant than the risk related to alcohol or smoking.[68]

An important study published in the *Journal of the American Medical Association* found that fetal loss (their term for the baby dying in utero) was directly and powerfully related to caffeine consumption *before* pregnancy. Women who consumed more than 321 milligrams of caffeine per day before they became pregnant had nearly twice the risk of fetal loss compared to those who consumed less than 48 milligrams per day. Obviously, the risk became worse if the mother continued drinking caffeine during pregnancy. In that case, a 200 percent increase in risk was associated with any caffeine intake over 163 milligrams per day.[69]

Caffeine is also a major risk factor in late spontaneous abortions, i.e., those occurring at the end of the first trimester or thereafter. The data from the definitive study will surprise you. In all, 80 percent of the women in the study were consuming caffeine, and nearly 30 percent were consuming more than 150 milligrams daily. Women in this group were far more likely to lose their babies (73 percent increased risk), and in women who had suffered a previous miscarriage, there was over a four-fold (400 percent) risk of spontaneous abortion associated with *any* intake of caffeine.[70]

Action/Inaction

In 1976, the Center for Science in the Public Interest (CSPI) sent a brief to the Department of Health urging the department to "immediately inform doctors and pregnant women that caffeine may cause birth defects or miscarriages and that women in the first three months of pregnancy should minimize their consumption of . . . caffeine." They cited new and compelling data reported in *Medical World News* that thirteen of fourteen women who drank seven or more cups of coffee per day had experienced "problem pregnancies," including miscarriages and stillbirths.[71]

In 1981, the FDA issued an advisory warning that "pregnant women should avoid caffeine-containing foods and drugs, if possible, or consume them only sparingly."[72]

But seventeen years later, this advice is still nearly impossible to follow. Why? Because the caffeine industry refuses to place warnings on their products, and in fact will not even list the caffeine content of foods and beverages.

In fact, the most common advice in print and in person today regarding caffeine and women's health is still "Caffeine is okay *in moderation.*" A 1994 medical review of animal and human data actually states that:

> Maternal coffee or caffeine consumption . . . does not seem to have measurable consequences on the fetus or the newborn, as long as ingested quantities remain moderate. Therefore, pregnant mothers should be advised to limit their coffee and caffeine intake to 300 mg caffeine/day.[73]

As you have certainly learned by now, this advice is dangerous, erroneous, and absurd: dangerous because what is moderate for one woman may be clearly excessive for another; erroneous because we know that as little as 100 milligrams of caffeine may increase risk for miscarriage; and absurd because women are consuming foods and beverages with undisclosed amounts of caffeine added to them.

Many members of the medical community refuse to take even a halfhearted stand, as illustrated by this summary published in *American Family Physician* in 1995:

> When women become pregnant, they expect their family physician to answer many questions about potential risks during the pregnancy and possible effects on the developing

fetus. . . . In general, women can be reassured that allergy medications and most common food additives, such as caffeine and aspartame, are safe to use during pregnancy.[74]

As you have already discovered, nothing could be farther from the truth.

Low Birth Weight

Low birth weight doesn't just mean you have a small baby. A more accurate term is "fetal growth retardation." The child has not developed to the extent that he or she should have. Low-birth-weight infants usually have smaller head circumference and are a great deal more at risk for morbidity and mortality (illness and death). This increased risk can extend through infancy, and some say even into adulthood. Babies with fetal growth retardation are often premature, but a baby can be born at term and still have a low birth weight. Caffeine has been shown conclusively to cause fetal growth retardation.[75–78]

Birth Defects

This is a hotly debated issue. Unlike delayed conception, miscarriage, and low birth weight, there is no clear-cut relationship between caffeine consumption and birth defects. Still, there is evidence on both sides, and the only sensible choice for a pregnant woman is to err on the side of caution and avoid caffeine. After all, data from animal experiments shows a clear relationship between caffeine intake and fetal malformations, especially of the brain and heart. These effects are dose-dependent and detectable at relatively low concentrations.[79]

There is also the issue of unseen defects that would elude detection but still affect the baby's health, such as decreased thymic weight (affecting immunity) and degeneration of the lens of the eye. In one animal study, these adverse effects were found in every one of the offspring born to caffeine-fed mothers.[80]

Equally hidden would be nutritional defects, and the likelihood of this occurrence is very significant. Caffeine fed to female animals causes marked decreases in the iron, copper, and zinc content of their milk.[81] This could have serious consequences beyond iron deficiency, in that copper and zinc are critically essential to a newborn's immune system.

But perhaps the most important (and nondebatable) point to be made regarding caffeine and birth defects is that caffeine potentiates the known teratogenic (defect-inducing) effect of other substances, such as tobacco and alcohol. In addition, it amplifies the blood-vessel-constricting effect of a number of medications (such as headache remedies) and can seriously reduce oxygen delivery to the fetus.[82]

Caffeine's Effects on Infants

Infants of mothers with high caffeine consumption often look like newborns withdrawing from other drugs. One study showed that infants born to mothers who were heavy caffeine users during pregnancy exhibited unusual behavior in the immediate newborn period. Predominant symptoms were irritability, jitteriness, and vomiting. The infants had extensive diagnostic studies, and none of the usual causes for such symptoms could be identified. Blood tests, however, revealed the presence of caffeine, and in half of the cases, caffeine was also found in the urine. The symptoms ultimately resolved without medication, indicating that the infants were suffering from a caffeine withdrawal syndrome after delivery.[83]

Newborn babies are extremely sensitive to coffee, from whatever source—breast milk, food, or beverages—because they lack the enzymes that break it down. Case studies show that life-threatening poisoning can result from ingestion of less than one gram of caffeine.[84]

Caffeine and SIDS

Sudden infant death syndrome (SIDS) is the leading cause of death in children between one month and one year old. Once again, there are numerous factors and, once again, caffeine may top the list. I started researching the issue ten years ago when I learned that caffeine was being used, in massive amounts, to treat neonatal apnea. Here is a condition where the newborn has lapses of breathing; and, lo and behold, caffeine stimulates the breathing mechanism and "cures" the apnea.

By now you ought to be pretty good at detective reasoning. We know that when mothers consume caffeine, children can be born with a chemical dependence on the drug. When they are moved to neonatal observation and don't get the caffeine, they go into withdrawal, which may include . . . you guessed it, apnea. Then doctors discover that caffeine effectively treats the apnea and marvel at how wonderful this drug is—when all along it's the cause of the problem!

This scenario is not far-fetched. In fact, recent research has confirmed that in a significant number of cases, this is precisely what's going on. A report published in the *Archives of Disease in Childhood* has found that pregnant women who drink more than twenty-four ounces of coffee per day (or the equivalent in soft drinks, tea, and coffee) are far more likely to give birth to infants who succumb to SIDS. The lead researcher, Dr. Rodney Ford, theorized that maternal caffeine use may stimulate the fetal respiratory system unnaturally. Then after birth, when this stimulation is withdrawn, the baby's respiratory drive may be inadequate to withstand infection or other stresses.[85]

Wake Up and Dump the Caffeine!

There's no denying that women today are pushed to the limit. It's a rare family that can "make it" on one paycheck. Unfortunately, to cope with the enormous pressures of juggling work and home life, women are turning to caffeine in ever-increasing numbers—and consuming ever-increasing amounts of this "legal" drug.

As this chapter has shown, a mountain of evidence proves that women—and their unborn children—are being seriously harmed by the caffeine habit. Still, the caffeine industry, and much of the medical community, holds to the contention that "moderate" caffeine intake poses no health risk to women. Loosely defined, "moderate" intake turns out to be 150 to 250 milligrams of caffeine per day. Surveys vary as to how much caffeine American women are actually consuming, but one group of researchers found that the mean intake of their study population was 588 milligrams per day![86]

What you need to remember is that the danger threshold is different for each woman. Caffeine's effects depend on body weight, body composition, menopausal status, menstrual history, and personality. And caffeine is never a single factor. The effect it has (and the damage it does) depends on your stress level plus your diet, lifestyle, and exercise habits.

The bottom line remains: *Reducing or eliminating your intake of caffeine can only benefit your overall health and well-being.* And there's only one way to find out: Try it for yourself. My Off the Bean program in Chapter 10 has already worked for hundreds of women, who now find that they enjoy better health and get more done, without the stress and destructive effects of caffeine.

A Word about Stress Management

Remember the equation at the beginning of this chapter? Caffeine = Stress. In this chapter I've also presented conclusive evidence of the connection between caffeine and depression. So what can you do about it? Simple. Reduce your intake of caffeine.

Every day of your life, you deserve to feel the best you can possibly feel. Amazingly, both medical and popular advice regarding stress management and depression seldom address the issue of caffeine. I believe that all the support groups and stress management techniques in the world will have limited effectiveness unless you directly confront one of the root causes of the problem: your caffeine intake.

I challenge you to disabuse yourself of the notion that coffee is a relaxing treat you use to reward yourself. The same goes for caffeinated tea and soft drinks. Far greater rewards are yours to discover when you live your life caffeine free.

CHAPTER 7

Politics and Pushers

The highest use of capital is not to make more money, but to make money do more for the betterment of life.

—HENRY FORD

A Marketing Dream Come True

If all you wanted to do was make money, how would you design the perfect product? Well, it would be incredibly cheap to make, and the market would be enormous: basically every man, woman, and child. It would be consumable, something people would buy every day. But to be the perfect product, it would have to be addictive. People would crave the product for its effect but, more important, they would suffer if they did not buy it. Importantly, this addiction would be firmly established by age seven or eight for maximum lifelong consumption. With a product like that, one could make billions.

Did you know that two of the most profitable companies in the world are the leading cola companies? And that some of the fastest-growing corporations today are the coffee bar chains? These companies produce mostly beverages with no nutritional value—and yet the explosion in the caffeine industry is unparalleled in the history of commerce. It has to do with the fact that caffeine is addictive, unregulated, and cheap.

Which is why companies are tripping over each other trying to get more caffeine-containing products on the market. Nineteen ninety-seven was a banner year, with the launching of coffee sodas, canned and bottled coffees, caffeinated water, and even coffee beer. It seems that America's thirst for caffeine is nearly unquenchable and, as the success of caffeinated water illustrates, it's fueled by addiction more than by taste. In a way, these are the perfect products, brought to you by companies whose only concern is that you keep buying their brands day after day, who are confident you'll feel miserable if you don't.

The True Nature of Addiction

Research has proven that people acquire tastes and preferences based on the psychopharmacological action of caffeine.[1] In other words, people may wax poetic about the aroma and taste of coffee or the flavor of a particular soft drink, but it appears that these preferences are formed subsequent to and based upon the addiction phenomenon. You may tell yourself that the craving you feel for a cup of coffee is based upon discriminating taste, but that's simply the rationale your mind has created to move you toward getting your fix. Research suggests that the beverage could taste like dirty socks and you would ultimately enjoy the taste. Why? Because consuming the beverage alleviates the adverse effects of withdrawal, even if the period of abstinence has been just a few hours.[2] Notice that the strongest craving for coffee is in the morning, corresponding to the longest period (overnight) of caffeine abstinence.

In the Name of Science

Caffeine industry corporations are listed as sponsors of numerous nutrition-related institutes and foundations, even though most of their products provide no essential nutrients—and even though their products have clear, well-defined, and proven *antinutrient side effects*. These nutritionally worthless products replace nutrient-rich beverages in ever-greater amounts for ever-increasing numbers of people. Their influence is pervasive. The caffeine industry funds "public service" programs and prints brochures ostensibly to "educate" the public about caffeine. The relationship between coffee and colas is a strong one because the decaffeination of coffee provides the caffeine for sodas. Keep those consumers addicted to caffeine and, whether they like it hot or cold, one or the other of these very compatible bedfellows will get the business.

Serving Size Shenanigans

You may recall from Chapter 1 that the caffeine industry would like you to believe a serving of soda equals six ounces and a serving of coffee equals five ounces. *So-called safety recommendations are therefore based on consumers drinking half a can of soda or half a cup of coffee.* Another tactic used by caffeine promoters is to translate dose amounts incorrectly. For example, they will report that a caffeine dose of ten mg./kg. (milligrams per kilogram body weight) causes significant harm to a rat. But then they claim that such a dose is the equivalent of twelve cups of coffee to a seventy-kilogram (165-pound) man. The reader (including other scientists, who do not question the data) therefore reasons that there is little risk.

In fact, you *cannot* simply compare the weight of a rat to the weight of a man and arrive at an equivalent dose. Rats and men have far different metabolic rates. Scientists working on this problem long ago arrived at a more accurate way of comparing people to rodents using what is termed metabolic weight.[3] When this important factor is considered, the ten mg./kg. dose translates to four six-ounce cups of coffee, or two mugs—quite a different story. One leading researcher made the assertion that these errors (intentional or unintentional) "perpetuate misleading impressions about the safety of caffeine."[4]

RESEARCH CAPSULE

A study titled "Caffeine-containing Beverages and the Prevalence of Hypertension" appeared in the *Journal of Hypertension*.[5] Ninety percent of readers only skim the summary or abstract, which states:

> We found evidence that caffeine intake was positively related to an increased blood pressure but the effect was small. . . . There was no evidence

that regular caffeine intake increases the risk of being classified as hypertensive.

This information is then picked up by the media, and millions of people read that "regular caffeine intake" is not a risk factor in hypertension. But what did the study really prove? Nothing, except that poor research can get published in good journals.

A careful read of the entire document reveals that the investigators in this study did not measure "normal" caffeine intake at all. The mean intake of their subjects was calculated to be only 181 milligrams per day (the equivalent of one strong mug of coffee), far below the 250 to 300 milligrams per day considered "normal" by other researchers and surveyors. What's more, there is no reason to believe that this calculation is anywhere near accurate. That's because they didn't measure caffeine intake at all, but rather intake of coffee—and they did not discriminate between regular and decaffeinated coffee!

Reliable data from other surveys tells us that approximately 20 percent of these subjects were actually drinking decaf. No wonder the increase in blood pressure was "small." The final flaw in this research is revealed when you learn that blood pressure readings were taken without determining the time of the subject's last intake of caffeine.

The FDA and the Caffeine Industry

Imagine if the FDA allowed manufacturers to put an undisclosed amount of a mild amphetamine in foods and beverages. Think of the wide range of sensitivities and reactions that would arise in a population consuming such products if everyone from toddlers to seniors were eating and drinking these products with no knowledge of how much or even if the amphetamine were present. Sound absurd? This is exactly the situation with caffeine. Because it has been scientifically acknowledged that caffeine is addictive, the FDA is coming under pressure to rein in the "carte blanche" permission for manufacturers to dump caffeine in whatever food, beverage, or over-the-counter drug they choose at whatever dose they desire.

In July 1997, on the heels of revelations about how tobacco manufacturers have manipulated the level of nicotine in cigarettes to increase consumption, the Center for Science in the Public Interest (CSPI) filed a petition urging the FDA to force manufacturers to label their products for caffeine content. (Although FDA was obliged to act within six months, as of March 1998, they were still evaluating the issue.) CSPI pointed out that a cup of Dannon Light Coffee Yogurt has as much caffeine as a twelve-ounce can of Coca-Cola, while Dannon Light Cappuccino Yogurt is caffeine free. Sunkist Orange Soda, according to CSPI, has more caffeine than a Pepsi, while Minute Maid Orange Soda has none. If you thought root beer was safely caffeine free, think again. Some brands contain a significant amount. Coffee ice cream can have as much as forty milligrams of caffeine per serving, and the drug is showing up in more and more foods and beverages, none of which disclose to consumers (who may be pregnant) how much caffeine they are ingesting.

Joining CSPI in support of this petition were ten health and consumer groups, as well as thirty-four scientists from Johns Hopkins, Yale, Harvard, Duke, the University of Michigan, the University of California at Berkeley, and other institutions. John Hughes of the department of psychiatry at the University of Vermont organized a coalition of scientists concerned about caffeine, and in a separate action, the American Medical Association has called upon the FDA to require caffeine-content labeling.

Will it happen? Don't hold your breath. In 1981, after legal action by CSPI, the FDA finally issued an advisory warning: "Pregnant women should avoid caffeine-containing foods and drugs, if possible, or consume them only sparingly." That "if possible" is the problem. How can you avoid a substance that is hidden, whose bitter flavor is masked, and that appears in products you wouldn't suspect? It certainly seems logical to me that the FDA, whose mission is to protect the health of American consumers, would finally issue some controls regarding caffeine, the last unregulated addictive drug in our food supply. Hopefully that day will come sooner rather than later.

Diet Pills: Caffeine and Its Cousins in Capsules

The Controlled Substances Act of 1970 put most amphetamine manufacturers out of business—and with good reason. Amphetamine "pep pills" were being abused by large numbers of people, with disastrous consequences. Amphetamines are powerful central nervous system (CNS) stimulants that suppress appetite and give one the feeling of being "wired." The street name for these drugs is speed. Truck drivers and students used them to stay awake. Housewives and businesspeople used them to get through the day, and countless thousands used them for weight loss.

The problem was that speed damaged the adrenals and nervous system. When users stopped taking the drug, they experienced a "crash" rebound of profound fatigue and almost uncontrollable depression. Most who made it through this withdrawal eventually regained their health, but many others did not.

After amphetamines were banned, manufacturers started producing a combination of caffeine and related stimulants like ephedrine, together with a popular appetite suppressor found in diet aids known as phenylpropanolamine (PPA). All of these drugs are adrenal and CNS stimulants, and when combined, they produce effects and dangers very similar to those of amphetamines.[6] In 1982, the FDA caught on and banned the triple combination of caffeine, ephedrine, and PPA.

Manufacturers continued to market caffeine-PPA combinations until 1991, when this combination was also banned. Importantly, the reason given for the ban was safety and lack of efficacy. People were experiencing dangerous side effects, such as increases in blood pressure, anxiety, insomnia, and heart palpitations. Reports in the medical literature presented cases of cerebral hemorrhage from these products.[7] Regarding efficacy, it was determined that caffeine does not foster weight loss.

In the 1990s, in a cat-and-mouse game with the FDA, manufacturers started marketing caffeine-ephedrine combinations as *herbal* weight loss and energy pills. Herbal sources of caffeine include guarana, bissy nut, maté, and kola nut. The herbal source of ephedrine is ephedra, also known as ma huang. Some manufacturers hide these ingredients even further by using the botanical name of the herb in Latin, such as *Ilex paraguayensis* instead of maté. Manufacturers have also tried to claim that maté doesn't contain caffeine, and that the caffeine in guarana is somehow "different" from that in coffee. These assertions are patently false and disregard the chemical composition of the plants. How do manufacturers get away with this?

Remember, the FDA doesn't require labeling of caffeine content.

These manufacturers take advantage of the popular notion that herbs are somehow safe because they're "all natural." But whether you use herbal sources or the refined drug, these stimulants will still stress your adrenals and nervous system. They still increase your heart rate, blood pressure, and your risk for stroke, heart attack, and other disorders. Ephedra, which has been used in China for thousands of years, dries the mucous membranes so effectively that it brings relief to people suffering from upper respiratory problems such as asthma, bronchitis, and sinus congestion. But combined with caffeine (which acts as a catalyst for ephedrine's stimulating properties) and taken at high dosages for weight loss, ephedra-caffeine combos cause extreme jitters, muscular and nervous tension, accelerated and abnormal heartbeat, and insomnia. Concerning these stimulant combinations, an important medical study noted: "This finding ... clearly suggests that these caffeine/phenylethylamine combinations are potent CNS stimulants with behaviorally disruptive effects and abuse potential similar to that of amphetamine. ... In addition, it strongly suggests that there is a potential for dangerous interactions among these drugs when *any combination* of caffeine plus phenylethylamines are ingested together."[8]

Caffeine Does Not Help Weight Loss

While there are studies suggesting that CNS stimulants can enhance weight loss, there is no long-term evidence of benefit. In fact, recent research shows that they may instead foster weight gain. Dean Krahn, M.D., lead researcher in a study conducted at the University of Michigan Medical Center, explains that people are more prone to binge-eat when they are anxious, and CNS stimulants cause anxiety.[9] Recent research supports Krahn's concern. In a study evaluating caffeine intake among patients with eating disorders, caffeine consumption was associated with an increased tendency to binge and abuse laxatives and diet pills.[10] Moreover, data published in the medical journal *Brain Research Bulletin* shows that people tend to crave fat when their stress hormone levels are elevated.[11]

Is caffeine a "fat-burner"? Only insofar as stress accelerates the conversion of fat to fatty acids. Remember, this reaction is part of the fight-or-flight response. But unless that conversion is followed by strenuous exercise, the fatty acids will simply be redeposited in adipose tissue when the caffeine wears off.

What about the claim that caffeine raises metabolic rate? Once again, caffeine promoters are using half-truths to push their product. Caffeine will increase metabolic rate, but only to the extent of burning an extra fifty to seventy-five calories a day. And even that effect requires more caffeine than most people would normally consume.

Still, to this day, manufacturers continue to make weight-loss claims for caffeine combination pills and a variety of caffeine-ephedrine teas. As usual, the FDA has been monitoring reports of adverse effects. The March 2, 1995, issue of *Food Labeling News* reported an FDA action against a company selling a caffeine (source: kola nut) and ephedra combination. According to the article, the FDA determined that:

The product can cause severe injury or death in some people who consume them. . . . Reported reactions range from serious, life-threatening conditions such as irregular heartbeat, heart attack, stroke, seizures, hepatitis and psychosis to relatively minor and temporary conditions such as dizziness, headache and gastrointestinal distress. Several deaths have been associated with the products. FDA and outside medical experts have determined that the products represent a threat to health because the combination of Ma Huang, a source of ephedrine, and kola nut, a source of caffeine, can cause severe injury to people even under conditions of usual or recommended use.[12]

The Health-Food Hustle

I have watched the shift in the health-food industry with amazement. Instead of providing a "natural choice," there is, in some cases, a wholesale endorsement of caffeine and other CNS stimulants. It's now common to find coffee bars in health-food stores and shelves of herbal pep pills loaded with caffeine and ephedra. Herbal weight-loss programs, often accompanied by very scientific-looking literature, keep their adherents hyped up on quasi-legal stimulants to produce appetite suppression. When the users decide to stop taking the pills, their appetites return with a vengeance, and the lost pounds are rapidly regained. In the meantime, their health may suffer tremendously.

Until the 1990s, caffeine was one of the no-nos of the health-food industry, like sugar and white flour. Caffeine-free herbal teas got their start in the health-food industry, where caffeine-free products have traditionally been the hallmark of natural food choices. Now those same stores have huge display bins full of coffee beans and many have coffee bars serving pumped-up caffeine concoctions. How did this happen?

It began in the early 1990s, when consumers started to buy organic foods in earnest. The fledgling organic industry accelerated at a rate of 25 percent per year to reach sales of $4.2 billion in 1997. Natural food companies began to look at every agricultural product—including coffee—to see if an organic source could be found. At first there were only one or two small brands of packaged organic coffee grown on estates in Mexico, where the owners adhere to traditional organic practices such as improving the soil with compost and using natural pest control techniques. But then it was discovered that much of the high-altitude coffee in Central America is grown by small landholders living in very rural communities with limited funds for commercial fertilizers and pesticides. These farms were declared "organic by default." In other words, no fertilizers or pesticides had been used on the coffee beans, so the crop was labeled organic.

Unfortunately, the tenets of organic agriculture—conservation, soil improvement via compost and companion planting, and natural pest control—were not part of this scenario, nor are they likely to be given the difficult conditions under which the small landholder ekes out a living.

Natural food companies saw the opportunity to provide consumers with an organic version of their favorite addictive product, and they invested significant capital to develop the market. At the same time, natural food supermarkets were built with space aplenty and a broader mix of consumers than the original die-hard health devotees. The face of the industry changed as the original visionaries sold out to conglomerates for whom profit superseded health principles. The proliferation of organic coffee bins in natural food stores took off, and before you knew it, manufacturers of health-food products discovered what the food and beverage industry has known for decades: Caffeine sells.

Know the Coffee You Drink

The purpose of this book is to give readers the information they need to make informed choices about both the amount and the type of caffeine products they consume. In this regard, it's important to note that there are very significant differences among the caffeinated products available today. As it turns out, the choices you make can have a significant influence on the fate of the planet.

Pesticides Travel a Long Way to Your Coffee Cup

Commercially grown coffee is the most heavily sprayed food or beverage crop in the world (overall third, behind cotton and tobacco), and the chemicals that are liberally used include some of the most dangerous herbicides, pesticides, and fungicides.[13] In fact, many of the chemicals sprayed on coffee plants are banned in the United States, and there is evidence that these chemicals are present at high levels on coffee beans.

A report published by the Natural Resources Defense Council (NRDC) explains the problem. First of all, FDA surveillance of imported food is spotty. Only a small fraction of shipments is analyzed. Secondly, analysis does not cover all possible pesticides, herbicides, and fungicides. Thus, chemicals that are not included in the analysis may be present in high amounts.

Then there is the problem of analytical methods. While FDA analysis may show low levels of pesticide residue, more sensitive analysis provides a much different picture. In one such testing program, multiple pesticide residues were found on *every sample of green coffee beans tested.*[14] For example, Brazilian coffee beans (the most common type sold in the United States) were found to contain residues of DDT, BHC, lindane, aldrin, and chlordane, all known carcinogens.[15]

Now, the common claim is that these deadly chemicals are "burned off" in the roasting process, but this also may be inaccurate. Careful testing by NRDC found that roasting did in fact reduce most chemicals to below detectable levels. But the key word here is *most.* The toxic metabolite of DDT (known as DDD) remained at nearly the pre-roasting level.[16]

The Other Side of the Issue

Whether pesticide residues are a major health risk for those who drink coffee is a continuing debate, but that is only half of the pesticide issue. The other half concerns the chemical exposure of the growers and processors, as well as the horrific environmental impact of this massive quantity of deadly chemicals. We may be safe from harm as we sip our cappuccinos at a sidewalk café, but the picture at the other end of this commodity chain is anything but rosy.

Studies by international health agencies have documented rampant misuses of pesticides and herbicides throughout coffee growing regions, with little or no protection given to agricultural workers who spray, dust, and in some cases apply by hand chemicals that would require a full protective suit and breathing apparatus if used in the United States.[17-19]

"[Developing countries] suffer from illiteracy, overpopulation, and low standards of living. Their deficient economy and infrastructure hinder their ability to regulate efficiently registration of pesticides. Their inhabitants are at high risk due to the acute and chronic adverse health effects induced by pesticide exposure. . . . Their legislations, regulations, technical capabilities, and medical care need to be upgraded to a reliable standard. This is essential for the global welfare because any hazardous pesticides dumped or released in the environment in these countries will not be dissipated but can reappear as residues in imported raw foods or by destroying terrestrial and aquatic life, through their transportation within the atmosphere, or in liquid discharges to soil and water."

Source: A. H. el Sabae, "Special Problems Experienced with Pesticide Use in Developing Countries," *Regulatory Toxicology and Pharmacology,* June 1993;17(3):287–91.

Pesticides that seem easy to regulate in the first world can get completely out of control in the third world due to illiteracy and lack of government regulations. I'll never forget watching a villager in a small rural community in Mexico grind her corn. She was nearly covered in white powder that looked almost like flour. Because of the characteristic smell, I looked at the bag on the floor of her hut and saw that it was a well-known pesticide. Apparently, the government had distributed the chemical to help villagers keep insects out of their stored corn. There was no warning label or instructions on the bag that this woman could read; not that it would matter, considering the high rate of illiteracy in that area. Pesticides to dust your corn? Who in the United States would dream of using deadly chemicals in their food?

The export of pesticides and fertilizers to developing countries is a huge business. Pesticides that have been banned in the United States due to their carcinogenic properties are still allowed to be exported to developing countries whose governments don't have up-to-date regulations. They end up in the hands of the least educated people who have the least amount of information about appropriate use. They then contaminate crops being grown for export and reappear in the first world countries on imported foods.

Fertilizers in the third world wreak their own destruction. Governments support the spread of fertilizers through free distribution programs to rural communities. But government programs are fickle. They may exist for one or two years and then not the next. In the meantime, the soil has been altered. Many fertilizers kill off the natural microorganisms that keep soil healthy, so humus is no longer broken down into plant nutrients. Chemical fertilizers used for a couple of years produce lifeless soil that will grow crops only if more fertilizer is added. You could liken the use of fertilizers to an addiction, with the soil and the farmer being codependent on chemicals in order to produce a crop. This dependency leads to the breakdown of plant health, in this case the coffee trees, which are negatively affected by poor soil nutrients.

Fertilizer-weakened plants are prone to insect infestations because their natural immunity is compromised, and now you need more pesticides. Then there is the runoff of excess nitrogen from the fertilizers, which is excessive on the steep slopes of coffee plantations in rain forest climates. The nitrogen kills fish in streams and lakes and eventually finds its way to the ocean. There, the pristine coral reefs that grace the coastlines of tropical countries slowly perish under the onslaught of nitrogen-stimulated algae overgrowth.

This pollution of the coastal waters is a tragedy of immense proportions. Coral reefs, often extending for thousands of miles, are like the ocean's rain forest in that they support an astounding abundance and variety of sea life. In fact, such habitats support nearly 25 percent of all marine species. But algae overgrowth is choking off the supply of light and oxygen to the coral polyps and the coral reefs are dying. In the last forty years, pollution of the oceans has devastated coral reefs that have existed for 260 million years. Environmental groups are fighting to reverse this trend, but without concerted action on the part of industry and government, experts fear that we may lose 70 percent of all coral reefs within the next fifty years.

The rise of organic agriculture using sustainable practices is the only program that can halt this terrible cycle and return the soil, plants, and we humans who depend on their harvest to a balanced relationship. If you intend to keep coffee in your diet after reading this book, I urge you to become a consumer who demands organically grown coffee from your retailer or your local coffee shop. Vote with your dollars for a more sane, safe, and healthy planet.

You Can't Eat Coffee

In addition to the exposure to pesticides and pollution, there is another perspective I would like you to consider regarding the people who grow our coffee. When you walk past the coffee display in your market and read the labels— Java, Kenya, Colombia, Guatemala, Brazil—what goes through your mind? If you're like most people who have never visited a coffee plantation, you may have the image of a tropical paradise dotted with coffee trees, with happy laborers picking the crop, receiving a fair wage and working in good conditions. In reality, this is rarely the case.

I remind my students that coffee is not indigenous to the countries where it is grown. People do not go picking coffee the way you might walk through a forest picking blackberries. Coffee is grown on huge plantations that arose during the colonial period when massive amounts of land were placed in the hands of a small aristocracy. Sometimes the landowners were the Europeans who "discovered" the country. Later, enormous tracts of land were apportioned to multinational corporations. No matter who the landlords are, the indigenous people of these nations have little choice but to pick coffee (or sugar, cotton, rubber, or bananas) under oftentimes slave-labor conditions for someone else.

Rain Forests, Songbirds, and Your Coffee Cup

I remember the moment when this realization hit me. It was in botany class and we were looking at the destruction of the planet's rain forests. Much of this devastation was due to logging, but the greatest cause of deforestation was due to agriculture and livestock. The professor talked about the growing world market for beef and how rain forests were being destroyed to raise cattle. But the agriculture issue was never explained, nor was it covered in the materials we were reading. I might have passed it off as well except for an agricultural table that showed massive acreage devoted to coffee plantations throughout the same region. I noticed that the latitude and elevation of these plantations matched the area previously covered by rain forest. In fact, the countries with the greatest loss of rain forest were those with the highest production of coffee. I thought I had been tuned in to the ecology movement. Why hadn't I heard about this before?

The Coffee Cover-up

When I contacted members of the coffee industry, I heard a familiar story. Coffee, they claimed, was actually *saving* the rain forests by providing the people with income other than logging. "Except," I replied, "that the coffee plantations appear to occupy the same regions that used to be rain forests." This of course set off a defensive reaction that went in circles. "Look," I said, "my question is really simple: Have rain forests been destroyed to plant coffee?" I was told that "minimal" clearing had been conducted, but that coffee plants grow well in the shade, so the rain forest did not have to be destroyed. This, I later learned, was only half true.

The Whole Truth

There are two types of coffee trees, commonly referred to as shade and sun coffee. Traditionally, coffee trees grew under the protection of taller shade trees. Plantations on rain forest land destroyed the understory part of the forest, but left the overstory or forest canopy intact. This forest canopy is essential for diversity in wildlife. Monkeys travel from tree to tree as they swing through the forest in search of fruit. Birds sip nectar as they pollinate flowers that later produce fruit for monkeys and other animals. If you've ever visited a rain forest, you know that most of the life you hear but can rarely see is happening high in the upper story of the rain forest's canopy. So coffee was relatively compatible with the rain forest. Coffee plantations would affect plant diversity and species on the ground, but at least the plantations would maintain the continuity of the canopy, allowing animals (who are often the carriers of seeds and pollen) to travel from one patch of undisturbed rain forest to another.

But in the late 1980s some of the large coffee growers started shifting to a new hybrid coffee that grows in full sun. Without competition from other trees and plants, these plantations were planted more densely. Yields from sun coffee plantations were three to four times higher than traditional shade coffee farms, resulting in greatly increased profits. Faced with competition from sun plantations, more and more growers started clear-cutting rain forest to increase their yields. This increased production coincided with two years of bumper crop production worldwide—and suddenly, in the early 1990s, there was a glut of coffee on the world market.

Prices plunged as importers bid lower and lower for an oversupply of green coffee beans. Exporters in developing countries went bankrupt by the dozens. But the real tragedy happened in the rain forest. Both plantation owners and small landholders couldn't afford to harvest their coffee beans for the pennies per kilo they were being offered by exporters. While more and more Americans were queuing up at trendy espresso bars, coffee plantations were being torn out all over Central and South America. The small farmer slashed and burned his coffee–rain forest hectares and planted corn and beans to feed his family. Finally, from a combination of poor harvests and the exhaustion of excess coffee inventories, prices began to climb again. But by that time, not only was the damage already done to the rain forest canopy, but farmers were advised to replant their land with sun coffee. No more graceful tall shade trees keeping the forest canopy intact. Sun coffee was here to stay.

The loss of forest canopy has devastating effects on plants, animals, birds, and insects alike. To get a sense for the loss of life, let's look at just one small group of birds that are near and dear to North American hearts: songbirds such as orioles, warblers, and thrushes, the birds who usher in the return of warm weather to the woods of North America with their songs. These birds, along with hummingbirds and many other species, traditionally spend their winters in the rain forests of Central America dining on tropical flower nectar, insects, fruit, and seeds. The Smithsonian Migratory Bird Center discovered that between 1966 and 1996 the numbers of these songbirds have been drastically reduced. By studying the number of species inhabiting small plots of shade coffee trees versus large plantations of sun coffee, the Smithsonian discovered that the population of songbirds has been dramatically affected by the switch from shade to sun coffee. In the scientific literature, sun plantations have been referred to as "biological deserts."[20]

Many tropical countries face the almost complete elimination of natural forest cover by the end of the century. Few countries will have any substantial tracts of moist tropical forest left by the middle of the next century if present trends continue.

Source: Marcus Colchester and Larry Lohmann, *The Struggle for Land and the Fate of the Forests*.

The bottom line regarding rain forest destruction was put succinctly by a university ethnobotanist. "South American nations such as Brazil and Colombia were once predominately rain forest. Now, tens of millions of acres have been turned into coffee plantations. You do the math." In Brazil alone, more than half a million square kilometers of Amazonian rain forest were destroyed between 1975 and 1995.[21]

Silent Death: Water Pollution from Coffee Processing

If you've been reading environmental journals, you may have heard about rain forest destruction for sun coffee plantations or the reduction of wildlife species and songbirds. What you haven't heard about is the deadly pollution caused by the processing of the fresh coffee "cherry" in large and small coffee-washing facilities that dot coffee growing regions. Most of these facilities are quite rudimentary, since the process is not complex. The idea is to remove the pulp of the coffee cherry from the bean and dry the green bean. The process takes large amounts of water over several washing steps. There are two main end products: coffee beans ready for export and coffee pulp.

The beans go off to market, but what happens to coffee pulp and the processing water? This water, now laden with pesticides, fungicides, and nitrogenous waste, goes directly into local streams, rivers, and lakes. With no filtration or reconditioning, the water pollution harms aquatic life as well as the health of people who live alongside those same bodies of water. And the coffee pulp? It sits in huge, rotting piles, leaching out its high nitrogen discharge into the groundwater and eventually into the same polluted waterways. You can't stand downwind of one of these piles if you visit a coffee-washing facility. You'll gag. Sadly, the pulp could be turned into rich compost to feed the coffee trees. But that takes money, labor, and transport—three elements in short supply in rural areas where people are preoccupied with survival.

The Power of One

It always comes down to you, the choices you make for your own health and your family's health, and the information and motivation that guides those choices. My task is to give you the best information so you can make the best decision. My hope is that you will use this information to look at your life, see if you've fallen victim to caffeine addiction and whether it is serving or harming you.

If you decide to drink coffee, then look for organically grown coffee from shade groves that you can feel good about putting in your coffee cup. If you decide to drink caffeinated soft drinks, your task is harder because you can't control how the coffee that produced the caffeine in soft drinks was grown. But at least you don't have to be swayed by the latest brand advertised as providing youth and sex appeal. And you can teach your children not to become bamboozled consumers.

Coffee Doesn't Have to Leave a Bitter Taste in Your Mouth

The difference between exploitation and fair market boils down to the way profits are divided. In regards to coffee, all significant profits are made by the processors who export, roast, and grind the various blends, including instant and decaf products. Until recently, they have all been owned by foreign corporations, not the people on whose land the coffee is grown. Thus, third world peoples have been forced to sell their crops for what is often little more than the cost of production.

Today, there is a viable alternative to agribusiness. Rural cooperative ventures, in which growers participate in the ownership and profits from coffee production, are starting to take hold, providing decent working conditions and a fair wage to the people who grow and pick coffee and other export crops. Environmental groups work with the co-ops to teach conservation, assuring a sustainable future for the land and the people. Importantly, some U.S. marketers of organic coffee return a percentage of their profit to the co-ops, creating a truly equitable production and distribution system that works for everybody. (See Appendix B.) Obviously, coffee from these sources costs more, but it's worth every dime, and it's the only way I know to *truly* enjoy a cup of coffee.

If you drink coffee, I encourage you to look for fair market or organic brands. You can also choose to support organic agriculture in many other ways by supporting your own local organic farmers. There are many steps each of us can take—and while they may seem small, they are right in front of us and they may just change the world.

CHAPTER 8

The Hard Truth about Soft Drinks

Of particular concern is the fact that children are often the targets of marketing activities designed to promote the consumption of caffeine-containing foodstuffs such as cola-based soft drinks and chocolate, and that increasing numbers of children may be consuming caffeine in sufficient quantities to be detrimental to health. It is noteworthy, for example, that a 375 ml [twelve ounce] can of one of the more popular cola drinks has a caffeine content approximately equivalent to an average-sized cup of instant coffee.

—JACK E. JAMES and KERYN P. STIRLING,
British Journal of Addiction

Picture yourself walking through a primordial forest about 10,000 years ago. It's a beautiful warm day, and you've been out with your friends gathering food. You're thirsty, so you make your way to a crystal pure spring. You kneel beside the clear, cool water and drink deeply. Immediately, the water starts to replenish the cells of your body, and you feel completely refreshed.

Now, fast-forward to the present. Your body, its needs, and its functions are exactly the same as they were 10,000 years ago. But instead of that pure clean water, you reach for the pull tab on a can of cola. You take a long drink of an artificially colored, chemically flavored mixture of carbonated water, phosphoric acid, sweeteners, preservatives, and caffeine. To add insult to injury, some of the aluminum from the can may have leached into the beverage—despite the can's so-called protective coating.[1]

If it's a "regular" cola, your body is jolted by about nine teaspoons of sugar. (When was the last time you put nine teaspoons of sugar in a beverage?) In response, your blood glucose levels rise quickly and your pancreas pours out insulin. Both the elevated glucose and insulin foster weight gain. Plus the sugar sticks to your teeth, feeding the bacteria that cause cavities, and the soft drink's acidity weakens tooth enamel.[2–4]

If it's a diet cola, your brain registers the intense sweetness of aspartame and instructs the intestinal tract to prepare for an enormous intake of calories. Your body creates enzymes to convert future calories to fat, just like it did 10,000 years ago. So even though the beverage contains only one calorie (a concept your brain and body do not understand), you remain primed to create fat as soon as you eat some real food. That's why the more artificial sweeteners you consume, the more likely you are actually to *gain* weight—as confirmed by a study of 80,000 women over a period of six years.[5]

Then there's the caffeine. It gives you a slight adrenal "buzz," but the stress causes your body to lose calcium, magnesium, and B vitamins. The caffeine also impairs your absorption of valuable iron. After this scenario plays out, your body is finally able to separate usable water from the additives, preservatives, and other chemicals, and your cells are replenished—somewhat.

Cola Wars

The term *cola wars* is often used to refer to the rivalry between the two major soft drink companies. But the real war is being waged against your health. *Cola beverages have absolutely no nutritional value*—in fact, they have been shown to increase risk for a number of health disorders significantly. Yet the two leading colas are America's top two favorite "foods," measured by total volume of grocery store sales. Today Americans are drinking more soft drinks than any other beverage, including water—and it's not only because colas are the most successfully marketed consumer products in history. Cola beverages have something else going for them: They are delivery systems for an addictive drug, namely caffeine.

The Soft Drink Drug Lords

In 1886, a pharmacist named John Pemberton invented Coca-Cola. The word *cola* was derived from "kola nut," the name of the source plant for one of the flavors. *Coca* referred to another ingredient in Pemberton's recipe: cocaine, derived from the coca plant of South America. When it became clear that cocaine was a destructive and addictive substance, the cocaine was replaced with caffeine. The only problem is, we now know that caffeine is also an addictive drug, whether it is delivered via soft drinks or a coffee mug.[6]

Numerous researchers have established that caffeine can create a dependence syndrome (see Chapter 3). In fact, in the most conclusive study, subjects exhibited all of the behaviors of classic drug dependence—and *nearly half of those found to be addicted were consuming mainly soft drinks.*[7] The authors of that study state:

> The existence of a caffeine dependence syndrome, which includes evidence of continued caffeine consumption despite medical or psychological problems from caffeine consumption and unsuccessful efforts to quit caffeine use, provides a further similarity between caffeine and classic drugs of dependence.
>
> Source: E. C. Strain, G. K. Mumford, K. Silverman et al., "Caffeine Dependence Syndrome," *Journal of the American Medical Association,* 1995;273:1418–19.

In response to studies showing conclusively that people can and do become dependent on caffeine, spokespeople for the National Soft Drink Association sprang into action, pointing out that "the destructive antisocial behavior provoked by drugs of abuse is clearly not associated with caffeine consumption."[8] In fact, this party line is often repeated by the caffeine industry, but it is a weak and absurd defense. If a drug is harming people and in spite of that people find it impossible to stop consuming that drug, does it really matter if the drug (caffeine) is so affordable that addicts don't have to rob others at gunpoint to get the cash for their fix?

Of course, soft drink manufacturers will never admit to a marketing strategy of addicting children to caffeine in order to create lifelong customers. When asked why they use caffeine at all, the standard reply is, "It's a flavoring agent." But anyone who has ever tasted caffeine will tell you that it's a bitter, foul-tasting substance, and including it in a beverage requires extra sweeteners just to *mask* the taste. The flavoring argument also falls apart when you remember that both of the major cola companies make caffeine-free products that taste just like the caffeinated versions, yet relatively few people buy them.

Still, since calling caffeine a flavoring agent is the only possible excuse they can use, cola companies have developed a legal rationale, claiming that the FDA definition of a cola beverage mandates inclusion of caffeine. This is simply not true. FDA label regulations specify only "caffeine from a natural extract." The fact is that this kola nut extract required in a "cola" beverage contributes less than 10 percent of the total caffeine present in soft drinks today.[9] The remaining 90 percent is added by the manufacturers, usually in the form of pure caffeine obtained as a by-product of the production of decaf coffee. The question remains, Why?

How Soft Drinks Suck You Dry

The fallback position of some cola promoters is to admit that their products produce a dependency, but that it's a "good" dependency. After all, they reason, soft drinks don't harm anybody. Wrong again. Health experts have long lamented the effects of skyrocketing soft drink consumption. Their main concern: malnutrition.

Because most soft drinks contain zero nutrients and are consumed in place of nutrient-rich beverages, regular use of soft drinks contributes to insufficient intake of calcium, magnesium, riboflavin, vitamin A, and vitamin C.[10] But it's not only that these worthless beverages replace nutritious alternatives. Caffeinated soft drinks actually have antinutrient properties that affect the absorption and metabolism of the entire diet.

We learned in Chapter 3 that caffeine causes an increased loss of B vitamins in the urine.[11] Because the B vitamin status of many Americans (especially teenagers) is borderline to begin with, regular consumption of soft drinks can contribute to deficiency and a raft of symptoms, including neurological damage. Widespread use of soft drinks has been shown to contribute to outbreaks of beriberi among teenagers. Beriberi is a serious thiamine deficiency disease that usually occurs only in the most malnourished of populations.[12]

We also know that caffeine interferes with iron absorption, and this is a critical factor in women's health. In the United States, more than 8 million women will spend their entire lives iron deficient,[13] and the health consequences can be devastating (see Chapter 6).

Caffeine of course, is not the only culprit. There are the sweeteners, either sugar or aspartame. The high sugar content of "regular" soft drinks (approximately nine teaspoons in a twelve-ounce serving) contributes to blood sugar problems, metabolic stress, and malnutrition via loss of B vitamins, calcium, copper, and chromium. The aspartame (brand names NutraSweet and Equal) in diet soft drinks has been associated with neurological and behavioral problems, even though most studies show that aspartame is safe when consumed in amounts within the acceptable daily intake (ADI) established by the World Health Organization. It is important to note that aspartame was originally approved only for use in beverages. Since it is now approved and found in more than a dozen types of foods—including breakfast cereals, chewing gum, candy, and desserts—individuals who consume large amounts of these foods and beverages can easily exceed the ADI. The long-term effects of excessive aspartame intake are unknown, but a condition known as aspartame intolerance has been identified.[14]

"In the United States, no matter where you are, you're never more than a three-minute walk from a soft drink."

Source: Frederick Mails, PepsiCo executive, quoted in *Investment Vision* magazine.

Those Most Vulnerable: Our Children

Health experts are most worried about the effects of soft drink consumption on children. After ingesting soft drinks, they may have high blood levels of caffeine for many hours. The cumulative effects derived from consuming soft drinks throughout the day are completely unknown, but it may be no coincidence that cases of hyperactivity and attention deficit disorder (ADD) have grown to epidemic proportions at the same time soft drinks have become the dominant fluid intake for many children.

Recently, a group of preschool boys with ADD participated in a ten-week, placebo-controlled study that included the avoidance of sugar, artificial flavors, artificial colors, preservatives, and caffeine. Over half of the subjects showed reliable improvement on the experimental diet as compared to no improvement in the placebo period.[15] Clearly, the elimination of soft drinks from the diet contributed to the success of this treatment.

Soft Drinks and Depression

In Chapter 4, I presented evidence that caffeine contributes directly to depression. But the combination of caffeine and aspartame may be even worse. We have long known that the amino acid tryptophan is critically important in maintaining normal mood. That's because the brain converts tryptophan to a biochemical known as serotonin, which in turn contributes to feelings of pleasure and relaxation. When serotonin levels fall (due to metabolic or dietary reasons), just about anyone can feel depressed and anxious. As a result, drugs that raise brain serotonin levels (like Prozac) are presently among the most widely prescribed medications in America.

It turns out that phenylalanine (one of the ingredients in aspartame) competes with tryptophan for absorption, and may therefore contribute to reduced serotonin levels. In one study, researchers found that depressed patients had lower tryptophan levels compared with people who were not suffering from depression. Most important, there was evidence that the cause of the tryptophan deficiency was high levels of competing amino acids such as phenylalanine.[16] Given this data, it is not unreasonable to conclude that "diet" soft drink consumption may contribute to depression.

And on Top of Depression, How About Fatigue?

The connection between caffeine and sleep disturbance is covered thoroughly in Chapter 3. What's worth mentioning here is that soft drinks are implicated in reports of fatigue and sleep disturbance as well as coffee. One study coordinated by the World Health Organization examined tiredness and sleep disturbance among eleven-, thirteen-, and fifteen-year-olds, as well as the relationships between their sleep habits and use of caffeine, tobacco, and alcohol. Not surprisingly, a direct relationship was reported among caffeine intake, disturbed sleep, and reported tiredness during the day.[17] It's important to remember that while the caffeine intake of preteens and teenagers may come from multiple sources—including coffee, chocolate, and soft drinks—soft drinks are overwhelmingly the primary source. Clearly, soft drinks do nothing to enhance the performance of these youngsters at any level—rather, just the opposite.

How About Depression, Fatigue, and Decreased Learning Skills?

Caffeinated soft drinks are often portrayed as a "think drink" for the younger set. Solid scientific research, however, tells a different story. In Chapter 4, I presented evidence that caffeine decreases learning skills in a number of ways. It constricts blood vessels in the brain, leading to a marked reduction in cerebral blood flow, and interferes with brain biochemistry. As little as 100 milligrams of caffeine (two colas contain that much) can cause a significant decrease in recall and reasoning.[18] What's more, caffeine contributes to anxiety, irritability, and anger, feelings that are certainly not conducive to scholarship and learning.

Recently, investigators at Johns Hopkins School of Medicine discovered yet another way caffeinated soft drinks can interfere with learning. This could be called the iron connection. Studies show that more than 25 percent of all adolescent girls in the United States are flat-out iron deficient. And remember, this is determined by serum ferritin, not the presence or absence of anemia. Iron insufficiency (which typically occurs years before anemia) is believed to impair the activity of enzymes necessary for brain functions associated with memory, learning, and mood.

The Johns Hopkins team gave an iron supplement or placebo to high school girls with lower-than-average serum ferritin levels. After eight weeks, the girls given iron scored much better in memory, attention, and learning ability tests.[19] Since caffeine interferes with iron absorption (reducing the iron absorbed from a meal by as much as 50 percent), it is no stretch to conclude that caffeinated soft drinks contribute to the mood swings and learning deficits experienced by millions of high school and college women.

Soft Drinks Linked to Childhood Obesity

According to a report by the New York Hospital–Cornell Medical Center's Nutrition Information Center, childhood obesity has as much to do with what kids drink as with what they eat. The study claims that between 1978 and 1994, the average U.S. teenager's soft drink intake tripled to 64.5 gallons per year. Over the same time period, soft drink intake for children aged six to eleven doubled. High-calorie soft drinks are implicated in weight gain among children in these age groups.

Soft drink intake is linked to a number of other conditions, including bone fractures due to deficient calcium, tooth decay, tooth tissue loss, and dehydration. The report said, "We believe it is high time to help children and adolescents break the high-calorie fruit drink and soft drink habit."[20]

Yesterday's News

There is more evidence than ever before that caffeinated soft drinks have tremendous potential for harm, especially in growing children and in adults when consumed to excess. Yet this conclusion is nothing new. In 1977, a U.S. Senate subcommittee investigated the issue thoroughly, gathering hundreds of pages of testimony from leading experts. The report noted that

> Doctors, particularly pediatricians, have reported signs—including irritability, headaches and nervousness—of what has come to be known as "caffeinism" among cola-guzzling youngsters whose total caffeine intake may be boosted by cocoa or hot chocolate and chocolate bars.[21]

The Senate report distilled a mountain of data into some very clear recommendations, including a reduction in soft drink consumption. But since that report was published in 1977, soft drink sales have skyrocketed to an astounding fifty-five gallons per year for every man, woman, and child in America.[22] Of course, that doesn't tell the whole story, since some people consume few or no soft drinks, while teenagers and young children consume even higher amounts. Alarmingly, peak consumption has been reported among children at ages three, thirteen, and seventeen.[23] The tragedy, of course, is that these are the years when diet is most important, and instead of nourishing our children we're pushing them toward illness and degeneration.

You Are What You Watch

Researchers at the University of Minnesota spent more than fifty hours viewing Saturday morning kids' shows and advertising. Most of the foods advertised were candy, soft drinks, cookies, chips, and cakes. Not one ad promoted the eating of fruits and vegetables, and fewer than 5 percent advertised milk or other dairy products.

Source: "Saturday Morning Pyramid," *Current Health 2*, vol. 21, issue 9;May 1995:2.

Anatomy of an Addiction

The degree to which someone becomes dependent upon caffeine is related to the blood level of the drug to which they become accustomed. In children, blood levels of caffeine can remain high for five to six hours after a single dose. There are two reasons for this: their small body size and the limited ability of their liver to detoxify caffeine. To be precise, a sixty-pound child consuming three cola beverages and a few candy bars in a day would be ingesting more than eight milligrams of caffeine per kilogram of body weight. (A kilogram equals 2.2 pounds.) That is the equivalent of eight cups of strong coffee for a 165-pound man.

Remember also that there are two aspects to any drug addiction. First is the reward sought by the user. In this case, it is the "buzz" of adrenaline, the heightened caffeine state that is so often confused with energy. The second aspect is the desire to avoid the pain of withdrawal. It's hard to say which is more motivating, but one thing is certain: Children easily fall prey to the addictive properties of soft drinks and their relentless marketing campaigns—a juggernaut that seems virtually unstoppable.

Of course, as I mentioned, soft drink manufacturers would never admit to a marketing strategy of addicting children to caffeine. Nevertheless, studies have found that the caffeine withdrawal effects experienced by children are very similar to those experienced by adults: fatigue, headache, malaise, anxiety, and depression. And these effects can begin after a very short period without a caffeine "hit," even as simple as a child missing their lunchtime or after-school soft drink.[24]

While leading health experts issue warnings that caffeine is creating early addiction with lifelong consequences,[25, 26] soft drink sales have never been better, and sales increase every year. The next time you're in a supermarket and see two-liter bottles of soft drinks on sale for forty-nine cents or when you're in a fast-food restaurant or convenience store that offers unlimited refills on soft drinks, remember this: *Soft drinks may be the most success-*

fully marketed product in the history of the world, but they owe their success to your addiction.

Bad to the Bone

In addition to the caffeine, sugar, and artificial flavors in soft drinks, many health experts are concerned about phosphoric acid. Optimum bone health requires a certain ratio of calcium to phosphorus, and each can of cola contains about seventy milligrams of phosphorus. This amount of phosphorus can adversely affect bone strength unless it is balanced by a higher intake of calcium.[27-29] But soft drinks (which contain no calcium) are replacing milk, the major source of calcium in the American diet. The scenario gets even worse when you remember that caffeine also tends to increase calcium loss in the urine.

The effect of caffeine on children's growth is nearly impossible to evaluate because it would be unethical to dose children with caffeine in order to measure changes in growth rate. But in some South American cultures children drink a significant amount of coffee. One recent study in Guatemala found that taking children off caffeine for just five months resulted in 22 percent gains in length compared to the group that continued drinking coffee. More important, the caffeine-free group registered a 46 percent greater weight gain and decreased incidence of illness.[30]

The caffeine habit is a terrible legacy to give our children. During adolescence, there is a window of opportunity to form strong bones, and those bones must last a lifetime. Once a child's skeleton is fully formed, very little can be done to increase its mineral content. And at this all-important moment when every gram of calcium and magnesium count toward either future health or the pain and crippling of osteoporosis, we hand our kids a can of pop.

RESEARCH CAPSULE

What's Wrong with This Picture?

In the April 1, 1996, issue of *Family Practice News*, I was surprised to see an article titled "Carbonated Beverages No Threat to Bones."[31] Numerous studies show an undeniable association between high soft drink consumption and increased risk for bone fractures. Was the present study really debunking the cola connection? You be the judge.

Point 1. The chief researcher announced that five colas have "about the same amount of caffeine as one strong cup of coffee." In fact, a twelve-ounce cola contains 45 to 72 milligrams of caffeine, so five soft drinks will deliver at least 225 milligrams and as much as 360 milligrams of caffeine. A strong cup of coffee contains 120 milligrams of caffeine per six ounces.

Point 2. The mean age of the women in the study was seventy-two.

Point 3. Soft drink intake was determined by lifetime recall, a technique notorious for error.

Point 4. The average soft drink intake of the women in the study was one serving per day.

Conclusion: This study proves only that elderly women who remember drinking approximately one soft drink per day do not have weaker bones than elderly women who remember drinking less than one soft drink per day. It never tested the real question as to whether soft drinks in amounts commonly consumed today contribute to bone loss or fracture. Nevertheless, this study became a news item, reducing concern regarding the soft drink–osteoporosis connection.

The Truth: A careful review of the effects of soft drinks on bone health was recently conducted and published in the journal *American Family Physician.* The researchers conclude that "excessive consumption of carbonated and cola-type beverages, combined with low dietary calcium intake, is a major public health issue that predisposes female adolescents to bone fracture and perhaps increases the likelihood of osteoporosis later in life."[32]

Soft Drinks Promote Hypertension

It has long been known that decreased intake of calcium and magnesium directly and significantly increases the risk for hypertension in adulthood. But recent research with children shows that suboptimal intake of these important minerals is also associated with something that was unheard of a generation ago: pediatric hypertension.[33] Once again, by foisting soft drinks upon our children, we are setting them up for a serious lifelong disorder. That's because caffeinated soft drinks:

1. Provide no calcium or magnesium;
2. Replace other nutritious beverages that normally provide these important minerals;
3. Actually deplete calcium and magnesium from their bodies; and
4. Contribute directly to hypertension.

Soft Drinks Have Invaded Our Schools

Many studies show widespread suboptimal nutriture in American schoolchildren.[34] How did this happen? Amazingly enough, a large part of the answer lies in our schools.

More than thirty years ago, when soft drink consumption was nothing compared to what it is today, the Council on Foods and Nutrition of the American Medical Association issued a statement expressing its strong opposition to the sale of carbonated beverages in school lunchrooms.[35] Then, in the 1970s, carbonated beverages were allowed to be sold, but only after the lunch period had ended.

In 1983, soft drinks were prohibited only during the actual service of food, the rationale being that the U.S. Department of Agriculture considered such beverages to be inappropriate in nutrition education settings. But today there are soft drink machines in high schools across America, and average teen consumption is pushing three cans a day. Here's how it happened.

Imagine you're a school administrator and budget cuts have forced the cancellation of your junior varsity sports program. Then you receive a visit from a cola company representative, who expresses concern that you are under such tight financial constraints and suggests a solution. If you authorize the placement of cola vending machines throughout your campus and sign a contract granting exclusive sales rights (for about ten years), the cola company will pay a commission on each can sold—and, in time, you'll get your sports programs back. Suddenly, cola machines appear all over the school—in the lounges, cafeteria, and, in some cases, the hallways.

An article on this subject in *The New York Times* on March 9, 1998, quoted Larry Jabbonsky, a spokesman for Pepsi-Cola, as saying, "They [the schools] need to generate funds. At the same time, we are constantly looking for new ways to broaden our exposure among young people. It's a pretty natural independent fit."[36] Though neither Coca-Cola nor Pepsi (the two biggest players) will say how many schools have signed deals, this movement is exploding across the nation. In November 1997, the Colorado Springs, Colorado, school district signed a ten-year deal with Coca-Cola for $8 million, and more if it exceeds the "requirement" of selling 70,000 cases of Coke products annually.[37]

"While soft drink giants have long fought to be designated the official beverage of professional sports and college campuses, only recently have they turned their sights on the kindergarten-through-high-school set."

Source: *The New York Times,* March 10, 1998, page C1.

Money from the cola companies is funding not only sports programs, but new computer programs and more. The schools are delighted with the easy money and apparently have no issue with treating the students as a commodity to sell to the highest bidder. *Meanwhile, the issue of our children's health has fallen completely by the wayside.* In *The New York Times* article quoted above, health issues surrounding soft drinks were not even mentioned. Consumers Union decries the practice of soft drink deals, not because of the health hazards, but because it is "using taxpayer space to promote commercial messages and give over these audiences to corporations."[38]

While school administrators and cola executives are congratulating themselves on a win-win deal, the real losers are the children. They lose critically essential nutrients at a time when every vitamin and mineral counts toward a life of health or illness. They lose the freedom to choose what beverages they want to consume, and they lose an environment that encourages free thinking, as schools plaster contract-mandated advertising on the buildings, scoreboards, cups, banners, and vending machines. One Texas school district has cola brand logos painted across the rooftops of its two high schools. And, of course, the kids lose a measure of self-determination as they become addicted to caffeine.

"You want to get them started young and hopefully keep them for life—that's what brand loyalty is all about."

Source: Ira Mayer, publisher of *Youth Markets Alert*.

Of course, universities have been signing exclusive soft drink deals for years, and they're proud to point out that much of the cola money goes to fund women's athletic scholarships.[39] The irony is that caffeine increases a woman's risk for anemia, PMS, osteoporosis, fibrocystic disease, anxiety, and depression (see Chapter 6), making cola beverages the very antithesis of peak sports performance.

And It's Not Just the Schools

Even as more children every day become casualties of the cola wars, soft drink manufacturers are going out of their way to promote their products through youth service and educational organizations. Some point out that these deals usually involve significant donations, but does that justify promoting products that harm children?

The New York Times recently reported that the Boys and Girls Clubs of America and the Coca-Cola Company would jointly raise $60 million over the next decade for a youth development program sponsored by the clubs.[40] Seems like the cola giants are only too willing to lend a helping hand to our kids, all the while creating a whole new generation that will grow up addicted to caffeine.

And Just When You Thought It Couldn't Get Any Worse . . .

Soft drink manufacturers today are rushing to bring products to market with greatly increased caffeine levels—as much as 168 milligrams per twelve-ounce serving! In 1996, Pepsi brought out Josta, which combines two sources of caffeine, and Coca-Cola quickly responded with their own supercharged brand called Surge. As this book was going to press, more than a dozen companies were jumping on the high-caffeine bandwagon with product names like Guts, XTC, Krank, Jolt, Power Kid, Boost, and Zapped. Once again, the trend is being fueled by an illusion, created by manufacturers, that such products provide energy. In fact, the caffeine in these beverages produces nothing more than metabolic, biochemical, and emotional stress.

School administrators are witnessing this firsthand as manufacturers fill school vending machines with high-caffeine products. In a recent *New York Times* article, Margaret Mohrman, headmistress of the Academy, a school for gifted students in Little Rock, Arkansas, explained that the school banned Surge from its snack bar after students drank themselves into a caffeine frenzy. "I just couldn't believe it," she said. "The kids were holding two in their hands and drinking one after another. When they weren't jumping up in the bathroom, they were climbing the walls."[41]

For parents, these high-caffeine products present a real dilemma because they are sold in schools and convenience stores everywhere, and kids are under tremendous pressure to "get their kicks" from a can. Indeed, the manufacturers' trademarked slogans are all geared toward a drug-oriented "high" with caffeine as the drug of choice. Below are a few examples:

Beverage	Slogan
Jolt	"America's most powerful cola."
Krank 20	"Water with caffeine, lots of caffeine."
XTC	"A carbonated slap in the face."
Surge	"Feed the rush."
Go Go	"It'll blow your mind."
Josta	"Unleash it."

The point that needs to be remembered is that these products are not only being marketed to teens and the twenty-something age group. In fact, sales are geared to children as young as seven, using cartoon characters as enticements. *The New York Times* reports, "Market research shows that Mountain Dew [the original high-caffeine soda] is more than twice as popular as other soft drinks among children younger than 6."[42]

There is no doubt that the "rush" induced by these products is harmful to children. Caffeine affects their brains and growing bodies in ways that have never been evaluated because no one would dare administer high amounts of caffeine to a child in a controlled study. Tragically, there is no safety data, and the marketing campaigns that flood the airwaves are reprehensible in light of caffeine's well-known negative effects on the body and mind.

The Relentless Push Continues

Recently, cola companies hit upon yet another strategy to increase consumption. In case you haven't noticed, twelve-ounce cans are gradually being replaced with twenty-ounce bottles, thus increasing the serving size by 65 percent. These twenty-ounce bottles deliver an astounding fourteen teaspoons of sugar and enough caffeine—seventy-five milligrams—to produce quick addiction and severe withdrawal.

Clearly, caffeine is a drug being administered as a food. No scientist or health professional would deny this. Yet the only guidance that the public receives regarding soft drinks is to consume them "in moderation." At the same time, the soft drink industry has made every effort to thwart even this modest goal. They refuse to put warning labels on their products, refuse to disclose the amount of caffeine in their products, and then create products with ever higher levels of caffeine in ever larger servings.

To make matters worse, the FDA has literally stood by and watched the drugging of America take place. Their inaction has led many people to assume that caffeine is harmless and perfectly fine for children. Now that the truth is known, the question is: What shall we do?

I believe that the pendulum is about to swing. The proliferation of high-caffeine beverages is already having a serious effect on the nation's health, and it is only a matter of time before people start to take action. From my point of view, we need to begin with efforts to protect our children. For starters, I believe that soft drink machines have no place in schools, that soft drinks should list their caffeine content, and that people should be educated concerning the real and significant consequences of caffeine addiction. Only then will we be able to consume soft drinks "in moderation," or not at all.

CHAPTER 9

Options and Alternatives

If your life revolves around caffeine, be it in a coffeepot, teacup, or soda can, don't despair. The purpose of this book is not just to give you the bad news about caffeine. The good news is that there are plenty of delicious, caffeine-free beverages that will enrich your life and at the same time support optimal health. Fortunately, we live in a time when our global society offers us an unprecedented choice of foods and beverages from all over the world. After reading this chapter, you will be fully informed about a wide selection of alternative beverages to taste and explore.

Developing new lifestyle habits takes experimentation and time. Importantly, your taste buds will readjust as you make changes in your diet. Beverages that were once strange and unfamiliar will become more satisfying and delicious than your old caffeinated beverages. You'll feel better physically, and life will hold more possibilities. If "variety is the spice of life," then read on to discover the diversity of beverages that can help you successfully reduce or eliminate your caffeine intake.

Decaf versus No-caf

Many of you who are coffee drinkers might be thinking, Why don't I just switch to drinking decaffeinated? First, you have to remember that decaf doesn't mean no-caf. Decaf coffee beans have undergone an extraction process to remove the majority of the caffeine, but there is still some left. A twelve-ounce cup of decaf typically contains at least 10 milligrams of caffeine, and possibly more depending on how it's brewed.

Second, you have to look at your own health reasons for reducing or eliminating caffeine. For example, if your liver can't properly detoxify caffeine or your adrenals are completely exhausted, 10 milligrams multiplied by several cups per day may still aggravate your condition. If your body reacts to coffee with allergic responses such as skin rashes or mood swings, or if you suffer from any of the problems listed in Chapter 5, even decaf coffee may be a problem.

DECAF AND YOUR STOMACH

The acidity of coffee is higher in decaf because robusta beans are commonly used to produce decaf coffee. Robusta beans have a higher caffeine content and a stronger acidity than arabica beans, so more of the coffee flavor survives the extraction process. But the acids and oils that carry the flavor can be harsh on the intestinal tract and are often a problem for sensitive individuals.

If you suffer from digestive and gastrointestinal disturbances (especially ulcers), eliminating coffee altogether is the healthiest choice for you. Coffee often causes a hypersecretion of stomach acid, which is why many people have to eat something with their coffee or suffer from acid indigestion. Moreover, decaf still frequently causes the malfunction of the lower esophageal sphincter, the valve between your stomach and esophagus. This malfunction allows the acidic contents of your stomach to reflux into the sensitive tissue of the esophagus, producing heartburn. If you commonly use antacids, gastroenterologists recommend that all coffee, decaf or regular, should be avoided.

CHEMICAL RESIDUE

The method of extracting caffeine from coffee beans may leave behind chemical residues. Unless you're buying a higher-priced decaf coffee brand that is marketed as Swiss Water Process or CO_2 extracted, you are exposing yourself to the residues of methylene chloride, the solvent used to extract caffeine in the great majority of decaf products. There is disagreement as to how much of a health risk this represents, but here is how I see it: (1) Testing shows small but significant methylene chloride residues in decaffeinated coffee and tea;[1] and (2) methylene chloride is carcinogenic.[2, 3]

CHOLESTEROL

Decaf coffee appears to raise cholesterol levels higher and faster than regular coffee, a fact that most of us can't afford to ignore. Even worse, it is the LDL fraction of cholesterol (commonly known as "bad cholesterol") that appears to be affected the most. In one Stanford University study, drinking decaf for only two months raised LDL by 7 percent. Statistically, that represents approximately a 12 percent increase in heart attack risk in just two months.[4] If you are suffering from a heart condition, you may also want to consider that the amount of caffeine remaining in decaf can still increase the heart rate of sensitive individuals.

BLOOD SUGAR

People who are hypoglycemic or diabetic shouldn't risk the blood sugar swings that caffeine causes. Decaf can still affect a sensitive person's blood sugar levels. Diabetics can run a simple experiment on themselves by testing their blood sugar before and after a cup of decaf coffee and watching the blood sugar rise then fall within several hours. Hypoglycemics need only to observe their energy levels dip one to two hours after drinking decaf to realize that no coffee is the best choice for them.

DETOX-ABILITY

As you age, your tolerances change. Many people find that coffee, both regular and decaf, becomes difficult to metabolize as they pass the age of fifty. They'll often recall that they could drink as much coffee as they liked in college, but now they suffer from indigestion, insomnia, tension, and the jitters. The liver no longer detoxifies the oils, acids, and caffeine the way it once did, and they find themselves looking for coffee alternatives.

There is only one way to find out if coffee, regular or decaf, is compromising your health. You can conduct your own experiment by simply giving it up for sixty days. Before you do, fill out the questionnaire in Appendix C to note any discomforts, mood swings, or health problems from which you may suffer, no matter how subtle or obscure. Then follow my Off the Bean program detailed in Chapter 10 and make your comparison after two months. You may be surprised to note a number of symptoms improve or disappear that you never would have suspected were exacerbated by caffeine.

AND REMEMBER . . .

When not at home, you can't be sure what they're serving you for decaf in food-service establishments. In fact, many times when ordering at a restaurant or café, decaf drinkers find that they are served regular coffee by mistake.

New Choices for Coffee Drinkers

NO-CAF SOLUTIONS

Fifteen years ago when I realized I had to find a substitute for coffee, there were not a lot of alternative choices. Postum, of course, had been around for nearly a century, and there were a few herb teas that produced somewhat of a hearty brew. I found Celestial Seasoning's Roastaroma to be quite good.

For decades, though, "coffee substitute" was synonymous with "instant grain beverage." Postum was joined by Pero, Cafix, and Roma, all variations on the wheat, rye, barley, and chicory powder theme. And while these were good when in a hurry (you just mix a spoonful of powder in boiling water), I missed my coffee making ritual and the deep, full-bodied flavor and aroma that only a brewed product can deliver.

My prayer was answered recently in the development of herbal coffee. Herbal coffee is naturally caffeine-free because it doesn't contain coffee beans. But unlike the powdered "substitutes," herbal coffee is brewed just like coffee, and produces the same deep, rich flavor and aroma. The way I see it, a coffee drinker needs three things in order to be satisfied without coffee. First is taste and aroma. A coffee drinker wants deep, full-bodied flavor— forget this light tea-water stuff! A coffee drinker isn't satisfied with weak, leafy infusions. It's got to have the mouth-feel that gives you substance and a variety of flavor notes that hit your taste buds from front to back. When I brewed my first cup of herbal coffee, I tasted surprising richness and was enticed by the aroma. The flavor isn't identical to coffee, but I enjoyed it just as much.

Secondly, a coffee drinker wants to keep his or her same brewing ritual. For many, it's an essential part of the enjoyment of coffee. Maybe you like to wake up to the aroma of coffee dripping in your automatic drip coffeemaker, or perhaps you're a French press devotee who likes to make sure a full five minutes has allowed the grounds to steep into the richest brew. If cappuccinos are your thing, only a frothed cap of steamed milk on top of dark espresso from your espresso machine will do. In fact, if you can keep your same brewing ritual, it won't seem like you are making such a radical lifestyle change. Herbal coffee allows you to make your customary brew any way you desire. So don't worry; the only change you need to make is what you put in your coffeemaker.

Third, let's face it. Coffee, which most people find unpleasant upon first taste, has become a fixture in our lives because of one thing. It is an excellent drug delivery system for caffeine. A coffee drinker wants, expects, and has grown to require an energy lift. When a coffee drinker quits caffeine, he or she misses the drug-induced jolt that gave the sensation of having enough energy to get going. What coffee drinkers really need is a true natural energy lift.

I get that from herbal coffee, although I don't know exactly why. Herbal coffee does provide some energy from its ingredients: herbs, grains, fruits, and nuts that contain valuable nutrients. Herbal coffee is also naturally high in potassium, an electrolyte mineral that plays an important role in the muscle and nervous systems. Potassium is added to sports drinks to help athletes recover after workouts. Herbal coffee has twice the potassium of Gatorade, and the potassium comes naturally from the ingredients rather than being artificially added.

Importantly, you don't need to sweeten herbal coffee because it's naturally sweet from dates and figs. The absence of refined sugar and caffeine means you won't experience an energy crash after drinking a cup of herbal coffee.

WHERE TO FIND HERBAL COFFEE

There is presently only one product on the market, known as Teeccino. I suspect more will follow quickly because just as herbal tea revolutionized tea drinking in the seventies, herbal coffee is going to do the same for coffee drinkers. Right now, you may have to ask your natural food stores to order it for you (see Appendix B), but I expect that soon you'll be able to stop into your corner espresso bar for a cup of caffeine-free herbal coffee. Fortunately, Teeccino comes in seven flavors, so whether you're a flavored coffee drinker or a purist who only drinks regular coffee, you'll quickly discover your favorite blend. I recommend both Java and Original for people who don't like flavored coffee. Java has natural coffee flavoring that makes it the most coffee-like of all. But if you sweeten your coffee, you'll find that Original allows you to skip the sugar because the dates, figs, and orange peel give it a naturally sweet flavor with a subtle, fruity top-note. If you relish nutty coffee flavors, like Hazelnut, Vanilla Nut, and Amaretto, Teeccino (which actually contains roasted almonds) comes in your favorite nut flavor extracted from all-natural ingredients. For chocolate lovers, there is Mocha, that superb combination of cocoa and natural coffee flavor, and Chocolate Mint, whose minty coolness comes from real peppermint leaves.

Sound delicious? See, I told you that I wouldn't ask you to give up your favorite brew without something equally satisfying to take its place. In the next chapter, where I describe my Off the Bean program, I'll tell you how to reduce or eliminate your intake of caffeine by using a variety of coffee alternatives, including herbal coffee.

Healthful Ingredients in Herbal Coffee

Carob pods, roasted: Carob is a nutritious, naturally sweet food, often used today as a healthy substitute for chocolate. Carob's antidiarrheal properties were discovered by a Spanish physician who observed that children of the poorer class who ate large quantities of carob pods had fewer digestive problems than children of the wealthy, even though their living conditions were less hygienic. Carob is high in calcium and vitamin A.

Chicory root, roasted: Used for more than twenty centuries, chicory was first roasted and consumed as a coffee substitute during Napoleon's Continental Blockade in 1806. Chicory is naturally high in potassium, calcium, and FOS, a valuable carbohydrate that contributes to the health of the gastrointestinal tract. Chicory has a stimulating effect on digestion and is often combined with coffee to cut the caffeine and reduce coffee's acidity.

Barley, roasted: The nutritious staple grain of the early Mediterranean cultures, barley is valued for its high potassium and iron content. Barley roasts dark brown like a French roast and gives a deep, nutty flavor to herbal coffee.

Figs: This sweet fruit has been enjoyed for over 5,000 years for its nutritious and slightly laxative properties. It is high in potassium and contributes a natural sweetness to herbal coffee. Figs are used in Turkey to impart a rich flavor to coffee.

Almonds: Rich in calcium, magnesium, and protein, almonds have been used in baked goods and beverages for their nutritious value and nutty flavor. Golden roasted almonds impart a rich, savory flavor to herbal coffee.

BREWING TIPS FOR HERBAL COFFEE

Herbal coffee can be made from as many as eight different ingredients. Unlike coffee, where one bean is ground to different sizes for each type of brewing method, herbal coffee is a composite grind that can work in all types of coffee brewing equipment, including drip coffeemakers, French press pots, percolators, and espresso machines. The following tips will help you brew a delicious cup of herbal coffee:

- Adjust quantities of herbal coffee to your own preferences. Just like coffee, some people like it strong while others prefer it weak. You may make a couple of cups before you find the dosage that is perfect for you.

- Drip coffeemakers brew herbal coffee best with a "gold-tone" or metal filter. Paper filters tend to brew slowly because the composite grind in herbal coffee may have some fine particles that can clog the paper. The good news is that gold filters save trees and produce a better-flavored brew because paper absorbs flavor. Gold filters are easy to rinse clean and are available for both cone and flat-bottom coffeemakers. Once you switch to gold filters, you'll never run out of paper filters again!

- Think about purchasing a French press pot. If you don't already have coffee brewing equipment, you'll find French press pots work just like a teapot with a built-in filter. They are great for brewing loose-leaf teas as well. Steep herbal coffee in a French press pot for five minutes to develop a deep, dark, roasted flavor with a stronger bitter note.

- You can make cappuccino without an espresso machine. It's simple to make a delicious, rich, frothy cup at home using the following steps: (1) Brew a strong cup by doubling the amount of herbal coffee you normally use, and (2) heat milk, froth in a blender or with a whisk, and add ½ cup of foamy milk to ½ cup of brewed herbal coffee.

The Good News and the Bad News for Tea Drinkers

Lately the media has been full of good news for tea drinkers. You may have been reading reports about the polyphenols in tea bringing you antioxidant health benefits. Tea sales have begun to climb as a result, and specialty tea companies have introduced a variety of teas that were previously unknown. Most people are familiar with black tea packed in tea bags, and, until recently, the names orange pekoe (denoting a quality of tea, not a type) and Earl Grey were as exotic as tea got. Then came the nineties, and interest in unique varieties of tea such as Darjeeling, Assam, Lapsang souchong, and oolong. Flavored teas appeared, with names like ginger peach and jasmine.

All Flavors Are Not Created Equally

If you love flavored tea or coffee, then you'll want to be sure that the brand you are buying uses natural flavors. Coffee and tea companies often use artificial flavors for two reasons: They are much cheaper, and the flavor may taste stronger. I didn't say better, just stronger. Natural flavors are derived from extracts of natural ingredients and taste real compared to the fake and perfumy quality of artificial flavors. Compare the difference between the flavor of artificial vanilla, called vanillin, to real vanilla extract and you will see that the difference in flavor complexity is dramatic. Instead of the single flavor molecule used for artificial vanilla, real vanilla has hundreds of components creating a superb flavor profile brought

---

to you by the unsurpassed artist of all time, nature. As always, buyer beware. Read the label and if it isn't clear, call the manufacturer to get the information you have a right to know.

Recently, green tea has started to appear on the grocery shelves as scientific studies verify its health benefits. Once, green tea was that strange-tasting brew you were only served at a Chinese restaurant. Now the sales growth of green tea is accelerating as people acquire a taste for its lighter, mellower flavor. So what is driving this newfound interest in one of the world's oldest brews? That's a story that takes a bit of telling.

A Brief History of Tea

Tea, the young leaves harvested from the *Camellia sinensis* plant, has been consumed ever since the Chinese emperor Shen Nong accidentally discovered the virtue of tea, according to legend, when some leaves fluttered into his pot of boiling water in 2737 B.C. Tea didn't make its way to Europe and Britain until the early 1600s. Interestingly, only green tea was originally available and drunk in both the American colonies and in Europe. Green tea is made from the unfermented young shoots, which are quickly pan-fired or steamed after harvest to stop fermentation. Black tea is created by a fermentation/oxidation process that begins after the leaf is rolled. The breakage of the leaf's cell walls begins an enzymatic process that changes the chemical composition, the flavor, and color of the leaf. It is during this stage that caffeine develops more fully in the black tea leaf. Oolong tea is partially fermented to develop its characteristic flavor and aroma and thus has less caffeine than black tea, but more than green tea.

Organically Grown Tea

The exposure of tea leaves to pesticides, fungicides, and herbicides is frightening. Unlike coffee, where the cleaning and roasting process helps to remove residues from the coffee bean, tea leaves are directly sprayed with these chemicals right before their harvest and end up in your teacup with potentially high levels of residue. On top of that, plants fed nitrogen fertilizers have higher caffeine contents by up to 40 percent![5] Responsible companies have now started testing for pesticide residues, but the technology is young, and results vary widely from lab to lab. The Europeans, whose governments have the strictest residue standards in the world, have influenced several large tea-growing estates in India to grow tea organically. These estates are using compost to improve their soil and are employing natural pest prevention. Just like coffee bean harvesters, tea pickers in developing nations are vulnerable to unprotected exposure to such chemicals as gramaxon, 24D, klaask, malathion, demicron, ethion, kelthen, aldrin, metasystox, and glyphosate. Help protect your health and theirs by buying organically grown teas. (See Appendix B.)

All About Polyphenols

Tea abounds with naturally occurring chemical compounds called polyphenols, which are powerful antioxidants or free-radical scavengers, and anticancer warriors. Often incorrectly referred to as tannins, polyphenols have nothing in common with the tannic acid used in leather preparation, though they do give tea its astringent flavor. While polyphenols are chemically similar to tannins, there are no tannins in tea.

Over thirty-five polyphenols have been identified to date. They include flavonoids, flavanols, flavanol glycosides, flavandiols, and phenolic acids. The dominant polyphenols in tea are known as catechins, and it is to them that most of the health benefits in tea are ascribed.

Scientific studies have shown that both animals and humans absorb catechins directly into the bloodstream, providing beyond a doubt that they are actually used by the body in various organs.[6, 7] In fact, catechins have been shown to glow as they go about their business of neutralizing free radicals![8] As antioxidants, in vitro studies show that catechins have the ability to halt enzymes that produce carcinogens and to inhibit cancer cell growth.

A study that measured catechins in tea extracts showed that green teas contained the highest percentage (26.7 percent), followed by oolong teas (23.2 percent), with black teas (4.3 percent) showing a dramatically decreased content.[9] While instant teas have still fewer catechins, they nevertheless continue to exhibit some antimutagenic and antioxidant properties.[10]

Tea catechins may help to protect tea drinkers from several chronic health problems such as high blood cholesterol and high blood pressure.[11, 12] Catechins make blood platelets less prone to abnormal clotting, a benefit that may reduce risk for both heart attack and stroke.[13]

Read Your Studies Carefully

As a nutritional biochemist, I am exposed to an endless stream of health-care "breakthroughs." It seems like every week someone takes a substance (an esoteric biochemical found in kumquats, for example) and adds it to a test tube containing a colony of cancer cells. When the cancer cells stop growing, people make the totally unscientific assumption that eating kumquats will cure cancer.

Remember that adding gasoline to a colony of cancer cells will stop cancer growth too, but that doesn't mean we should drink gasoline. Besides, even if a substance is safe to ingest, you still need evidence that test-tube results will be duplicated in the human body. After all, few substances make it through the digestive system intact, and then there is the question of whether the active ingredient is even absorbed through the intestinal wall.

That's why I carefully review all research concerning the health benefits of tea. When you read in the media that tea has just been shown to prevent cancer, it is important to examine the original research on which these claims are based. Much of the information concerning anticancer benefits from tea polyphenols is derived from animal studies in which mice or rats are inoculated with certain types of cancer. Some are then given tea extract to see if it helps prevent the development of tumors. These studies often use extracts with polyphenol concentrations much greater than one would obtain from drinking tea.

Recently, there was great fanfare concerning the ability

of tea to reduce risk for skin cancer. Newspaper reports suggested that readers start drinking green tea before exposure to summer sun. But in the actual research, the tea concentrate was applied topically.[14] It's also important to remember that tea can inhibit iron absorption enough to cause anemia.[15] Likewise, it has been shown to inhibit thiamine (vitamin B-1) absorption and increase the loss of this vital nutrient enough to produce frank thiamine deficiency and signs of beriberi.[16, 17] Tea has been shown to lower blood cholesterol levels, but to obtain any significant cholesterol benefits, you'd have to consume more than ten cups a day![18]

Dig Deep Before You Leap

Can positive results from animal studies be generalized to humans? Perhaps, but to be sure, we need evidence that groups of people drinking tea have lower incidence of cancer compared to similar groups who don't drink tea. The important word here is *similar* because, as I will explain, comparing people with different diets will give you meaningless information.

Epidemiologists are medical researchers who track the incidence of disease in various populations or geographic regions. Their studies regarding tea and cancer risk show mixed results, prompting the Working Group of the International Agency for Research on Cancer to conclude that the evidence for a cancer risk reduction from tea was inconsistent and inconclusive.[19] Studies in Japan have shown that communities that consume large amounts of green tea daily have lower rates of stomach, esophageal, and liver cancer.[20] But a study in China showed this protective effect only in women and not men. Confused, the Chinese group removed from their data anyone who smoked or drank alcohol. When this variable was eliminated, consumption of green tea was associated with reduced risk for esophageal cancer.[21] What's going on?

I believe that this research illustrates a critical point regarding purported health benefits from herbs, foods, or beverages. We human beings are desperate to find substances that will protect us against disease. And let's face it, there are also plenty of people looking for a way to make money. Thus when research suggests that something as simple as drinking tea will reduce your risk of cancer, everyone jumps on it. Sales of tea skyrocket, articles are printed in newspapers and magazines, and all the while, the epidemiologists are saying, "Hey wait a minute. . . ."

So why don't people who smoke or drink appear to benefit from green tea? I believe it's because green tea is a weak agent. It provides benefit to people whose diets are low in antioxidant fruits and vegetables, but it doesn't provide sufficient antioxidants to protect someone who smokes or drinks. Thus, the accurate message here is not "Run to your grocery store and stock up on green tea," it's "Eat plenty of fruits and vegetables, and if you're going to drink tea, make it green."

Not to belabor the point, but a similar scenario resulted in the United States when Harvard researchers found that consumption of tomato sauce was associated with decreased risk for prostate cancer.[22] The popular interpretation of that data (reflected in newspaper headlines) was "Run out and eat pizza." The more accurate message is, "The standard American diet is so pathetically low in antioxidants that even the tomato sauce on a pizza will confer some benefit."

Now, I'm not saying that tomato sauce and green tea are not valuable. But they are weak agents, and we should not stake our hopes for avoiding cancer on these substances. The more prudent and proven approach is to reduce your intake of saturated fat and consume at least five servings of antioxidant-rich fruits and vegetables daily. And if you want more protection, throw in a comprehensive nutritional supplement that provides the full range of antioxidant vitamins, minerals, and botanical extracts.

One More Perspective

Think of the British versus the Chinese. If the British, who have the largest per capita consumption of tea in the world, were experiencing lower rates of cancer, we'd have heard about it loud and clear. There are lots of studies showing the Chinese to have lower rates of certain cancers compared to Westerners, but once these same Chinese move to the West and start eating a Western diet, lo and behold, their cancer rates increase dramatically. Does tea help prevent cancer? Green tea might, but black tea probably won't, and in fact may be associated with *increased* risk for cancer of the colon, rectum, and lung.[23]

A Tip for Better Taste:
Consider Brewing Loose-Leaf Tea

People have become dependent on brewing tea using tea bags because they think it is easier. But tea leaves and herbs have to be cut very fine in order to fit into these small filter bags. These fine cuts, known as

---

"fannings" or "dust," are considerably lower in grade and quality than whole leaves. Black, green, and herb teas all suffer the same rapid loss of volatile components once they are cut so fine. Thus, the flavor you want in your tea cup tends to evaporate into the air long before you ever open your box of tea bags.

In the tea renaissance of the nineties, there has been a revival of brewing loose-leaf teas, and a variety of tea filters is now available. There are filters for single cups of tea and ones for teapots. There are French press pots originally designed for coffee but that work perfectly for tea. I bet you'll find it is just as easy to brew loose-leaf tea, and you won't believe the difference in flavor. Tea bags are great for traveling, but brew your tea from loose-leaf teas at home. (See Appendix B for sources of tea filters.)

Caffeine Is Still Caffeine

The good news about green tea is that it is lower in caffeine than black tea. The caffeine content in black tea is made more bioavailable during the fermentation process. The longer you brew your tea leaves, the more caffeine a cup of tea will have. A five-minute brew of black tea typically contains sixty to ninety milligrams of caffeine per six-ounce cup. A three-minute brew has about half that amount. A cup of green tea has approximately twenty-five milligrams per cup. The caffeine content is also affected by the cut size of the leaf you brew. If you use tea bags versus whole-leaf tea, you'll end up with a lot more caffeine because the caffeine is released more readily from the smaller-cut leaf. By choosing what type and cut of tea you drink and how long you brew it, you can modify how much caffeine you ingest.

Green and Herbal Tea Blends

Suddenly everyone is marketing green teas blended with herbs. Why? The flavor of green tea is unappealing to the American palate, which is conditioned to expect tea to taste like black tea. Herbs enhance the flavor of green tea and add their own healthful properties. Most importantly, the addition of caffeine-free herbs to green tea cuts down on the amount of caffeine that ends up in your teacup.

Try some of the following blended green teas:

- The Republic of Tea: Organic green teas, Morrocan Mint, and Tea of Inquiry
- Yogi Tea: Wake Me Up Tea
- Tazo: Zen, Om and Green Ginger
- Celestial Seasonings: Green Tea with Antioxidants

Caffeine is caffeine no matter where you get it, and everything reported in this book regarding health disorders associated with caffeine applies to tea as well. Review the study presented in Chapter 6 in which women consuming high amounts of tea suffered 80 percent more PMS. If you are dependent on tea to get you going in the morning or give you a lift during the day, chances are you may be abusing caffeine and should reduce your daily intake.

Decaffeinated Tea

Unlike decaf coffee, decaf black tea has not been readily adopted by tea drinkers, and it seems to be simply a matter of taste. Coffee beans are decaffeinated before roasting, which reduces the flavor significantly, but not nearly as much as tea. The caffeine from tea is extracted after fermentation, and the dull, flavorless leaves are disdained by true tea lovers. Usually decaf tea is sold blended with flavors to give it some character. Unfortunately, because there are no standards set by the FDA for decaffeinated tea, manufacturers will sometimes add black tea to the decaf tea leaves to give them flavor, thus spiking the caffeine levels.

What concerns me a great deal more than the loss of taste, however, is the presence of chemical residue in decaf tea. There is no Swiss Water Process for decaffeinating tea leaves, so at this point, the only method available is the solvent process. One study showed that residues of methylene chloride (a known carcinogen) were four times (400 percent) higher in decaf tea compared to decaf coffee.[24]

Caffeine-free Herbal Teas

While herbal teas became popular in the seventies with the introduction of delicious herbal blends, people have been brewing leaves, fruits, flowers, roots, barks, and berries for millennia. The word *tea* is now commonly thought of as a hot brewed beverage and no longer is it the exclusive domain of the *Camellia sinensis* plant. Instead we have black tea, green tea, and herbal tea, which comes in a great diversity of types and flavors. Of the three, only herbal tea is caffeine free, but you still have to be careful. Some herbs, like maté (yerba maté), kola nut, bissy nut, and guarana, contain caffeine and may not be labeled as such.

Although there are over 3,000 varieties of black tea, most people's taste buds couldn't tell the difference between many of them. With herbal teas, though, you get quite a range of flavors. There are several hundred different leaves, fruits, flowers, roots, barks, and berries in commerce that an herb tea company can use to create its blends.

A true medicinal tea that is used to produce a specific effect on one's health is usually brewed differently than the herb teas you buy in the grocery store. For instance, if you visit a Chinese herbalist for help with a medical condition, you'll be given a bag of roots, barks, leaves, or even mushrooms to take home and simmer on your stove for up to a half an hour depending on the herbs. You can imagine that this brew, which is called a decoction by medicinal herbalists, won't be pleasant tasting or smelling, but you'd only have to drink it for a period of time until your health improves. Herbal teas, on the other hand, with their smaller dosage of herbs per cup of tea, have more generalized health-promoting properties. They are designed to be drunk daily if desired without producing any side effects. Herbal teas can be soothing when you're suffering from minor symptoms, but they are primarily formulated for taste enjoyment and general health enhancement.

Since there is such a wide variety of herb teas sold on the market, it is helpful to classify them according to type. Once you know what's available, it's easier to make a selection of the kind of tea you might want to drink. You'll find that it's great to have a variety of herbal teas on hand to suit different moods, weather, and occasions. Here are some of my favorites. Enjoy them hot or iced!

IMMUNE-STIMULATING BLENDS

This is the type of herbal tea I drink most frequently. After all, on a day-to-day basis, we mostly need to keep our good health intact. If I feel "immune challenged" or I want to start my day with an immune boost, I'll drink a cup of a blend that contains any of the following tonic herbs, known as adaptogens (herbs that strengthen or enhance the immune system, nervous system, and/or glandular system while they help the body cope with stress): Siberian ginseng, Panax ginseng, astragalus, shizandra, echinacea, ashwagandha, reishi mushrooms, licorice. Some of my favorite brands include:

- The Republic of Tea: Ginseng Peppermint and Organic Temple of Health
- Traditional Medicinals: Echinacea Plus, Reishi Defense, and Double Ginseng
- Celestial Seasonings: Emperor's Choice, Echinacea Herb, and Ginseng Plus
- Yogi Tea: Ginseng NRG Tea and Echinacea Special Formula

DIGESTIVE TEAS

One of the main reasons people started experimenting with herbs was to help their digestion. Fortunately, many herbs have digestive-stimulating properties. They can help relieve gas and heartburn, stimulate the flow of gastric juices, relax spasms and cramps, and dispel nausea or queasiness. Look for digestive blends that have any of the following herbs: ginger, anise seeds, thyme, chamomile, hyssop, peppermint, spearmint, lemon balm, fennel, coriander, chicory, catnip, and cardamom. Bitter herbs such as genetian, artichoke, dandelion, and angelica are often found in herbal digestive bitters but not in tea. My favorite digestive teas feature ginger and/or mint, like the following brands.

- The Republic of Tea: Orange Ginger Mint and Organic Mint Fields
- Traditional Medicinals: Ginger Aid and Eater's Digest
- Celestial Seasonings: Grandma's Tummy Mint and GingerEase
- Yogi Tea: Lemon Ginger, Stomach E-Z, and Ginger Tea
- Tazo: Refresh

SEDATIVE TEAS

The number-one best-selling herbal tea in the United States is Celestial Seasonings, Sleepytime herb tea. Why? I guess after a day filled with caffeine and stress, Americans need help slowing down enough to fall asleep. Sedative teas are mild in action, again due to dose. You can't make a drinkable herb tea with a significant amount of sedative herbs because most don't taste very good. However, sedative teas can help you relax, and if you need extra help, try herbal extracts made from sedative herbs, too. The classic sedative herbs include: chamomile, hops, linden flowers, lavender, passion flower, skullcap, and valerian. Some lesser-known sedative herbs are tilia buds and white zapote from Mexico. I recommend:

- The Republic of Tea: Chamomile Lemon
- Traditional Medicinals: Nighty Night
- Celestial Seasonings: Sleepytime
- Yogi Tea: Bedtime Tea

STRESS-RELIEF TEAS

These teas differ from sedative teas because they are designed to help you cope with stress but not become sleepy. Two herbs stand out in this arena that have completely different actions from one another. Siberian ginseng, also called eleuthero ginseng, has been shown in both animal and human studies to help the body cope with stress.[25] Kava, a muscle relaxant with a long tradition of use in the South Pacific, can actually help relieve overtense muscles.[26] Kava is one of the new stars on the herbal market, and you'll find it in nutritional supplements and herbal extracts as well as teas. You may want to drink Siberian ginseng tea frequently, but kava should be saved for those times when you really need help relaxing and letting go.

For starters:

- The Republic of Tea: Ginseng Peppermint
- Celestial Seasonings: Tension Tamer
- Yogi Tea: Kava Kava Special Formula and Calming Tea

STIMULATING SPICE TEAS

Spices have long been valued for their flavor and stimulating properties. The spice trade fueled world exploration as

Europeans competed to find exotic flavors and dominate spice-growing regions. Once spices were as rare and dear as gold, but now, who could imagine a kitchen without cinnamon, black pepper, and ginger? Spicy herbal teas will warm you internally and stimulate your digestion and elimination. Spice teas have been popular for a long time, but the latest entries into the marketplace are the spicy "chai" teas inspired by Indian's custom of drinking black teas heavily sweetened and flavored with spice and milk. Chai teas come both as liquid concentrates and as teas to brew. Some chai brands are marketing all-herbal blends that are caffeine free. Spice teas in general require a longer brewing time and are best simmered for ten minutes to bring out their spicy flavor. They can be mixed with milk just like black tea.

- Yogi Tea: The original spice tea on the market. Look for their various blends either Original (loose pack) or in tea bags with flavors such as Tahitian Vanilla and Hazelnut Creme.
- The Republic of Tea: Rainforest Tea, Cardamom Cinnamon, and Cinnamon Chai. Their Republic Chai is black-tea based.
- Celestial Seasonings: Bengal Spice
- Tazo: Spice
- Sattwa Chai: Herbal Chai Spicy Peppermint Concentrate and Shanti Herbal
- Oregon Chai and Celestial Seasonings Mountain Chai are both black-tea based, but offer decaf versions.

Sweet Herbs That Save You Calories

There are several herbs whose natural sweetness makes herb tea blends sweet without added calories.

- Licorice is one of the oldest herbs, used by the Chinese for thousands of years to harmonize and balance their herbal formulas. The sweet component of licorice is glycyrrhizin, which is fifty times sweeter than sugar, so a little goes a long way. If you have high blood pressure, however, you shouldn't drink large quantities of licorice tea, as it can cause the retention of sodium.
- Stevia, also called sweet herb, is from Paraguay, where the Guarani Indians have used it for centuries to sweeten their food. Stevia's sweet glycoside, called stevioside, is 300 times sweeter than sugar! With nearly zero calories, it actually appears to help balance blood sugar levels— great news for diabetics and those with hypoglycemia. Stevia is now available as a nutritional supplement, although inexplicably it is banned in the United States as a sweetener (to protect the artificial sweetener industry?). Presently, you'll find stevia in teas where its sweetness helps bring out the flavor of other herbs.
- Sweet blackberry leaves come from a special variety of blackberry that grows in China. Its leaves are sweet only when picked at the right time of the year, but not as sweet as stevia or licorice. It has a little more astringency to its flavor. A recent introduction to the market, sweet blackberry hasn't been studied as extensively as stevia or licorice.

Fruit Teas

In Europe, fruit teas are the most popular type of herbal tea blends. Fruit teas usually have hibiscus flowers, orange peel, rose hips, and sometimes lemon grass in their base. The teas can contribute significant vitamin C to your diet, and they are delicious iced. Because they usually have a strong citrus accent, they are refreshing and thirst quenching. There are so many flavors of fruit teas, with multiple brands marketed by the same company, that you'll have to experiment to see which are your favorites. Here are some of mine:

- The Republic of Tea: Alpine Flowers Tea, Lemon Wintergreen, Kid's Cuppa, and Organic Flowering Fruit herb tea
- Tazo: Passion and Wild Sweet Orange
- Celestial Seasonings: Any of the Zinger blends in the fruit flavor of your choice

Rooibos Tea

This caffeine-free herb tea deserves a category of its own because it is unique in the herb-tea world. Rooibos (which means "red bush" and is pronounced "roy-boss") grows only in the tip of South Africa and was first discovered by the indigenous Khoisan peoples, the Bushmen and the Hottentots. It is the only herb tea that is fermented like black tea, producing a deep red color and body similar to black tea but without black tea's astringency. You can add milk to rooibos just like black tea. In fact, it is so similar to black tea that consumer taste panels in Britain were fooled into thinking it was black tea. (Personally, I like its flavor better.) Rooibos contains polyphenols just like green tea, giving it similar antioxidant properties. In vitro tests comparing rooibos to green tea, black tea, and oolong showed fermented rooibos to have slightly less antioxidant activity than green tea, but more than black or oolong tea.[27] Rooibos also contains vitamin C, minerals, quercetin, luteolin, rutin, and numerous other flavonoids that contribute to its antispasmodic, hypoallergenic, and antioxidant properties.[28] Studies in Japan indicated anticancer, anti-inflammatory, and even antiviral activity for rooibos tea.[29] In South Africa, it is clinically used for people who suffer from nervous tension, allergies, and various stomach and digestive problems. Rooibos is gentle, soothing, and delicious.

Sounds like green tea, doesn't it? So why doesn't everyone know about this herb? Well, rooibos simply hasn't yet had its moment in the media spotlight like green tea has had over the last two years. Also, rooibos is limited in supply due to the prohibition on the export of seeds or plants by the South African growers. But there are indications that its time is coming. Since the lifting of sanctions against South Africa, more and more tea manufacturers are using rooibos as a base in their herbal teas. Two major South African manufacturers are considering introducing their brands of rooibos tea to the American market. If you're a black-tea drinker who is not fond of the taste of green tea and wants to be off caffeine completely, I highly recommend looking for rooibos at your local herb shop or trying any of the following herbal tea blends that have rooibos in their base:

- The Republic of Tea: Rainforest Tea and Desert Sage
- Select Tea: Ruby Burst in three flavors

Herbal Teas on the Horizon

The movement in the herbal tea world is toward "nutraceutical" teas, teas that provide stronger medicinal properties by combining good-tasting herbal blends with herbal extracts and other nutritional supplements like vitamins, minerals, and natural hormones like melatonin. Watch for ginkgo-fortified teas, beverages, and foods. *Ginkgo biloba* has been in the media spotlight lately due to studies showing its effectiveness in helping Alzheimer's patients. Ginkgo increases the flow of oxygen to the brain by dilating the blood vessels, which is just the opposite of caffeine's vasoconstrictive effect. Ginkgo is valued for its ability to enhance memory and cognitive processes, so you'll find it in herb teas whose names suggest optimal thinking. Other examples of nutraceutical herbal tea blends are those specially designed for the male or female, teas for colds or flu, teas for mood improvement featuring St. John's wort extract, and teas for weight loss, which usually provide only diuretic effects.

Organically Grown Herbs

Herbs are grown or wildcrafted all over the world in many developing nations where labor is abundant and cheap. Harvesting herbs, especially flowers and berries like hibiscus and rose hips, is still done by hand, even though hibiscus is planted and rose hips are collected in the wild. Leaves, on the other hand, like the mints and lemon balm, can be harvested mechanically and because of this, the best qualities now grow in the United States. Due to the pioneer-

---

ing work of a visionary herb grower, Lon Johnson, an increasing supply of organically grown herbs is now available in the United States. Efforts are underway to help exporters in developing nations grow their herbs organically or certify their wild-crafted herbs growing in areas where no commercial activities spoil the environment. A few manufacturers have taken the risk of marketing herbal teas with organically grown herbs whose steady supply can be variable. Help support those tea brands and you contribute to increasing organic agriculture all over the world. (See Appendix B.)

Alternatives to Caffeinated Soft Drinks

The simple solution is to switch to caffeine-free sodas. Even the cola companies have finally seen the light and are offering caffeine-free versions of their normally caffeinated colas. Of course, at the same time they are sneaking in more heavily caffeinated sodas than ever before. I would like to propose a much healthier alternative. For all the reasons listed in Chapter 8, "The Hard Truth about Soft Drinks," you should consider replacing those cans of soda with healthier versions that actually contain nutrients, not just empty calories and sugar added to filtered tap water and accompanied by a host of chemical additives.

If you look at the Nutrition Facts box on a can of soda, you'll see that most contain upward of thirty-five or forty-five grams of sugar. You'd be amazed at how much sugar that is if you were to see it on your plate. Although your taste buds may now be accustomed to that level of sweetness, I guarantee you that you can gradually adjust them downward by choosing beverages that have lower and lower quantities of sugar. Your first step might be to choose a blended juice beverage. My favorites use sparkling mineral water as their base and have only juice concentrates added to them, no high-fructose corn syrups or artificial sweeteners. Juice is a natural source of antioxidants and vitamins, but it is high in sugars itself. When mixed with mineral water, blended juice beverages have under thirty grams of sugar. Still plenty sweet enough, but now you're getting some nutrition along with a superior source of water from natural mineral springs. When you're at home, you can make your own blend of mineral water with a splash of your favorite juice. Gradually, you'll find that you can cut down on the juice and drink more and more mineral water.

There are a variety of herbal tea and juice beverages on the market now that also make healthful replacements for soft drinks. Some are carbonated and some are not. Some have additional vitamins and herbal extracts that place them in the growing category of nutraceutically enhanced foods and beverages. Several ginger beverages that give you a naturally stimulating effect have grown in popularity. Once you start to look around, you'll find more and more tasteful beverages that provide you with a healthy alternative to sodas.

If you do this for a period of several weeks, your taste buds will no longer find that sugary sweet sodas taste that good. In fact, if you cut down on other sugars in your diet, you'll find you gradually lose the taste for anything that is overly sweetened. And if you are drinking artificially sweetened sodas, remember this: Research suggests that people who use artificial sweeteners tend to *gain* weight compared to those who do ..ot use these substances.[30] Why take the risk of consuming artificial sweeteners with their possible side effects if they are working against your goal to maintain ideal weight?

Some recommendations:

- Crystal Geyser: Juice Squeeze in a variety of flavors
- Tazo: Lemon Ginger and Wild Orange
- Reed's: Ginger Brew
- R. W. Knudsen: Fruit Teazers and Spritzer Light

Water, the Source of Life

Water is the point of all this, isn't it? Whether you're drinking coffee, tea, or sodas, your goal is to rehydrate your body using nature's perfect product. Our bodies are 70 percent water, which seems astonishing when you consider it. Since water permeates every tissue in our bodies and is the medium that carries all our nutrients to our cells, shouldn't we be rather careful about what kind of water we drink. Coffee, tea, and sodas are ways to make the rehydration process tastier. But we now know that caffeine contributes to dehydration through its diuretic effect. Thus, we are working against ourselves and against what our bodies need for optimal health. If we are supposed to drink eight to ten glasses of water a day, then let's make sure that what we drink is helping to accomplish that goal. Herbal coffee, green and herbal teas, juices with mineral water: these are all good-tasting, healthy ways to rehydrate our bodies and gain the benefit of their special health-promoting properties that only nature can provide.

CHAPTER 10

Off the Bean and On to Vitality

If the sum total of deleterious effects attributed to habitual caffeine use in any way approaches that which is suggested by the extensive literature on the subject, then an untold number of individuals in the community would appear to be in dire need of the assistance of an effective intervention to control caffeine intake.

—Jack E. James and Keryn P. Stirling,
British Journal of Addiction

There *Is* a Way!

You may have tried to quit caffeine already, but come face-to-face with a pounding headache that quickly drives you back to your coffee cup. Or you may have heard stories from others who became depressed and tired when they tried to quit caffeine. Don't worry—there *is* a pain-free path to kicking the caffeine habit, and it's easy to implement. My clinically proven Off the Bean program uses a gradual weaning off caffeine that allows your brain to get

used to its normal flow of oxygen again. Most importantly, this program is designed to help you reach this goal
without the splitting headache, depression, and fatigue
normally associated with caffeine withdrawal.

Headache isn't the only side effect you may experience
from quitting caffeine. It's just the most obvious. Your
body, which has become accustomed to drug-induced
stimulation, needs to recover its natural abundant energy
supply. After all, most people consume caffeine to boost
their energy levels, so restoring natural energy production
once you're off the bean is critical. If you find yourself
unable to muster the oomph to face the day, or crippled
by "brain fog" that won't clear, you'll get discouraged
quickly. Any program for quitting caffeine must provide a
variety of successful methods to deal with fatigue so you
don't go running back to caffeine.

By now, you're certainly aware that vitality does not
come from a coffee cup or a soda can—but where exactly
does it come from, and how can you get more of it? This
chapter will show you how to increase your vitality without the crutch of caffeine. The ultimate reason for quitting
caffeine is to restore optimal health to your body. If you've
been consuming caffeine for a decade or more, your body
will need to undergo a significant amount of repair. Fortunately, it's never too late to begin. Following my Off the
Bean program will reward you richly with health benefits
and enable you to enjoy high-level wellness.

Dealing with Caffeine Withdrawal

Caffeine withdrawal symptoms differ from person to person, but can include up to several weeks of misery. For the
most part, the withdrawal reaction has to do with the sud-

den change in your circulation brought about by the absence of caffeine. Blood vessels no longer constricted by caffeine suddenly open up and allow greater amounts of blood to flow through. And while this is a very good thing, when it comes to the blood vessels in your brain, the sudden increase in circulation can cause splitting headaches.

Other symptoms of caffeine withdrawal, like rebound constipation, are related to decreased muscular stress. With caffeine no longer contracting your intestinal muscles, you may experience sluggish elimination. It may take several months to restore the natural rhythm and function of your colon.

And then there's fatigue, depression, and "brain fog" resulting from caffeine withdrawal. Even though your nervous system is infinitely better off without high levels of stress hormones coursing through your veins, the adjustment period is often perceived as a "letdown." Perhaps you always reach for caffeine when you need to perform in a meeting and can't get your thinking in gear. My Off the Bean program will give you nutritional and herbal support to help you rebuild your mental vitality and recover your natural energy production.

Most importantly, all of the negative reactions associated with caffeine withdrawal can be avoided. How? By decreasing your caffeine intake in stages while you increase a variety of health-promoting habits. That's the secret behind this program.

Recovering Your Natural Energy

When we were children, we blasted out of bed in the morning, eager to explore the world and express ourselves in the new day. As adults, our experience of waking up in the morning is radically different. We *assume* that it's normal to drag ourselves out of bed feeling as though we've been hit by a bus. We *accept* as normal the absurd notion that it's okay to need a powerful adrenal stimulant—caffeine—to "get going." And then we *wonder* why life seems to require more than we have to give. No matter how much caffeine we drink, we don't seem to be able to recapture the exuberance of our youth. Sadly, one day we stop trying. Our dreams fade, and we just *resign* ourselves to a life that no longer sparkles.

What if you could change all that? What would your life be like if you could truly restore your energy and vitality to youthful levels? Well, you can—and that's not just my wish or opinion. It's a clinically proven fact. Thousands of people have already experienced this renewal, and you can, too.

Sure, most people are tired. Fatigue is one of the most common complaints that doctors hear. The problem is that doctors are tired too, and so they look at the patient (who may be forty years old) and say something like, "Well, Ms./Mr. Jones, you're just getting older."

Now that response is a terribly unscientific opinion because it is based on beliefs, not facts. We believe it because someone with authority in a white coat tells us that it's normal to lose our sense of vitality; we're "over the hill." Why do doctors believe this? Because that's what they see, day in and day out. Healthy, vital people aren't trekking into their offices with complaints. All day long doctors see people who are dragged down, and they themselves may be suffering the same loss of energy and vitality from their own caffeine abuse. What's more, they were never taught the importance of nutrition. They were trained only to offer you prescription drugs like antidepressants.

If you're feeling weary and burned out and your physician tells you that there's nothing you can do about it, what hope do you have? With no solution in sight, you can only look forward to the remainder of your life as a downward spiral of limitations, degeneration, and decrepitude.

Hogwash! There is no scientific rationale for "over the hill." In fact, science tells us exactly the opposite: that the human body is designed to last about 120 years, and that it is quite capable of sustaining a high level of energy until the very end. No matter where you look in human physiology, from organ systems to the musculoskeletal, brain, and nervous systems, you find tremendous resiliency, astounding capabilities, and even spare parts (you have two of many organs and need only one).

So why don't we feel this sense of vigor and vitality? It's not because we lose it. We throw it away. We fall into the trap of sedentary living, poor diet, and caffeine. When we stop moving, we lose metabolic efficiency. Remember, life is a "use it or lose it" arrangement. The body only produces as much energy as you create a need for. When you stop moving, your body takes the easier metabolic route of creating fat. With poor dietary habits, the body becomes malnourished. It can't maintain high energy or even adequate repair without the necessary raw materials. And then there's caffeine. At first it's a temporary crutch to get us through periods of fatigue, but caffeine quickly becomes an addiction, setting up a chain reaction of stress, illness, and fatigue that accelerates the downward spiral.

To recover your natural energy, you must take three important steps: Eliminate caffeine abuse, boost your nutritional intake, and develop a habit of regular exercise. The order in which you take these steps is also very important. You may have already learned that jumping into an exercise program can prove disastrous. While everyone else in the gym is exercising energetically, you feel like you're going to die. That's because you first need to restore your metabolic efficiency. You then take that renewed energy and use it to build up an exercise program that feels good and works. When I describe this sequence of events to patients, their most common response is "Of course. That makes perfect sense."

Boosting Your Metabolic Efficiency

In a very real sense, lack of energy is a problem of a sedentary lifestyle. Have you ever noticed that people who exercise regularly seem to have an abundance of energy? It's common to think that they exercise because they have energy, but it's more accurate to say that they experience energy because they exercise. Once again, it's use it or lose it. When you exercise regularly, you are placing a demand on your body, and your body will respond by creating energy. But if you do not make the demand, your body will not create a great deal of energy. Why should it?

Now, in order to generate consistent energy, exercise must also be consistent. And that's a problem because exercise for most people is arduous and painful. Who would willingly repeat a painful experience day after day? Only those who are fit can *really* enjoy exercise. So here's the catch-22: You can only enjoy exercise if you're fit, but you can only become fit by exercising. It seems like the unfit are doomed.

To find the way out of this dilemma, you need to understand why exercise feels bad to a sedentary person.

It's a phenomenon known as adaptation. You've seen it a hundred times (and perhaps experienced it yourself). Sedentary individuals get inspired to begin an exercise program, maybe even pay a handsome membership fee to a health club. They go to their first workout, but instead of feeling invigorated, they feel exhausted. The same thing happens on the second day, and by the third day they can barely move because every muscle and joint in their body aches. In frustration, they quit, assuming they just don't have what it takes.

What they were experiencing was adaptation, the painful period between the unfit and the fit state, the time when you're making new demands on your body but your body hasn't quite figured out where to get the energy you need. The sad part is that if these individuals had stuck with it through adaptation, they would have experienced a whole new level of energy. But adaptation takes time—from several weeks to months—and it is the rare person who has that kind of dedication.

Getting through (or Eliminating) Adaptation

I spent years studying the biochemistry of human performance. I have been an adviser to members of the U.S. Olympic team and served on the faculty of the American College of Sports Medicine. In helping to train world-class athletes, I developed a formula of what I termed *bioenergetic nutrients*. These substances are critically important for the body's creation of energy. They exist in every cell of the body, but most people don't have levels that will support peak performance.

I realized that the same substances I was using to help

athletes maximize performance could be used by unfit people to get through adaptation. That's because in both cases, the need is to enhance metabolic efficiency. Athletes benefit from these bioenergetic nutrients because they're using them up faster than they can be replaced. Unfit individuals benefit because their bodies have (temporarily) stopped making them in sufficient quantities.

In effect, raising tissue levels of bioenergetic nutrients tells the unfit (or semifit) person's brain that this body has been exercising. The brain then responds by directing the body to create more enzymes (such as fatty acid oxidase) to fuel energy production. The result? Greater vitality in a very real and natural sense, because the body itself generates the energy. And at that point, adaptation is no longer an issue.

The Energy Scams

In today's "you can have it all" world, the part that everyone forgets is that you have to do it all. That's why energy is a hot topic and a hot commodity. Leafing through a health magazine, you'd think that getting more energy was as easy as taking a few pills—but as much as we would like that to be true, it doesn't happen that way. Any pill that purports to give you instant energy is very likely to be just another stimulant like caffeine, the drug you're trying to avoid.

Energy pills abound at the checkout counter of your convenience store, in catalogs, and at the gym. But look at the ingredient list. Guarana, maté, bissy nut, kola nut, or green tea extract are simply herbal sources of caffeine. Ma huang and Chinese ephedra are herbal sources of ephedrine, another central nervous system stimulant. If you see botanical names of plants (such as *Ilex paraguayensis* or *Paulinia cupana*), the manufacturer is using the Latin nomenclature to further hide the fact that the product contains stimulants. I have even seen the chemical name for caffeine (trimethylxanthine) used on a product label! (See Chapter 7, "Politics and Pushers," for a detailed discussion of this ruse.)

What Will You Do with the Extra Energy?

What would you do if you won a million dollars? Chances are you'd spend some of it and invest the rest. In other words, money is useful for the things it can buy now and also for producing extra money for future needs. Likewise, when people start to experience greater energy, they naturally feel like spending it—usually in the form of exercise and activity. Soon they find that not only do they have more energy to spend, but for the first time they have an *energy reserve* that they can call upon when they most need it.

This energy reserve marks the difference between caffeine abuse and real energy. It also highlights an important difference in motivation. Whereas before you might have motivated yourself to exercise through guilt and condemnation (not very effective in the long run), now you exercise because you have abundant energy—and because you enjoy it!

When you win the energy lottery, your life can change dramatically. The amount of time it takes depends on how much caffeine you've been consuming. Tissue levels of bioenergetic nutrients are not restored instantly, but be patient—it doesn't take long. Most people start to feel better within a week. The full range of bioenergetic benefits won't be experienced until you've detoxified the caffeine in your body and normalized stress hormone levels. As we've learned, that may take three to four weeks.

Off the Bean

STRATEGIES FOR COFFEE DRINKERS

There are basically three ways to get off coffee:

1. Cold Turkey: This is a mistake. Don't do it. Remember that the crushing headache and other withdrawal symptoms are triggered by rapid changes in caffeine blood levels. Cold turkey (quitting all at once) is a surefire way to suffer the worst withdrawal reaction possible.

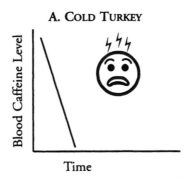

A. COLD TURKEY

2. Replacement: Some people find that this works, but it has to be done carefully. If you consume four cups of coffee a day, don't assume that you can have your first two cups and simply replace the last two cups with herbal tea.

That will still produce a radical drop in blood caffeine levels, triggering a withdrawal headache. For the replacement method to work, you have to figure out how to maintain a normal (for you) level of caffeine in your blood while you gradually reduce that level over a two-week period. That's most easily done by alternating coffee and caffeine-free beverages.

Example: Many people have two cups of coffee in the morning, another at midmorning, and their final cup with lunch or afternoon coffee break. A rapid drop in blood caffeine levels can be avoided by having cup #1 at the customary morning time, but replace cup #2 with decaf, herb tea, coffee substitute, herbal coffee, or hot soup. The midmorning coffee would be continued, and the alternative would be used at the afternoon coffee break.

Then, of course, one needs to reduce the caffeine intake at the morning and midmorning time points. Here are a few tips:

A. *Brew your coffee with 50 percent decaf.* Some companies produce coffee blends with a fifty-fifty mix of decaf and caffeinated coffee. After a week or so, you will need to add increasing amounts of decaf until you are ultimately using 100 percent decaf. Don't forget, decaf still contains some caffeine, as well as harsh acids and oils inherent in the coffee bean (see Chapter 9). You might do better by ultimately switching to herb tea, herbal coffee, or another coffee alternative.

B. *Get a smaller coffee mug.* One client of mine had a revelation when we were exploring the cause of her fatigue and anxiety. She started noticing increased fatigue shortly after turning thirty, and of course she (and her doctor) attributed it to "getting older." But as she and I looked at a possible coffee connection, she burst out laughing. "That's it," she cried. "For my thirtieth birthday, a friend gave me a coffee mug with one of those cute 'Now that you're over the hill. . . .' inscriptions. This new mug was huge, but I filled it and drank it twice a day as I had with my old mug." Unknowingly, this woman had nearly doubled her caffeine intake and was suffering the consequences.

Well, it works the other way, too. Most of us just want to have a mug of some good-tasting, hot beverage, and the size of the mug doesn't matter all that much. So downsize your mug (avoid refills) and that will help reduce your caffeine intake.

C. *Make your coffee weaker.* Whether you brew your coffee or use instant, you can gradually decrease the amount you use.

D. *Add more milk.* If you already take milk with your coffee, simply add more. If this is not your habit, give it a try. Adding low-fat milk reduces the amount of coffee in the cup and therefore decreases your caffeine intake. Plus the milk provides a valuable source of calcium and protein.

B. REPLACEMENT METHOD

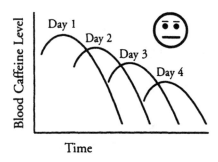

3. Weaning: The No-Headache, No-hassle Method. This is my recommended method for people who don't want to mess with the complex replacement technique. It also works great when more than one person is trying to get off the bean, because everyone can drink from the same pot. Here you simply brew or mix your coffee with small amounts of herbal coffee or coffee substitute, and continue drinking the same number of cups. Over a two-week period, you gradually increase the amount of herbal coffee or substitute while decreasing the coffee. Thus there is no dramatic decrease in blood caffeine levels and no headache.

Importantly, this method enables you to get used to new tastes, and if you're using herbal coffee, these tastes will be surprisingly rich and enjoyable. You can do this easily in a drip coffeemaker or a French press pot. Use a scoop or tablespoon as a measurement and mix your regular coffee with herbal coffee as follows: Begin by mixing approximately three-quarters regular coffee to one-quarter herbal coffee. After three to four days, reduce your regular coffee to two-thirds and increase the herbal coffee to one-third. Begin Week 2 by blending your regular coffee half-and-half with herbal coffee. After three days, reduce the regular coffee to one-quarter and increase the herbal coffee to three-quarters. Over the next few days, gradually taper off the regular coffee until you are drinking 100 percent herbal coffee. (See Appendix B.)

Here's an example of the measurements you can use if you make a ten-cup pot of coffee in your home or office:

Days 1–3	4 scoops (or tablespoons) regular coffee
	1 scoop (or tablespoon) herbal coffee
Days 4–6	3 scoops regular coffee
	2 scoops herbal coffee

Days 7–9	2½ scoops regular coffee
	2½ scoops herbal coffee
Days 10–11	2 scoops regular coffee
	3 scoops herbal coffee
Day 12	1 scoop regular coffee
	4 scoops herbal coffee
Day 13	½ scoop regular coffee
	4½ scoops herbal coffee
Day 14	5 scoops herbal coffee

Many people have found that blending herbal coffee with their regular coffee is the most painless way to kick the caffeine habit. However, if you use instant coffee, you can also blend it with an instant coffee substitute. These grain-based beverages are sold in your natural food store or supermarket. Blend each cup of coffee you make using both the instant coffee substitute and your regular brand of instant coffee just as described above. Over the two-week period, keep lowering the amount of regular coffee you use and increasing the amount of instant coffee substitute.

C. WEANING

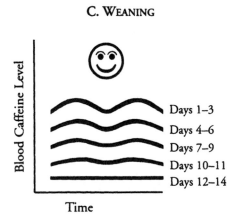

Strategies for Tea Drinkers

Begin by steeping your black tea for less time, such as one minute instead of three or four. Alternate every other cup of tea with either green tea, green tea mixed with herbs, or herbal tea. Try some of the stimulating herbal teas such as spice or ginseng blends. Gradually cut down the number of cups of black tea you drink over a two-week period while substituting low-caffeine or caffeine-free teas. Explore the many varieties of green and herbal teas suggested in Chapter 9, "Options and Alternatives."

Strategies for Cola Drinkers

Your task is to reduce both your caffeine intake and your sugar consumption. You will need to read the Nutrition Facts box on a variety of cola brands and start slowly pushing your sugar consumption downward as you wean yourself off caffeine. For the first week, alternate each can of your normal soft drink brand with a juice/mineral water combination that has under thirty grams of sugar. In Week 2, start substituting caffeine-free colas for some of your cans of caffeinated cola.

Depending on how many cans of soda you consume, you'll need to calculate a gradual reduction. Start blending mineral water with juice at home. Try some of the herb tea and juice blends recommended in Chapter 9. By Week 3, you can be off soda altogether and enjoying healthful beverages while you continue to get used to less and less sugar. After a month of being soda free, if you've successfully reduced your sugar intake too, you won't even like the overly sweet taste of colas anymore.

ADVICE FOR "COMBO" DRINKERS

Like many people, you may be drinking both coffee and colas, or tea and colas. In that case, the best approach to getting off caffeine is to eliminate coffee first, if you're a coffee drinker, or tea first, if you're a tea drinker. Your challenge is to keep from ingesting more soft drinks than usual during this process. Use the other substitute beverages recommended above. The good habits you establish during the coffee/tea phase-out will ultimately help you give up colas. Start cutting back on cola beverages only once you're comfortably off coffee or tea.

Tips for Traveling

When you're out of the house, it's easy to slip back into caffeine if there aren't any options available. I always have a selection of herb tea in my briefcase: Celestial Seasoning's Roastaroma for the morning, a ginseng or fruit-flavored tea for the afternoon, and chamomile or Celestial's Sleepytime tea for the evening. I look forward to the day when these options, as well as herbal coffee, are available in coffee shops.

Brain Defogging Aids

In the first stages of recovery from caffeine abuse, you may find that you can't stimulate and organize your thoughts as effectively as you did when you were on caffeine. Caffeine creates a highly alert phase during its onset, which is really a state of emergency induced by stimulating your adrenals to release stress hormones. When you first get off caffeine, you may benefit from some herbal support to overcome adrenal exhaustion. The following substances have proved helpful:

Ginkgo biloba: Ginkgo improves cerebral circulation, dilates peripheral blood vessels throughout the body, and increases memory retention and concentration.[1] As such, ginkgo's effects on the body are essentially the reverse of caffeine's. Moreover, the herb protects brain neurons against free-radical damage, and evidence suggests that it may be helpful in the prevention and treatment of Alzheimer's disease.[2] I recommend that everyone quitting coffee begin taking ginkgo extract, 24 percent standardized concentrate, in small dosages of thirty milligrams daily during the first two weeks of withdrawal. Increase the quantity of ginkgo to sixty milligrams after your system has been weaned off of caffeine, and continue a daily intake for one to three months.

Gotu kola: Gotu kola can help rebuild mental stamina, increase mental ability, and improve memory and learning retention.[3, 4] It can also help you overcome the negative effects of stress and fatigue. The herb has been used in India for centuries, where it is reputed to be a "rejuvenator." Gotu kola doesn't contain caffeine, although it has been confused with kola nut, which does contain caffeine. Gotu kola extract (one dropperful of liquid extract in juice) can be taken daily for the two-week period during which you are reducing your caffeine intake. Thereafter, continue taking gotu kola as needed.

Mood Support

Serotonin is one of the brain's pleasure and mood neuro-transmitters. Since caffeine can raise (and then lower) serotonin levels in the brain,[5] getting off caffeine too fast can affect some people's mood, especially if they've been drinking more than four cups a day. Using the Off the Bean strategy normally avoids this effect, but if you find that you're feeling blue, you might add a natural mood elevator to your postcaffeine routine.

St. John's wort is an herbal supplement that is extremely effective in raising serotonin levels. Look for a standardized concentrate providing twenty-five to fifty milligrams per dropper or capsule.

5-HTP is a natural tryptophan metabolite that helps to increase brain levels of serotonin. It is now available in health-food stores. Suggested dose is fifty milligrams per day.

Detoxification Support

The three eliminative organs most affected by caffeine abuse are the liver, colon, and kidneys. The function of all three will be improved when you get off of caffeine. However, there may be an interim period during which you can accelerate their recovery by giving them herbal assistance.

The Liver: In the section about aging in Chapter 5, we learned that the liver detoxifies caffeine via a group of enzymes known as the cytochrome P450 system. This group of enzymes is responsible for breaking down most foreign substances in our bodies, so it's called upon daily to remove from our bloodstream anything that might harm us. Long-term, high-dose caffeine use can tax this detox system. A herb known as milk thistle (silymarin) has been shown to enhance the activity of C-P450 enzymes so dramatically that it can be used as adjunct therapy in cases of liver disease.[6, 7]

The Colon: Because caffeine acts as a colonic stimulant, getting off the bean can result in sluggish elimination. In most people, this is easily remedied by increasing fiber intake. I recommend 100 percent pure psyllium powder without added dextrose. Psyllium in combination with a variety of brans (wheat, oat) is okay, but I do not recommend laxative ingredients such as senna or cascara because they work by irritating the lining of the intestine. Psyllium works by providing bulk and lubrication, which is more effective, safe, and gentle. Take a tablespoon mixed in juice in the evening.

The Kidneys: Here's the good news: All you need to do is drink eight glasses of pure water or herbal tea daily and your kidneys will be just fine. If you suffer from recurrent cystitis or urinary tract infections (often exacerbated by caffeine), you may find the herbs parsley and uva ursi to be of benefit.

Boost Your Energy with Nutritional Supports

The following seven bioenergetic nutrients have been clinically proven to boost your natural energy supply. Start taking them at the beginning of your Off the Bean program. After a week of taking these nutrients, you should find yourself naturally awake and alert, with ever-increasing energy that you can use to start an effective exercise program. These nutrients will also help you avoid the side effects of caffeine withdrawal. You can continue taking them indefinitely.

1. COENZYME Q10

Coenzyme Q10 (CoQ10) is one of a class of biochemicals known as ubiquinones. It is found in all living tissue and is essential for cellular respiration—that is, the conversion of fuel and oxygen to energy. As such, CoQ10 has been called the "sparkplug" of life. While we normally get CoQ10 from food, it is not considered a true vitamin because the liver can synthesize CoQ10 from various ubiquinones obtained in the diet. For that reason, it has received little attention from nutrition researchers.

But we now know that the modern Western diet does not always supply necessary amounts of ubiquinones, and the liver does not always manufacture optimal amounts of CoQ10.[8–12] That can affect the way you feel and limit the amount of energy produced by your cells. Foods vary widely in their ubiquinone content, and food processing and cooking can dramatically reduce availability of these vital nutrients. The refining of wheat and rice, for example, can result in the loss of 80 percent of the ubiquinone content of the grain.[13]

Interestingly, it appears that CoQ10 levels decline with age, and this may help explain why some people "run out of steam."[14] In placebo-controlled studies, middle-aged men given supplemental CoQ10 report greater feelings of vigor,[15] and, most important for this discussion, it has been found that the muscle content of CoQ10 is directly related to exercise capacity and sports performance.[16] Clearly, CoQ10 is a primary ingredient in any program to enhance energy or jump-start an exercise routine. Suggested use: twenty to sixty milligrams per day.

2. ALPHA KETOGLUTARIC ACID (AKG)

AKG is another essential nutrient that plays a critical role in the Krebs cycle. (Remember Biology 101: The Krebs cycle is the biochemical "assembly line" that converts carbohydrates, fats, and protein into energy.) Human volunteers given AKG supplements experienced improvements not only in stamina, but also in respiratory efficiency.[17] That means their bodies were extracting more oxygen (and thus more energy) from each breath. Surprisingly, AKG supplements for the most part have only been used by athletes and bodybuilders. But I have seen sedentary people gain significant energy benefits from this important nutrient, and when that happens, they do not remain sedentary for long.

Important Notes Regarding AKG

1. Alpha ketoglutaric acid is an important supplement to take while you are decreasing your intake of caffeine. I believe it can play a valuable role not only in enhancing natural energy production, but also in stress management due to its conversion by the body to glutamate and then

to gamma aminobutyric acid (GABA).[18, 19] GABA, you will remember from Chapters 3 and 4, is a natural anti-stress neurochemical synthesized by the brain, which produces feelings of calm attention. There is even evidence that raising GABA levels may help to overcome addiction, not only to caffeine, but to other substances as well.[20, 21]

2. GABA is available as a nutritional supplement, but taking a GABA tablet will not provide the benefits you want. That's because the complex molecule is quickly destroyed by the digestive system. Claims have also been made that supplementation with the amino acid L-glutamine can raise GABA levels, but this too is unlikely. One group of researchers termed glutamine a "metabolically remote" precursor for GABA.[22] Thus, research strongly supports the use of alpha ketoglutaric acid to optimize GABA production by the brain and body.

Suggested use: 200 to 400 milligrams per day.

3. VITAMIN B-6

Many of the B vitamins are involved in energy production, but I include B-6 specifically because it has been shown to work as a cofactor with alpha ketoglutaric acid in enhancing exercise ability.[23] This may be related to its role in the synthesis of hemoglobin and other oxygen transfer proteins.[24] Importantly, B-6 (pyridoxine) is often poorly supplied by the American diet.[25-27] A recent nine-year survey of American women revealed that regardless of income level, mean intakes by women were below the RDA for six nutrients, including B-6, calcium, and magnesium.[28]

Once converted by the body to pyridoxine 5 phosphate

(PLP), vitamin B-6 becomes an active coenzyme in literally hundreds of metabolic processes. For example, the utilization of any amino acid for energy production requires optimal levels of PLP. It is no surprise, then, to learn that exercise performance increased in a group of adolescents supplemented with B-6.[29]

Suggested use: 10 to 20 milligrams per day.

4. CHROMIUM

Although the hype surrounding chromium supplements has been largely overblown (it won't cause instant weight loss), the mineral is an important bioenergetic nutrient due to its cofactor role with insulin. In effect, insulin cannot do its job of delivering fuel to the cells of the body if there is insufficient chromium. Suboptimal chromium levels, therefore, will contribute directly to low metabolic efficiency.

Is chromium deficiency common? Studies conducted by the USDA show that the vast majority of those tested were obtaining less than adequate amounts of this essential nutrient.[30, 31] In another study of 216 healthy affluent American adults, more than 90 percent were receiving less than the minimum suggested amount of chromium in their diets.[32] It is no surprise to find literally dozens of studies showing that chromium supplementation can increase insulin sensitivity, improve glucose tolerance, and enhance the bioenergetic potential of the human body.[33–38]

Suggested use: 200 to 300 micrograms per day as chromium polynicotinate.

5. POTASSIUM AND MAGNESIUM ASPARTATE

Aspartic acid is a natural organic acid present throughout your body that feeds into the Krebs cycle, and it is best stabilized by potassium and magnesium for supplemental use. I have been using these mineral aspartates for decades, and there is impressive scientific support for their use as antifatigue agents.[39-41]

Suggested use: 200 to 400 milligrams per day.

6. GINSENG

Recommending ginseng is like telling someone to go buy some "transportation." What kind of transportation? A bicycle, car, and jet plane will all move you from Point A to Point B, but in vastly different ways. Likewise, there is a wide range of ginseng products available today, and some, using my analogy, would not even be considered roller skates.

Numerous plants are referred to as ginseng, but the two primary types are Siberian ginseng (*Eleutherococcus senticocus*) and Panax (or Korean) ginseng. Manufacturers have marketed a "new" botanical extract known as ciwujia, but this turned out to be a variety of Siberian ginseng. Just to confuse the issue, there is also American ginseng (*Panax quinquefolius*).

Looking at the scientific literature on ginseng, you will find conflicting studies whose results vary according to methodology and even the actual type of ginseng used. If I had not seen significant improvements using ginseng in hundreds of patients, I would be tempted to write it off. Here is the problem: Studies purporting to evaluate ginseng may be using a "roller skate" substance or even worse. In fact, one laboratory analysis of fifty-four commercially available ginseng products revealed that 60 percent were worthless, and 25 percent contained no identifiable ginseng![42] Using one of these substances would obviously show no benefit.

Fortunately, standardized extracts are becoming available that have demonstrated and verifiable benefits (see Appendix B). And while I am not willing to say that ginseng will greatly boost exercise ability (like AKG and CoQ10), the herb has been shown to have antifatigue benefits and may also improve mood and general health.[43–45] For these benefits, and especially since ginseng relaxes and dilates cerebral blood vessels,[46] the herb has proven to be extremely useful in my Off the Bean program.

Suggested use: Fifty to 100 milligrams of standardized 15 percent extract, preferably in divided doses. Ideally, this would be a mixture of Siberian and Panax ginseng.

7. DHEA

I have described in Chapters 3 and 4 how DHEA plays an important role in maintaining youthful energy and strength. Unfortunately, DHEA levels decline remarkably as we age, so that by age seventy, most people are producing only about 15 to 20 percent of prime peak (the amount produced at age twenty-five).

My book *The DHEA Breakthrough* (Ballantine, 1996) presents a comprehensive program for restoring and maintaining prime peak levels of DHEA in order to maximize the body's production of muscle tissue. It's not just a matter of popping a few DHEA tablets. For purposes of this discussion, let me simply say that it is important to know how much DHEA your body is presently producing. If you are getting off caffeine, wait a few weeks before you have a DHEA test, because getting off caffeine will in itself boost your DHEA levels.

After you've been caffeine free for three or four weeks, I suggest you have a saliva or blood test for DHEA (see Appendix B). If your levels are low, you may want to consult with your doctor and consider supplementing with DHEA. That's because low DHEA levels make exercise somewhat frustrating. You can lift weights for weeks and not see or feel much progress. With optimum DHEA levels, on the other hand, you will feel and see results in a matter of days. This doesn't mean that women will get bulging muscles. Rather, you will have a renewed sense of strength and power that can be quite significant and enjoyable.

Additional Nutritional Supplements

Multivitamin/mineral. This is nutritional insurance against the shortfalls of even a good diet. Look for a high-potency, multidose formula (one or more tablets with each meal) rather than a one-per-day.

Make it hot. Cayenne will help counteract the vasoconstrictive effect of caffeine. It decreases risk for cardiovascular disease and is energizing. Cayenne increases circulation (especially to the hands and feet), improves digestion, and may enhance immunity. Add sparingly to foods and beverages.

Antioxidants. Without a doubt, antioxidants comprise the most important category of nutritional supplements, protecting the body from the damaging effects of pollution, stress, injury, and metabolic toxins known as free radicals. I highly recommend a comprehensive antioxidant supplement containing vitamins C and E, beta-carotene, bioflavonoids, and extracts of pine bark, grape seed, and caffeine-free green tea.

Dietary Support

One of the reasons so many people require caffeine in the morning is that they have a low blood sugar reaction from breakfast. Today, breakfast typically consists of highly sweetened, refined carbohydrates such as commercial breakfast cereals, doughnuts, bagels, muffins, and croissants. Hitting your system with a whopping dose of carbos can raise blood sugar quickly, precipitating the release of insulin, which results in a blood-sugar crash shortly thereafter. This sets you up for midmorning fatigue, and the natural tendency is to reach for coffee.

Unfortunately, people getting off caffeine may try to get a replacement rush from sugar. Instead, try balancing protein with carbohydrates, and you'll experience sustained energy throughout the morning. *Don't skip breakfast.* Studies show that this common mistake leads to mood and energy swings and overeating later in the day.

Breakfast suggestions: Eggs are a good choice a couple of times a week. Pass on the sausage and bacon chock full of saturated fat and nitrates. There are excellent and delicious soy sausages that, combined with toast and orange juice, will keep you energized for hours. As an option to eggs, try scrambled tofu (recipe from your favorite natural foods cookbook).

Yogurt is another good choice, but be careful. Commercial varieties often contain high amounts of sugar or artificial sweeteners. I suggest low- or nonfat plain yogurt, to which you can add fresh fruit and whole-grain cereal.

Blender drinks (shakes) are also popular breakfast options, but once again, most are far too high in carbohydrates and low in protein. Many of my clients have used commercial drink mixes and found that they feel good for an hour and then become hungry and tired. This is a classic blood-sugar roller-coaster effect. When they replace the commercial shakes with a scoop of protein powder mixed in juice or low-fat milk, together with a banana or frozen fruit, their hunger is satisfied till lunch. For extra nutritional benefit, you can add some oat bran and/or a scoop of a multivitamin/mineral powder.

Adrenal Support

Just getting off caffeine will have a profound effect on your adrenal glands. When they are no longer hammered by the daily stress of caffeine, the strength of your adrenals will gradually be restored by your body's own healing power.

If you've been abusing your adrenals with caffeine for many years, you may need a little extra help. A group of herbs (mostly from Asia) have been used for centuries as adrenal support agents. Known as adaptogens, these herbs assist the body in dealing with physical, mental, and emotional stress.[47–50] These adaptogenic herbs include:

- Siberian ginseng (*Eleutherococcus senticosus*)
- Schizandra (*Schizandra chinensis*)

- Astragalus (*Astragalus membranaceus*)
- Ashwagandha (*Withania somnifera*)
- Ziziphus seed (*Ziziphus spinosa*)
- Withania extract (*Withania somnifera*)
- Gotu kola (*Centella asiatica*)

Look for herbal extracts, either liquid or capsules, that are standardized by their active ingredients. A dropperful of liquid extract, for example, can be added to your morning orange juice to start the day.

If you think you suffer from adrenal exhaustion, you may want to ask your doctor to order an Adrenal Stress Index Test, which uses your saliva to measure cortisol and DHEA over the course of a day. The lab then constructs a profile of your adrenal function and gives you and your physician specific information about therapeutic options and follow-up (see Appendix B). In addition, complementary therapies such as acupuncture may improve your adrenal function and provide additional support during the recovery period.

NUTRITION FOR ADRENAL SUPPORT

Potassium is an important mineral for optimum health of your nervous system and adrenals. A high-sodium diet exacerbates low potassium intake and may retard adrenal recovery. Good sources of potassium are avocados, bananas, tomatoes, fresh fish, and herbal coffee.

Vitamin C, pantothenic acid, and B-complex vitamins are all important for adrenal health.

Note: I do *not* recommend adrenal glandular supplements made from bovine adrenal gland.. There is no reliable scientific support for their use, and they may contain adrenal hormones. Thus, while these products can produce a short-term boost, the side effects and long-term risks are unknown.

Exercise: The Closest Thing to the Fountain of Youth

We are creatures made for movement. Every part of our bodies works better when we exercise consistently, including not only the cardiovascular and respiratory systems, but the immune system, skeletal system, and digestive system as well. Exercise will dramatically enhance the benefits you receive from the Off the Bean program, but remember that the operative word is *consistency.* Studies illustrate that when the brain learns the muscles will be requiring more energy on a daily basis, it kicks into gear a whole cascade of metabolic reactions that make that energy available.

And it's not just increased metabolic rate. Forget the charts you've seen showing that an hour of tennis burns only 200 calories. Who would be inspired by that? Those charts miss the point entirely, which is that: (1) your body will continue to burn additional calories for hours after the exercise is over; and (2) the enhanced metabolic benefits of exercise far exceed the number of calories burned.

Exercise increases muscle mass, and that's energy in action. A high muscle mass:

1. Increases metabolic efficiency. Food that you consume will be converted to energy to feed the muscles rather than be converted into fat.

2. Enhances immunity.
3. Looks great on you!
4. Ensures that you will be able to maintain your ideal weight without dieting. Dieting is a proven strategy for *gaining* weight, but that's another story.

START WITH WALKING

When all is said and done, walking is still the best overall exercise for the following reasons:

1. It's easy. Walking can be done just about anywhere by almost everyone.

2. It requires no special equipment other than a good pair of walking shoes.

3. Walking works the largest muscles of the body, the front and back of your thighs.

4. The rhythmic motion of walking (especially through an area you enjoy, like a park, forest, or the beach) helps you unwind and produces a naturally reflective mood. Walking has been shown to have significant antidepressant benefits.

Tips on Walking

Intensity: Make sure you don't get out of breath. That indicates oxygen debt. Although it's not dangerous for most people, it means that your muscles are not getting the oxygen they need to burn fat. Instead, you'll be burning primarily blood sugar (glucose), which may leave you feeling exhausted instead of invigorated.

Pace: Try to work up to a fifteen-minute mile. That means in thirty minutes, you will have walked two miles, a brisk but comfortable pace for most people.

Duration: A thirty-minute walk every day is a good start. But as soon as you can easily accomplish that, I recommend you increase the length of your walk as long as you comfortably can. If weight loss is one of your goals, duration is the key, as fat burning really kicks in after thirty minutes of walking.

The Mind-Body Connection

In the endeavor to regain your youthful vitality, you need to marshal all of your resources, including the power of your mind. I highly recommend listening to a "walking" tape that will help you get the most out of your exercise period. Music alone is fine, especially if it helps "pump you up," but there are special tapes available today that include guided visualization and embedded suggestions, as well as a new breakthrough in behavior modification known as neuroacoustic sound technology. This technology uses specific sounds and beat patterns that activate the mind to maximize the efficiency, power, and overall benefit of your walk. People using these tapes report that they walk faster and farther, and feel better than ever afterward (see Appendix B).

The Body-Mind Connection

We've all heard about how visualization, meditation, biofeedback, and prayer can strengthen the mind's positive influence on the body. But the opposite is also true. The body can exert a powerful influence on the mind, for good or ill. Chapter 4 described in detail how caffeine and tension can ultimately produce a level of stress and anxiety sufficient to cause emotional and mental illness.

Conversely, a discipline that produces ease and relaxation in the body can have a profoundly calming influence on the mind. Yoga is perhaps the most complete and time-tested system for developing and maintaining flexibility, strength, balance, and deep relaxation. There is no exercise, nutritional supplement, diet, practice, or program that can come close to providing the benefits that I have received from yoga over the last thirty years. For someone getting off the frazzling, chaotic influence of caffeine, yoga can be an extraordinary blessing.

Look for a yoga course designed for where you are. Explain to the teacher ahead of time that you are a beginner. It does no good to jump into an arduous or advanced class if what you need most is range-of-motion work and stress reduction. There are a wide variety of classes available in most areas of the country. I urge you to explore and enjoy this refreshing and relaxing practice.

Onward and Upward

The upward spiral of energy and metabolic efficiency is very real and exiting. We're cheated out of this experience by caffeine because the drug puts us on a continual roller coaster of artificial ups and downs. One of the most common responses I get from Off the Bean participants is, "So *this* is what real energy and vitality feels like!"

As you achieve higher levels of fitness and metabolic

efficiency from your walking program, it's time to expand your exercise into strength training. I highly recommend that you enlist the help of a certified fitness trainer, if only for a few sessions. I believe that it's impossible for a book to describe a safe and time-efficient strength-training program that will be appropriate for everyone.

Ideally, work toward performing a strength routine (with weights or machines or a combination) three times a week. This does not have to involve hours at the gym. Your fitness trainer will show you how to complete your training session in less than one hour, including a shower!

The advantages of strength training are by now well understood, and there's no age limit on who can benefit. For anyone from teens to seniors, added strength enhances overall health, protects the bones and joints, increases lean body mass, burns fat, and improves self-esteem. As we age, strength is one of the most significant factors in maintaining an independent lifestyle.[51]

> "Strength training enables individuals to maintain high levels of strength for many years and also provides individuals who have not been involved in strength training an opportunity to reverse many of the age-related deterioration processes that are observed in the muscles of sedentary people."
>
> Source: Waneen Spirduso, *The Physical Dimensions of Aging.*

The wonderful part of the upward spiral is that it is self-motivating. You feel so good that you just *want* to continue doing the things that support your new life. It's also self-perpetuating. The more you do, the more you are capable of doing. As your body improves, so does your mind. Recent studies have found that highly fit adults tend to have better cognitive (learning) skills compared to sedentary people matched for age and education.[52, 53] Part of that may be due to increased circulation to the brain, or the maintenance of certain neurochemicals or hormones.

Maximize the Rejuvenating Benefits of Sleep

In Chapter 3, I described the deep healing and rejuvenating benefits of sleep. Everyone knows from their own personal experience what it feels like to be truly rested. But most of us cheat on our sleep hours because of the pressure and deadlines we're under in our lives. You may find that after you quit caffeine, for a period of time it seems like your body needs an unusual amount of sleep. For one thing, you may have difficulty staying up late, because you won't have caffeine to keep you awake. Additionally, your body will require more sleep as part of its recovery from the sleep deprivation caffeine has caused. If you allow yourself to benefit from increased sleep hours during your first few weeks off caffeine, your body will more rapidly complete the high level of repair necessary in your organs and nervous system.

If you do not sleep soundly or awaken feeling tired, you may find that simply getting off caffeine solves your problem. If you need additional help, try the following suggestions to help produce a deep, restful, rejuvenating sleep.

1. *To improve sleep dramatically (and rejuvenate the body), exercise regularly.* Remember, the genes that control

every cell of your body have not changed at all in more than 20,000 years. That means your body is still designed for hunting and gathering and a very high level of activity. When you sleep, the brain queries the muscles to find out how much rest the body needs. If the muscles say, "Gee, boss, we haven't moved all day," the brain will set the sleep cycle differently than if the muscles are tired. I'm not saying that you have to be exhausted to get a good night's sleep, but well-exercised muscles send a sleep and repair message to the brain so that you enter a deeply restoring level of sleep.

Note: It is best *not* to exercise strenuously right before bed.

2. *Develop regular sleep habits.* Researchers from the Department of Psychiatry at the University of Arizona have demonstrated for the first time that sleep regularity (going to bed at the same time each night) can significantly enhance sleep quality in healthy people who are not sleep deprived.[54] In their study, two groups of students were asked to sleep at least 7.5 hours each night, but one of the groups was instructed to keep a regular sleep schedule. Compared to the sleep-only group, subjects in the regularity group demonstrated:

A. Decreased daytime feelings of fatigue
B. Greater and longer-lasting improvements in alertness
C. Greater sleep efficiency (they fell asleep faster and stayed asleep through the night).

Importantly, these benefits were realized after only four weeks.

3. *If you wake up earlier than you wish* and feel like going back to sleep, here are some suggestions:

- Make sure you can sleep for another ninety minutes. That will enable you to complete another sleep cycle. Going to sleep for thirty or forty minutes may result in your feeling more tired and cranky upon awakening.
- Try reading or meditating. Both will quiet the mind and keep busy thoughts from intruding when you're getting sleepy again.

4. *Take the TV out of the bedroom.* Some people use TV to fall asleep and keep it droning in the background while they sleep. The noise will keep you from deep sleep and may wake you up in the middle of the night.

5. *Developing good sleep habits starts with the setting.* You create the ambience for sleep and your body follows that train of association. Make your bedroom a place of retreat and privacy where you can forget the cares of the world.

6. *If you can't fall asleep, read a nonfiction book, not an action thriller.* Eventually, your brain will slow down if it's not overstimulated by an exciting novel.

7. *Eight hours of sleep beginning at 10 P.M.* do more to restore your body than eight hours starting after midnight. If you sleep from 10 P.M. to 6 A.M., you'll have more energy and vitality than if you sleep from 1 A.M. to 9 A.M. You'll get more done in the early morning hours than you will late at night after an exhausting day. Try it for yourself both ways and you'll see the difference!

8. *Try to eliminate noise.* I've found that a HEPA filter (high-efficiency particulate air filter) doubles as a white noise machine, effectively covering up the disruptive noise of traffic, barking dogs, and the neighbor's stereo. Heavy drapes are also a sound investment, again doing double duty by reducing both noise and light.

9. *Invest in a good pillow.* You spend many hours asleep, and you deserve a pillow that's just right for you. Many people also have favorite pillowcases, and some enjoy different materials, like flannel in the winter and satin in the summer.

10. *Women: If you go to sleep easily but wake up in the middle of the night,* you may be suffering from an estrogen/progesterone imbalance. Check with your doctor to have your hormones tested using a saliva test.

11. *Don't use alcohol to wind down at the end of the day.* One glass of wine with dinner is normally fine, but excess alcohol will disturb your sleep cycle. Typically, you'll fall asleep easily but awaken in the night. Getting back to sleep can then be difficult.

12. *Take a bath before bed;* relaxingly warm but not overly hot. Add your favorite bath oil or gel and soak your cares away.

13. *Use a deep relaxation technique or audiotape.* Tapes are available that combine soothing music or nature sounds with an effective guided relaxation voiceover (see Appendix B).

14. *Try one or more of the following just before bed to help induce sleep:*

- Melatonin: A natural hormone produced by your brain that sets your sleep/wake cycle. Start with a very low dose (0.25 milligrams) in a sublingual tablet twenty to thirty minutes before bed.
- Sedative herbal extracts: Valerian, hops, passion flower, and white zapote. Try a dropperful in a cup of hot, soothing tea.
- Kava: Kava is an herb from the South Pacific shown to help relax tense muscles.[55] Kava is also excellent

for decreasing anxiety.[56] Take a 200-milligram dose of kava extract standardized to 70 milligrams of kava lactones.

- Calcium citrate: 600 milligrams about thirty to forty-five minutes before bedtime.
- Magnesium citrate: 300 milligrams about thirty to forty-five minutes before bedtime.
- A mug of herbal coffee with milk: The natural potassium and calcium will help you relax, and you'll feel warm and full.
- A cup of sedative herbal tea: Look for suggestions in Chapter 9.
- A mug of hot milk and honey: The calcium helps you relax, and the honey is soothing.

15. *If insomnia still persists,* you may want to try certain prescription medications such as amitriptyline (Elavil) or doxepin (Sinequan). These are often prescribed to promote Stage 4 sleep. Note that these are not sleeping pills, but antidepressants. In low doses, these agents appear to enhance Stage 4 sleep, and if you are suffering from fibromyalgia or chronic fatigue, your physician may suggest using one of them. I don't recommend prescription sleeping pills, as these drugs interfere with deep sleep and dreaming.

In this book, I have often referred to evolutionary biology, what I call the "long view" of human history. The value of this approach is that it puts so much into clear perspective. Today, for example, there are dozens of conflicting theories as to what is the optimal diet. There is also widespread disagreement regarding exercise and other lifestyle factors. But the evolutionary biologist steps back and says, "How was the human organism designed? What have we been doing for the last 1.6 million years?" That line of inquiry cuts through all the theories and conjecture because you realize that we are, in every respect, natural creatures tied to nature in profound and powerful ways.

The fact that we have invented electric lights does not mean that sleep is no longer important for health and wellness. The fact that we have invented automobiles and television doesn't mean that we can become sedentary and not suffer terribly at some point. Sure, we have invented sugar, hydrogenated fat, caffeine, artificial colors, white flour, modified food starch, margarine, and a long list of chemicalized "foods," but that does not mean that these things are harmless when consumed day after day.

For 1.6 million years (possibly much longer), we ate nothing but whole, natural foods. We drank nothing but pure, clean water. We slept all night and kept active through most of the day. Those are the conditions for which we are designed, and to a great extent, our effort today to regain and maintain optimal health come down to duplicating these simple behaviors as closely as possible. The good news, of course, is that with exercise technology, nutrition science, and brain research, we have incredible tools that our ancestors never had. This secret is to take advantage of what can truly be the best of both worlds.

Conclusion

Thus we come to the coffee paradox—the question of how a drug so fraught with potential hazard can be consumed in the United States at the rate of more than a hundred billion doses a year without doing intolerable damage—and without arousing the kind of hostility, legal repression and social condemnation aroused by the illicit drugs.

The answer is quite simple. Coffee, tea, cocoa, and the cola drinks have been domesticated.

—Edward Brecher and associates,
Licit & Illicit Drugs

A Question of Balance

We are all very familiar with the idea of balance. We apply the concept to the color tones of our television sets, the bass and treble settings of our stereos, our tires, decor, and stock portfolios. But the balance that undoubtedly affects us the most, that determines to a great extent how well and how long we live, is the balance of our bodies and minds. In medical terms, this balance is known as homeostasis. It's the state of well-being characterized by a sense of peak functioning—physically, mentally, and emotionally.

And this is a state we all desire. It's the feeling that we are moving through life with a sense of control instead of being caught in an endless stream of events to which we must continuously react and adjust. Homeostasis is critical to life and survival, and so our bodies and minds are quite good at restoring balance. It is the essence of the self-regulating, self-repairing miracle that we are.

Our bodies have intricate and sophisticated systems for restoring and maintaining homeostasis: biological clocks, a complex system that continuously monitors and adjusts the pH of the blood, a vast array of hormones, coenzymes, and feedback information loops all designed for one thing: balance. The body as a whole is kept in balance because each individual system, and ultimately every one of our 75 trillion cells, is maintained in a balanced state.

Stress is the force that disturbs balance or homeostasis. Obviously, some stress is necessary and unavoidable. Accomplishing anything involves a measure of stress, and most of the time we know when we're out of balance and we know what we need to do to get it back. At the end of a particularly hectic day, we might use exercise and relaxation to wind down and restore our sense of peace. A warm bath and a few extra hours of sleep can work wonders.

But it is easy to see that most people today experience more stress than is desirable. And there comes a point where the sheer *quantity* of stress becomes unmanageable. You know this to be true, possibly because you've suffered from stress-related illness or perhaps because you've watched other people fall apart, unable to restore balance in their lives. It's extremely painful, and the point we have to remember is that it's *preventable*. Stress is not like a virus that we are exposed to from another person's sneeze. It's the result of decisions that we make on a day-to-day basis.

This book is about caffeine, a drug that induces and magnifies stress. I believe that we need to consider its effects carefully just as we consider all the other facets of life that affect our ability to maintain balance.

We make decisions about how many hours of sleep we get. We make decisions about what and when to eat, how much alcohol we consume, how many hours we are willing to work, what kind of music we listen to, and when to take a vacation. But the caffeine decision has been difficult for most people because they just didn't have the facts. And since everyone was drinking coffee, tea, and soft drinks by the gallon, it was hard to believe that these beverages could be harmful.

The Two Sides of Stress:
A Personal Anecdote

Caffeine Blues has focused a great deal of attention on the negative aspects of stress, but there is a positive side as well, and the key, as I understand it, is this concept of balance.

I was traveling through the islands of the South Pacific, sitting one afternoon on a hotel porch looking out across a stunningly beautiful bay. In fact, I was very sensitive at that moment to the feeling of serenity and balance that I was enjoying. Then one of my fellow travelers started musing about how far it was to the opposite shore and how long it would take to swim it. I guessed it was at least a mile, and he suggested a race across the bay. Within minutes, my perfect state of balance was altered. Part of me was excited about the challenge. Win or lose, it had to be a high point of the trip.

By the time we got to water's edge, I could feel my heart beating slightly faster. Already, you see, my body was responding to the stress of competition. We eagerly dove into the water, and I started a slow and steady pace. In the back of my mind there was a slight fear. After all, this was going to be a long swim across an unknown body of water. But the South Pacific breeze was gentle and intoxicating, and I was enjoying the rhythmic movement of my body through the warm sea.

As I swam, my body made continual adjustments to maintain balance. My muscles demanded more and more oxygen and my breathing increased to provide it. I was aware of breathing more rapidly and deeply but, unknown to me, biochemicals including coenzyme Q10 were pouring into my bloodstream to enhance the extraction of oxygen from each breath. Fatty acid oxidase enzymes were being mobilized to enhance the utilization of fat to create even more energy for the muscles. After about thirty minutes, I stopped to get my bearings. Looking back at the hotel, I was pleased to see that I had made it about halfway across the bay. Since my friend was nowhere in sight, I figured I must be way ahead or way behind. Since I was feeling good, I picked up the pace, making my way toward the opposite shore.

Suddenly I was seized by a terrible pain. I had swum right into a colony of jellyfish. Their stinging tentacles raked over my face, arms, and chest, and I felt as if my skin were on fire. Since the tentacles of a jellyfish can extend a hundred feet, there was no way to escape their poisonous sting but to swim harder and faster. The adrenaline rush sent enormous amounts of energy to my legs and arms to accomplish this.

But what followed was quite surprising. I was in incredible pain, but I was also aware of every facet of my existence, every minute detail of my surroundings. And this heightened sense was simply part of the stress response. In a split second, my brain had analyzed the situation, identified the problem, and was looking for solutions. My eyesight improved as I scanned the horizon for help. There were sailboats in the bay, but my brain instantly calculated that the opposite shore was closer. Since there was no one in sight, shouting was futile and would waste energy.

As I continued swimming, my mind raced through everything I had learned about jellyfish in marine biology. The poison released by the tentacles is actually a neurotoxin, only slightly less powerful than cobra venom. At that moment, my body was producing massive amounts of antibodies to this toxin, trying to keep it from circulating to my heart, lungs, and kidneys. With a shudder, I remembered that men have died from the stings of jellyfish. Still, I reasoned, as long as I remained calm and continued swimming, I would survive.

A minute later, however, I tasted blood and realized that the welts on my face and chest were raw and bleeding. A new fear swept over me, knowing that a shark can sense blood from a distance of nearly a mile. This sent a second rush of adrenaline through my body, and I have to say that I swam faster in those last 200 yards than ever in my life before or since. Fortunately, when I reached the shore, my friends were waiting to congratulate me. Instead, when they saw my condition, they rushed me to the local hospital.

Medically, there's not much you can do about jellyfish stings. Nurses applied a paste of ammonia and herbs that was supposed to neutralize the toxin but actually made the pain worse. My face swelled up like a boxer after a terrible beating, but other than that, it was just a matter of waiting for my body to restore balance.

Looking back, I am still amazed by the power of this survival mechanism. The stress response triggered the release of endorphins, which enabled me to continue swimming without being overcome by pain. The same adrenal hormones helped to create astounding amounts of energy. In the span of less than thirty minutes, my muscles used up all available carbohydrate, every gram of available fat, and even broke down protein to fuel the effort.

The adrenal response also created inflammation to localize the toxin and mobilize the immune system. It increased the clotting ability of my blood to minimize blood loss, and heightened every sensory organ to maximize my chance of survival.

Although I was released from the hospital that same evening, it took weeks for my body to recover fully. That was simply because my balancing mechanism and my "energy reserves" were exhausted. I felt like an invalid, hardly able to get out of bed for more than a few hours at a time. I was reminded of chronic fatigue patients who told me stories of simple tasks like grocery shopping taking half a day. Adrenal exhaustion is terribly debilitating.

I am going to suggest that we are all, to some degree, in this vulnerable state of stress response and recovery. It may not be jellyfish, mile-long swims, and the fear of sharks, but it could be job stress, bills to pay, crying children, and traffic jams. And in this modern world, there is a raft of additional stressors, including the pollution of our air, water, and food, all of which upset and tax our biochemical balance.

Each time we have to deal with one of these stresses, the body does its best to restore balance. My ocean ordeal ended happily, but for many people, the stresses of life accumulate over the years, and recovery takes longer and longer. If you add caffeine to this scenario, you have to understand that recovery may *never* take place fully. Under the biochemical influence of caffeine, the body concludes that stress is *always* going to be present and stops trying to restore balance. Blood pressure, heart rate, and cortisol levels remain elevated. What was meant to be a temporary emergency state becomes a way of life where the pleasures of deep relaxation, peace, and tranquillity are no longer available.

A Matter of Time

To a great extent, stress comes from the time crunch: the twelve-hour workdays and sixty-hour workweeks that have almost become routine in America. Surveys show that nearly half of all adults feel stressed for time due to business, personal, and family responsibilities. What are these people doing to meet the deadlines and make ends meet? They're cutting back on sleep and drinking more caffeine.

It's not hard to see how this happened. The business climate worldwide has changed radically in the last decade. There is no such thing as job security in many industries, and the fear of losing one's job means that employees are willing to put in extra hours, for free if necessary. A veteran of the corporate rat race recently told me that in his company "you're either overworked or unemployed."

Men and Women

Much has been made of the difference in the way men and women deal with the time crunch. Men, for example, tend to reduce time spent with their children and wives. Women, on the other hand, give equal time to job and family, sacrificing personal time to get everything done. On the surface, this implies that men are somehow better off, but the men I talk with feel terrible about this. The problem is that in today's cutthroat business environment, "family man" has taken on a whole new meaning, actually inferring that the man is not a serious player.

Unfortunately, there's someone on nearly every corner offering the harried worker, the busy mom, and stressed-out executive a cup of coffee. But this is like the frenzied man trying to put out the fire in his house by throwing on a bucket of gasoline. His explanation? He couldn't find a bucket of water, and he had to do something!

Saving Minutes, Losing Years

Look at the fast-food industry, still growing at an astounding rate because Americans don't have time to cook—and drive-through windows because we hardly have time to eat. If you look at the foods and beverages served at the rate of hundreds of millions of "meals" per day, you come to a startling realization. The foods, high in salt and saturated fat, combined with beverages laced with caffeine, are direct and powerful contributors to cardiovascular disease.

If such fare is a once-in-a-while thing for you, it's certainly not going to be a problem. But if you find yourself consuming fast food on a regular basis, you have to ask yourself if the minutes you save now will be worth the years you might lose if you die prematurely of a heart attack, stroke, or diabetes.

Then there's the "time management" industry. Don't get me wrong, I think it's important to budget your time and prioritize tasks. But all too often I see people trying to control time, an effort that is futile and stressful in itself. Real time management is not about cramming activities into every minute of every day. It is looking at the time we have in life and making the most of it.

That takes wisdom and vision. It requires that we get in touch with our core desires, and make decisions based on a firm understanding of what truly matters in life. I honestly believe that caffeine has no place in developing or maintaining that perspective. In fact, it supports the opposite mind-set, which is that we are incapable, without this drug, of accomplishing anything of value. In our quantity-oriented society, quality of life is completely forgotten, and at the root of this is a very unhealthy assumption that we are not sufficient, that we must constantly strive for more and more.

In my patient interviews, one of the most common responses regarding coffee was, "I could never do what I have to do without caffeine." People have a dependent relationship with the drug that goes deep into their self-image. The person who openly admits to a dependency on caffeine is saying, "I am not acceptable for who I am. I need to do more, sleep less, strive harder."

The irony of it all, of course, is that caffeine actually doesn't help at all. As I explained in Chapter 4, the drug reduces cognitive skills, impairs cerebral circulation, and hinders your ability to see the big picture. When you come right down to it, caffeine is desirable primarily because it alleviates the miserable feelings associated with withdrawal. No one has difficulty understanding this in relation to cigarette smoking. You take away a smoker's cigarettes and he or she feels terrible. If you give the smoker a cigarette, he or she feels much better. But no sensible person would conclude that smoking is therefore *good* for that smoker.

Likewise, caffeine produces some short-term improvements in mood and behavior, and we as a nation have become dependent on that "lift" with no thought to the long-term consequences. Yet the connection between nicotine and caffeine is closer than you might imagine, in terms of its psychopharmacology.

In one study, habitual users of tobacco and caffeine were asked to abstain from both products. In a short time, their performance on a variety of mental tests was remarkably impaired, even tasks involving simple addition and subtraction! The researchers noted increased ratings of irritability, muscular tension, and headache. The subjects felt "drowsy," "clumsy," and "feeble." All this was accompanied by altered brain wave patterns.[1] Obviously these are not enjoyable feelings, and so the temptation to continue consuming these substances is almost overwhelming.

The Road Less Traveled

More and more people today are realizing the true nature of the stress-caffeine-overwork beast. Books on simplifying one's life are becoming best-sellers, something I don't think could have happened a decade ago. People are starting to realize that, at a certain point, free time rather than economic gain brings value to their lives.

The yearning for a simpler, more relaxed life is very real and very deep. We look to developing countries and envy rural communities for their slower pace of life. They live by the rhythm of the seasons, have time for relationships, family, celebrations, and artistic endeavors. But, inexorably, the modern pace of Western efficiency is bearing down on these cultures, as alarm clocks, calculators, fax machines, and deadlines infiltrate their lives.

My point throughout this book has been that unless you eliminate caffeine, your chances of living a more relaxed and healthier life are practically nil. Life without the pressure of caffeine is definitely the road less traveled. Hopefully by now you're feeling inspired to give it a try. The three steps listed below will help you transform that inspiration into action.

Step One: Resist the Herd Mentality

I'm always amazed when someone tells me about a particular pain or condition in their body, and when I ask how long they've been feeling that way, they answer, "Oh two or three years." It could be lower back pain, depression, tension headaches, insomnia, or an involuntary twitch. People somehow don't tune in to the fact that such conditions are signals that they're *doing something wrong.* They choose instead to cope with the situation (usually with over-the-counter drugs) and continue living in the same way.

Of course, one only needs to watch TV for a few evenings to learn where this behavior comes from. There is certainly no shortage of manufacturers who will gladly help you cope, with pills to help you sleep, reduce your pain, calm your nerves, and settle your stomach. At times, I imagine a giant conspiracy where such pill manufacturers pay huge kickbacks to the caffeine industry for supplying so many suffering customers.

What I teach my students is that this behavior is abnormal. "If smoke started pouring into this classroom," I ask, "would you be concerned?" The next question: "What would you think if someone appeared in the smoke-filled door, saying 'Don't worry folks, I've turned off the fire alarm'?"

Now, my students all laugh because the scenario is absurd. We all know that smoke is a worrisome sign and disconnecting the alarm is not the same as putting out the fire. Yet Americans spend over $200 billion on prescription and OTC drugs every year, the vast majority of which do nothing to cure the underlying cause of pain and illness. And look at the top sellers: ulcer medications are number one, followed by antidepressants and tranquilizers. Clearly, the stress-caffeine factor is a *major* part of most people's illness and pain.

But you would never know that by looking around. Practically everyone you see is on caffeine at least part of the day, and they consider it to be perfectly normal and harmless. Hopefully, this book will help bring people to a clear understanding of caffeine's real effects and break the conspiracy of silence that has existed for so long.

A friend of mine related a very revealing story. She worked for a large metropolitan newspaper and was writing a story for the lifestyle section on stress management techniques. She covered the current understanding about visualization techniques and guided imagery, collected research on meditation, interviewed yoga teachers and biofeedback technicians. She also included her own story of how her life changed when she got off coffee. Her editor returned the rough draft with the coffee paragraphs Xed out in red. When she protested, he told her simply that people don't want to read bad things about coffee. "But," she protested, "this is an article about stress reduction. How can we not mention caffeine?" "Easy," he said, "we run this kind of story every year and we never talk about coffee. Accent the *positive.*"

The truth is, of course, that you can meditate, repeat a mantra, imagine yourself on a peaceful mountaintop, listen to soothing music—and not one of those techniques will relax you if there's caffeine and stress hormones in your muscles, brain, and bloodstream. If only the editors, journalists, and doctors would look at the big picture and acknowledge that reducing caffeine is the *first* essential step in any stress-management program, we'd all be much better off. In many cases, getting off caffeine determines the actual outcome of the stress-management therapy or technique. For example, individuals with high blood pressure who drink coffee do not achieve the same benefits from meditation as nondrinkers. It is, as I have said many times, like trying to fill a leaky bucket.

Step Two: Listen to Your Body

All of us at times get so caught up in the busyness and stress of life that we ignore clear warning signs of impending illness. For many people these warning signs are never heeded, and they end up in the hospital or funeral home. You've heard the phrase "Listen to your body," but you might be wondering exactly what that means. For me, it means taking an inventory a few times each week of how I'm feeling, both physically and emotionally.

I suggest you do this in a quiet place when you have a few minutes you can spend alone. Pay careful attention to any tightening in the chest, tension or pain in the stomach or solar plexus (your "gut" feelings), any clenching or pain in the jaw, tremor in the fingers or legs (restless leg syndrome), and involuntary twitching in limbs, eyelids, or face. These are all signs of accumulating stress, danger signals that need to be dealt with while they are still minor.

Watch your breath rising from the solar plexus up to your lungs. Feel the rib cage expand and the collarbones rise. Then watch the exhalation, feeling the relaxation and letting go of the breath and body. Take time to feel the sensations that come and go, and in a few minutes, you will have a clear connection to your emotional state.

If you're feeling anxious or worried at all, ask yourself what is the source of your discomfort or anxiety. Is it something you can resolve, and if so, what course of action needs to be taken? For many people, the source of discomfort and anxiety is vague and unclear. It's been described as "background stress," and I suggest that caffeine is at the core of such feelings.

It's important to understand that stress and anxiety *affect every part of you.* I've described in detail the impact that stress has on the body and mind, but on a more subtle level, it affects who you are. The sage advice to "know thyself" is an important part of self-mastery. It helps us tune in to what is truly important and meaningful. Life is short, and we really don't want to be "spinning our wheels," or wasting precious time on matters that do not enrich us.

I believe it is nearly impossible to gain this perspective

when you're amped out on caffeine. Scores of people have told me over the years that the most significant change they noticed when they got off caffeine was in their personality, how they related to their family, friends, and colleagues. This is the very essence of who we are as individuals and how we act together as a society.

Step Three: Start with What's in Front of You

In my clinical practice, I saw people who were for the most part highly motivated to improve their health and their lives. Often they were seeking guidance on exercise, nutrition, stress management, and human performance. I learned an important lesson in those years. When I sent them home with lots of things to do, they were often overwhelmed, and so, out of frustration, they did nothing. But the people who left with one or two changes to employ often made those changes and came back for more. These were the people whose lives were changed, who got on the upward spiral and never got off. Today, they are living proof that health and vitality can be enjoyed at any age, that life can be a wonderfully exciting and deeply fulfilling adventure.

So when it comes to change, I recommend you start with what's in front of you. Start with a single step that will improve your physical, mental, and emotional health in myriad ways. Get off the caffeine drug, and find out who you really are.

APPENDIX A

Fifty Proven Stress Reducers

1. A lot of things are "stressful" simply because we don't allow ourselves enough time to get them done. Look for ways to take the hurry out of your everyday tasks and responsibilities.
2. Get out of bed fifteen minutes earlier to avoid the morning rushing around.
3. Prepare for the morning the evening before. (Set out clothes, breakfast, sack lunch, etc.)
4. Write things down; don't rely on your memory. (Trying to remember not to forget is stressful.)
5. Ask questions, repeat back directions, repeat back what you heard the other person say, etc. Taking an extra minute to be sure you understand what was said can save time and prevent aggravation.
6. Keep a duplicate car key in your wallet; bury a duplicate house key in your garden.
7. Practice "preventive maintenance" on your car, appliances, teeth, personal relationships, etc., so they won't break down at the worst possible moment.
8. Add an ounce of love to everything you do.
9. Eat healthful foods. Don't overeat (always leave the table feeling a little hungry).

10. Procrastination is stressful. Whatever you want to do tomorrow, do it today; whatever you want today, do it now. Hard work is simply the accumulation of easy things you didn't do when you should have done them.

11. Organize your home and work area so that everything has a place. You won't have to go through the stress of losing things.

12. Plan ahead. Don't let the gas tank get below one-quarter full, keep a well-stocked "emergency shelf" of supplies at home and at work. Buy postage stamps and bus tokens before you need them, etc.

13. Schedule a realistic day. Allow ample time between appointments. Make a "to-do" list and cut it in half.

14. Relax your standards. The world will not end if the grass doesn't get mowed this weekend.

15. An instant cure for most stress: thirty minutes of brisk walking or other aerobic exercise.

16. Make everyday purchases by cash or check; save credit cards for major planned purchases.

17. Make friends with nonworriers.

18. Every day, find time for solitude and introspection. Seek out quiet places.

19. Resolve to be tender with the young, compassionate with the aged, sympathetic with the striving, and tolerant with the weak and erring—for sometime in life you will have been all of these.

20. Simplify.

21. Say "No, thank you" to projects you don't have time or energy for.

22. Always carry reading material to enjoy while waiting in lines or for appointments.

23. Remind yourself that Babe Ruth struck out 1,330 times.

24. For every one thing that goes wrong, there are 50 to 100 blessings. Count them.

25. Do nothing that, after being done, leads you to tell a lie.

26. Put brain in gear before opening mouth. Before saying anything, ask yourself if what you are to say is (1) true, (2) kind, and (3) necessary. If it's not all three, K.M.S. (Keep Mouth Shut).

27. If an unpleasant task faces you, do it early in the day and get it over with.

28. Do one thing at a time.

29. Donate extra belongings to your favorite charity. Getting rid of what you don't need will make what you do need easier to find.

30. Write your thoughts and feelings in a journal. This can help you clarify your ideas and put things in their right perspective.

31. When someone cuts you off in traffic, stops suddenly in front of you, etc., instead of getting mad, think of all the driving mistakes you've made in your life—and give the other guy a break.

32. Remember that everyone around you is carrying some kind of burden.

33. Get enough sleep. Use an alarm clock to remind you to go to bed, if necessary.

34. Set up contingency plans. "If either of us is delayed, here's what we'll do." "If we get separated in the mall, here's where we'll meet," etc.

35. To relax instantly, breathe as if you were trying in inflate an imaginary balloon in your stomach. Inhale slowly to the count of 10; then exhale slowly to the count of 10. Repeat.

36. Turn "needs" into preferences. Our body's basic needs are food, water, and keeping warm. Everything else is a preference.

37. Don't put up with things that don't work right. Get things fixed or replace them.

38. Stop worrying. If something concerns you, do something about it. If you can't do anything about it, let go of it.
39. Practice labeling situations differently. Are you really "furious" about something, or are you simply feeling angry or annoyed? Are you "crushed," or are you merely let down or disappointed? If World War II was "terrible," can you describe your flat tire as "terrible"? No, at worst, it was an inconvenience. Resisting the temptation to exaggerate situations, and labeling situations with the appropriate word, can reduce stress.
40. Live in the present.
41. Every day, do at least one thing you really enjoy.
42. Be kind to unkind people—they probably need it most.
43. Unplug your phone or switch on your phone answering machine while you take a bath, have dinner, etc.
44. Don't sweat the small stuff.
45. Laugh! It puts distance between you and your problems.
46. Make promises sparingly and keep them faithfully.
47. Remember that the best things in life aren't things.
48. Buy clothes and shoes that are: (1) comfortable, (2) easy and inexpensive to maintain, (3) easy to match with other clothes you have.
49. Using the TV or radio for background "company" can be surprisingly stressful. Learn to enjoy quiet.
50. Forget about counting to 10. Count to 100 before saying anything that could make matters worse.

Reprinted with permission. Hope Publications, Kalamazoo, Michigan.
www.hopepublications.com

APPENDIX B

Resources

PRIMARY RESOURCE

www.caffeineblues.com

OPTIONS AND ALTERNATIVES

Herbal Coffee

Teeccino Caffé, Inc.
P.O. Box 42259
Santa Barbara, CA 93105
800-498-3434
www.teeccino.com
e-mail: Teeccino@aol.com

Teeccino caffeine-free herbal coffee is available in seven flavors. The company sends out literature and a 50¢ discount coupon for free. They offer a Teeccino sampler consisting of four different flavors for $5. Teeccino is distributed to natural foods stores in the United States, Britain, and Canada. The company sells directly to consumers via catalog.

Instant Coffee Substitutes

Postum Instant Hot Beverage
Maxwell House Coffee Company
Kraft General Foods, Inc.
Box PR7
White Plains, NY 10625
1-800-432-6333

Instant grain beverage made from wheat bran, wheat, molasses, and maltodextrin. Available in grocery stores.

Kaffree Roma Roasted Grain Beverage
Worthington Foods, Inc.
900 Proprietors Rd
Columbus, OH 43805-3194
618-885-9511
www.wfds.com

Instant grain beverage imported from Germany made from roasted barley malt, barley, and chicory. Available in natural foods stores and some grocery stores.

Pero Instant Natural Beverage
Unifranck of Germany
Distributed by Alpursa
P.O. Box 25846
Salt Lake City, UT 84125-0846

Instant grain beverage imported from Germany made from malted barley, barley, chicory, and rye. Available in natural food stores and some grocery stores.

Herb Teas, Tea, and Organically Grown Tea

The Republic of Tea
8 Digital Drive, Suite 100
Novato, CA 94949-5759
800-298-4TEA
www.republicoftea.com

The Republic of Tea distributes its full line of teas, including eleven organic teas, to specialty stores and natural food stores nationwide. They sell direct to consumers via their catalog, which also features tea wares. Annual donations are made from the sales of their Rainforest Tea to local, nongovernmental organizations in Mexico that work to preserve the rain forest and improve the quality of life for people who live in fragile rain forest regions.

Seelect Herb Tea Co.
P.O. Box 1969
Camarillo, CA 93011-1969
888-273-3532

Seelect distributes single and blended herbal teas, including some organic herbs, to natural food stores in the United States and Canada. Upon request, the company sends out a sample and literature.

Traditional Medicinals
4515 Ross Rd
Sebastopol, CA 95472-2250
707-823-8911

Traditional markets its line of teas through natural food stores and some grocery stores in the United States and Canada. Call to request a free sample and catalog. The company adheres to socially and environmentally responsible business practices.

Long Life Herbal Teas
111 Canfield Ave, #B-6
Randolph, NJ 07869
800-645-5768, ext VT 1296

An environmentally conscious tea company offering many organic herbal blends. Sold in health-food stores nationwide.

Celestial Seasonings
4600 Sleepytime Dr
Boulder, CO 80301-3292
800-351-8175
www.celestialseasonings.com

Celestial Seasonings distributes its full line of teas through grocery and natural food stores worldwide. You can order merchandise and teas from their mail-order catalog.

Yogi Tea Co.
1616 Preuss Rd
Los Angeles, CA 90035-4212
800-YOGI-TEA
www.yogitea.com

Yogi Tea has made a commitment to source organically grown herbs whenever available for all of their teas. Call to request a free natural products catalog and a sample of Yogi tea. Yogi Tea is distributed in the United States, Europe, and Canada in natural food stores and some grocery stores.

Tazo
P.O. Box 66
Portland, OR 97207-0066
800-299-9445

Tazo distributes its full line of teas and microbrewed bottled tea and juice to specialty and natural food stores. They also sell direct to consumers via catalog.

Silk Road Teas
P.O. Box 287
Lagunitas, CA 94938
415-488-9017

Silk Road Teas offers a rich variety of white, green, oolong, black, and pu-erh teas, some of which are unavailable from any other source. Most importantly, they work with established tea gardens in China and help to develop organic practices. Call for catalog.

Brew Ware

French presspots, gold-tone filters, and loose-leaf brewing filters can be purchased at department stores, specialty coffee shops, and gourmet food stores or directly from some mail-order catalogs. The following brands are recommended:

- The People's Brew Basket from the Republic of Tea. Fits ten-ounce mugs.
- Swiss Gold Cup o' Tea Permanent Tea Filter. Fits any size mug.
- Swiss Gold One Cup Drip filter for coffee or herbal coffee. Great for making a single cup of coffee.
- French press pots and tea pots from Bodum
- Krups, Swiss Gold, and Mr. Coffee gold-tone filters for both cone and flat-bottom coffeemakers

Organically Grown Shade Coffee

Allegro Coffee Company
1930 Central Ave
Boulder, CO 80301
www.allegro-coffee.com
800-277-1107

Supports Coffee Kids, a nonprofit organization working to improve the life of the families and communities who harvest coffee beans. Distributed in natural foods stores and sells direct to consumers via mail-order catalog.

Cafe Altura
Clean Food Inc.
760 East Santa Maria St
Santa Paula, CA 93060
800-526-8328

Organically grown estate coffee. Biodynamic certification. Supports Natural History Chapter of Chiapas, Mexico, and private conservation endeavors in Mexico. Sold in natural food stores.

Equal Exchange
250 Revere St
Canton, MA 02021
781-830-0279
www.equalexchange.com

Follows fair trade principles, member of Fair Trade Federation. Offers preharvest financing to small-scale farmer cooperatives that are democratically run. Sells under brand name Equal Exchange Coffee in retail. Sells direct to consumers via mail-order catalog.

Frontier Cooperative
P.O. Box 299
Norway, IA 52318-0299
800-669-3275

Frontier organically grown coffee is purchased from co-ops.

Thanksgiving Coffee Company
Box 1918
Fort Bragg, CA 95437
800-648-6491
www.thanksgivingcoffee.com

Supports American Birding Association programs, which help fund Partners in Flight, a neotropical bird conservation project.

NUTRITIONAL SUPPORT AND INFORMATION

MaxCell Bioscience
100 Technology Drive
Suite 160
Broomfield, CO 80021
1-800-MaxCell
www.MaxCell.com
President: Stephen Cherniske

Bioenergetic nutrition, exercise and deep relaxation audio tapes.

Advanced Physicians Products
831 State Street
Suite 280
Santa Barbara, CA 93101
800-220-7687
President: Kenneth Frank, M.D.

TOOLS FOR RELAXATION, STRESS MANAGEMENT, AND CONFLICT RESOLUTION

Preventive Medicine Research Institute
900 Bridgeway #1
Sausalito, CA 94965
800-775-PMRI
415-332-2525
President: Dean Ornish, M.D.

Ojai Foundation
Education Retreat
9739 Ojai Santa Paula Road
Ojai, CA 93023
805-646-8343

School of Lost Borders
Box 55
Big Pine, CA 93513
760-938-1177
Attn: Virginia Coyle

The Association for Applied
Psychotherapy and
Biofeedback (AAPB)
10200 W. 44th Ave #304
Wheat Ridge, CO 80033
303-422-8336

Institute of HeartMath
P.O. Box 1463
Boulder Creek, CA 95006
831-338-8700

YOGA AND EXERCISE

White Lotus Foundation
2500 San Marcos Pass
Santa Barbara, CA 93105
800-544-FLOW
www.whitelotus.org

Yoga instruction, teachers' training, retreats, videotapes.

Satchidananda Yoga
Ashram
Box 172
Route #1

Buckingham, VA 23921
800-969-3121

Certifying Organizations for Fitness Trainers

American College of
Sports Medicine
P.O. Box 1440
Indianapolis, IN 46206
317-637-9200

Aerobics and Fitness
Association of America
15250 Ventura Blvd, Suite 310
Sherman Oaks, CA 91403
800-446-2322

IDEA International
Association of Fitness
Professionals
6190 Cornerstone Ct East,
Suite 204
San Diego, CA 92121-3773
800-999-4332

LABORATORIES— HORMONE SALIVA TESTS

Aeron Life Cycles
San Leandro, CA
800-631-7900
510-729-0383

Diagnos-Techs, Inc.
6620 S. 192nd Place
Suite J-104
Kent, WA 98032
800-878-3787
206-251-0596

APPENDIX C

Your Off the Bean Journal

A RECORD OF YOUR SUCCESS IN REDUCING OR ELIMINATING
CAFFEINE FROM YOUR DIET

Before you begin your Off the Bean program, answer the
following questions. Make a copy of this evaluation first
so that you can retest yourself at thirty-, sixty-, and ninety-
day intervals: DATE: _____

1. Using the information in Chapter 2, calculate how much
caffeine you consume daily.

<100 mg   200 mg   300 mg   400 mg   500 mg   >600 mg

2. Note any of the following symptoms you suffer from:

Score a "1" for occasional, "2" for frequently, and "3" for constant.

Emotions
___ Anxiety/nervousness
___ Irritability, anger, or
      aggressiveness
___ Mood swings
___ Depression
___ Panic attacks

Energy
___ Energy swings
___ Fatigue, sluggishness
___ Poor concentration
___ Restlessness
___ Hyperactivity

Digestion
___ Ulcers
___ Acid indigestion
___ Heartburn
___ Bloating/gas
___ Diarrhea
___ Colitis
___ Irritable bowel
  syndrome

Heart
___ Irregular or rapid heartbeat
___ High blood pressure

Skin
___ Skin rashes
___ Aging skin
___ Dry skin

General
___ Gout
___ Candida/yeast infections
___ Neck, shoulder, or back pain
___ High cholesterol
___ Bladder/Urinary tract infections

Other
___ _____
___ _____

Head
___ Tension headache
___ Migraine
___ Dizziness
___ Tinnitus (Ringing
  in the ears)

Blood Sugar
___ [Diabetics] Wide
  blood sugar swings
___ Low blood sugar

Sleep
___ Difficulty falling
  asleep
___ Difficulty staying
  asleep
___ Tired upon arising

Women's Health
___ Premenstrual
  tension (PMS)
___ Fibrocystic breast
  disease
___ Low iron

Men's Health
___ Enlarged prostate
___ Urinary symptoms

TOTAL SCORE: _____

3. Note any particular times of the day when your energy routinely slumps:

Upon arising	2–3 P.M.
8–9 A.M.	4–5 P.M.
10–11 A.M.	6–7 P.M.
12–1 P.M.	8–9 P.M.

4. How often do you exercise?   5. How long do you exercise?

    0–1 x week   10–15 minutes
    2–4 x week   15–30 minutes
    5+ x week   30+ minutes

6. How intense is your   7. How do you feel after you
    exercise?   exercise?

easy   medium   hard   exhausted   tired   invigorated

8. How would you rate   9. Are you alert upon
    your energy level?   awakening?

low   medium   high   never   sometimes   often

10. How would you rate   11. Do you experience
     your ability to cope   sugar cravings?
     with stress?

low   medium   high   frequently   sometimes   never

12. Rate your mental clarity.   13. Rate your overall
                                 emotional state.

foggy average   sharp   depressed   erratic   balanced

Retest yourself thirty days, sixty days, and ninety days after initiating your Off the Bean program. Compare your score and progress. Note below any observations or improvements you experience that aren't covered above:

NOTES

Introduction

[1]M. L. Arbeit, T. A. Nicklas, G. C. Frank et al., "Caffeine Intakes of Children from a Biracial Population: The Bogalusa Heart study," *Journal of the American Dietetic Association*, April 1988;88(4):466–71.

Chapter 1

[1]S. Y. Tse, "Cholinomimetic Compound Distinct from Caffeine Contained in Coffee II: Muscarinic Actions," *Journal of Pharmaceutical Sciences*, May 1992;81(5):449–52.

[2]World Health Organization International Agency for Research on Cancer, "Coffee, Tea, Mate, Methylxanthines, and Methylgloxal," *International Agency for Research on Cancer Monograph Evaluation of Carcinogen Risks in Humans*, 1991;51:1–513.

[3]R. M. Gilbert, "Caffeine as a Drug of Abuse," in R. J. Gibbins et al. (eds.), *Research Advances in Alcohol and Drug Problems* (New York: John Wiley & Sons, 1976), pp. 49–176.

[4]R. N. Warren, "Metabolism of Xanthine Alkaloids in Man," *Journal of Chromatography*, 1969;40:468–69.

[5]J. J. Barone and H. R. Roberts, "Caffeine Consumption," *Food and Chemical Toxicology*, 1996;34(1):119–29.

[6]A. Koczapski, J. Paredes, C. Kogan et al., "Effects of Caffeine on Behavior of Schizophrenic Inpatients," *Schizophrenia Bulletin*, 1989;15(2):339–44.

[7]P. B. Lucas, D. Pickar, J. Kelsoe et al., "Effects of the Acute Administration of Caffeine in Patients with Schizophrenia," *Biological Psychiatry*, 1990;28(1):35–40.

[8]B. Stavric, R. Klasses, B. Watkinson et al., "Variability in Caffeine Consumption from Coffee and Tea: Possible Significance for Epidemiological Studies," *Food and Chemical Toxicology*, 1988;26:111–18.

NOTES

[9]R. M. Gilbert, J. A. Marshman, M. Schwieder et al., "Caffeine Content of Beverages as Consumed," *Canadian Medical Association Journal,* 1976;114:205–08.

Chapter 2

[1]"Combating Caffeine's Arrhythmogenic Potential," *Postgraduate Medicine,* 1992;9(1):57–58.

[2]Food and Drug Administration, *Caffeine Content of Various Products,* FDA, Washington, D.C. Paper T80-45, 1980.

[3]"Coffee Craze Stirs Up Some New Headaches," *Family Practice News,* 1996;26(6):21.

[4]G. Bovim, P. Naess, J. Helle et al., "Caffeine Influence on the Motor Steadiness Battery in Neuropsychological Tests," *Journal of Clinical and Experimental Neuropsychology,* May 1995;17(3):472–76.

[5]M. J. Shirlow and C. D. Mathers, "A Study of Caffeine Consumption and Symptoms: Indigestion, Palpitations, Tremor, Headache and Insomnia," *International Journal of Epidemiology,* June 1985;14(2):239–48.

[6]V. Saano and M. M. Airaksinen, "Binding of Beta-carbolines and Caffeine on Benzodiazepine Receptors: Correlations to Convulsions and Tremor," *Acta Pharmacologica et Toxicologica,* Copenhagen, October 1982;51(4):300–08.

[7]B. H. Jacobson, K. Winter-Roberts, and H. A. Gemmell, "Influence of Caffeine on Selected Manual Manipulation Skills," *Perceptual and Motor Skills,* June 1991;72(Pt 2):1175–81.

[8]J. R. Hughes, S. T. Higgins, W. K. Bickel et al., "Caffeine Self-Administration, Withdrawal, and Adverse Effects among Coffee Drinkers," *Archives of General Psychiatry,* July 1991;48(7):611–17.

[9]H. Schroeder, H. Siegmund, G. Santibanez et al., "Causes and Signs of Temporomandibular Joint Pain and Dysfunction: An Electromyographical Investigation," *Journal of Oral Rehabilitation,* July 1991;18(4):301–10.

[10]C. J. Pierce, K. Chrisman, M. E. Bennett et al., "Stress, Anticipatory Stress, and Psychologic Measures Related to Sleep Bruxism," *Journal of Orofacial Pain,* Winter 1995;9(1):51–56.

[11]J. R. Hughes, S. T. Higgins, W. K. Bickel et al., "Caffeine Self-Administration, Withdrawal, and Adverse Effects among Coffee Drinkers," *Archives of General Psychiatry,* July 1991;48(7):611–17.

[12]E. C. Strain, G. K. Mumford, K. Silverman et al., "Caffeine Dependence Syndrome: Evidence from Case Histories and Experimental Evaluations," *Journal of the American Medical Association,* 1994;272:1043–48.

Chapter 3

[1]R. J. Thomas, "Caffeine and Arrhythmias: What Are the Risks?," *Your Patient & Fitness,* 1991;5(5):6–8.

NOTES

[2]M. Vincent-Viry, Z. B. Pontes, R. Gueguen et al., "Segregation Analyses of Four Urinary Caffeine Metabolite Ratios Implicated in the Determination of Human Acetylation Phenotypes," *Genetic Epidemiology,* 1994;11(2):115–29.

[3]J. Soto, M. J. Alsar, and J. A. Sacristan, "Assessment of the Time Course of Drugs with Inhibitory Effects on Hepatic Metabolic Activity Using Successive Salivary Caffeine Tests," *Pharmacotherapy,* November 1995;15(6):781–84.

[4]C. Stratton, "Fluoroquinolone Antibiotics: Properties of the Class and Individual Agents," *Clinical Therapeutics,* May–June 1992;14(3):348–75.

[5]A. H. Staib, W. Stille, G. Dietlein et al., "Interaction between Quinolones and Caffeine," *Drugs,* 1987;34 supplement 1:170–74.

[6]E. Tarrus, E. I. Garcia, D. J. Roberts et al., "An Animal Model for the Detection of Drug-Induced Inhibition of Caffeine Metabolism," *Methods and Findings in Experimental and Clinical Pharmacology,* May 1987:9(5):311–16.

[7]R. A. Upton, "Pharmacokinetic Interactions between Theophylline and Other Medication (Part I)," *Clinical Pharmacokinetics,* January 1991;20(1):66–80.

[8]J. O. Miners, "Drug Interactions Involving Aspirin (Acetylsalicylic Acid) and Salicylic Acid," *Clinical Pharmacokinetics,* November 1989;17(5):327–44.

[9]K. L. Rost and I. Roots, "Accelerated Caffeine Metabolism after Omeprazole Treatment Is Indicated by Urinary Metabolite Ratios: Coincidence with Plasma Clearance and Breath Test," *Clinical Pharmacology and Therapeutics,* April 1994;55(4):402–11.

[10]N. R. Scott, D. Stambuk, J. Chakraborty et al., "Caffeine Clearance and Biotransformation in Patients with Chronic Liver Disease," *Clinical Science,* 1988;74:377–84.

[11]J. A. Swanson, J. W. Lee, J. W. Hopp et al., "The Impact of Caffeine Use on Tobacco Cessation and Withdrawal," *Addictive Behaviors,* January–February 1997; 22(1):55–68.

[12]R. Garcia, "The Cardiovascular Effects of Caffeine," *Caffeine, Coffee and Health.* S. Garattini, (ed.), (New York: Raven Press, 1993).

[13]J. Ferri, "Under Pressure," *The Tampa Tribune-Times,* April 27, 1997, pp. 1–2.

[14]A. Nehlig, J. L. Daval, and G. Debry, "Caffeine and the Central Nervous System: Mechanisms of Action, Biochemical, Metabolic and Psychostimulant Effects," *Brain Research Reviews,* May–August 1992;17(2):139–70.

[15]W. Lovallo, M. Al'Absi, K. Blick et al., "Stress-like Adrenocorticotropin Responses to Caffeine in Young Healthy Men," *Pharmacology, Biochemistry and Behavior,* November 1996;55(3):365–69.

[16]J. M. Nash, "Addicted: Mounting Evidence Points to a Powerful Brain Chemical Called Dopamine," *Time,* May 5, 1997, pp. 68–76.

[17]G. R. Stoner, L. R. Skirboll, S. Werkman et al., "Preferential Effects of Caffeine on Limbic and Cortical Dopamine Systems," *Biological Psychiatry,* April 15, 1988;23(8):761–68.

[18]J. H. Boublik, M. J. Quinn, J. A. Clements et al., "Coffee Contains Potent Opiate Receptor Binding Activity," *Nature,* January 20, 1983;301(5897):246–48.

[19]J. Zhou, S. Olsen, J. Moldovan et al., "Glucocorticoid Regulation of Natural Cyto-

NOTES

toxicity: Effects of Cortisol on the Phenotype and Function of a Cloned Human Natural Killer Cell Line," *Cellular Immunology,* June 15, 1997;178(2):108–16.

[20]I. J. Elenkov, D. A. Papanicolaou, R. L. Wilder et al., "Modulatory Effects of Glucocorticoids and Catecholamines on Human Interleukin-12 and Interleukin-10 Production: Clinical Implications," *Proceedings of the Association of American Physicians,* September 1996;108(5):374–81.

[21]R. Glaser, J. K. Kiecolt-Glaser, R. H. Bonneau et al., "Stress-Induced Modulation of the Immune Response to Recombinant Hepatitis B Vaccine," *Psychosomatic Medicine,* January–February 1992;54(1):22–29.

[22]N. Christeff, N. Gherbi, O. Mammes et al., "Serum Cortisol and DHEA Concentrations During HIV Infection," *Psychoneuroendocrinology,* 1997;22 supplement 1:S11–18.

[23]J. Brind, "Spotlight on DHEA: A Marker for Progression of HIV Infection?" *Journal of Laboratory and Clinical Medicine,* June 1996;127(6):522–23.

[24]P. Salvato et al., "Oral Intake of DHEA Is Associated with Reductions in Viral Load," *International Conference on AIDS,* July 7–12, 1996.

[25]D. C. Mackay and J. W. Rollins, "Caffeine and Caffeinism," *Journal of the Royal Navy Medical Service,* 1989;75(2):65–67.

[26]D. J. Roca, G. D. Schiller, and D. H. Farb, "Chronic Caffeine or Theophylline Exposure Reduces Gamma-Aminobutyric Acid/Benzodiazepine Receptor Site Interactions," *Molecular Pharmacology,* May 1988;33(5):481–85.

[27]C. Stratton, "Fluoroquinolone Antibiotics: Properties of the Class and Individual Agents," *Clinical Therapeutics,* May–June 1992;14(3):348–75; Discussion 347.

[28]B. I. Davies and F. P. Maesen, "Drug Interactions with Quinolones," *Review of Infectious Diseases,* July–August 1989;11 supplement 5:S1083–90.

[29]E. B. Truitt, Jr., "The Xantjhines," in J. R. DiPalma (ed.), *Drill's Pharmacology in Medicine* (New York: McGraw-Hill, 1971), pp. 533–56.

[30]J. M. Ritchie, "Central Nervous Stimulants II: The Xanthines," in L. S. Goodman and A. Gilman (eds.), *The Pharmacological Basis of Therapeutics* (New York: Macmillan, 1970), pp. 358–70.

[31]A. Goldstein, L. Aronow, and S. M. Kalman, *Principles of Drug Action: The Basis of Pharmacology* (New York:Wiley, 1974).

[32]A. N. Nicholson, A. J. Belyavin, and P. A. Pascoe, "Modulation of Rapid Eye Movement Sleep in Humans by Drugs that Modify Monoaminergic and Purinergic Transmission," *Neuropsychopharmacology,* June 1989;2(2):131–43.

[33]H. P. Landolt, D. J. Dijk, S. E. Gaus et al., "Caffeine Reduces Low-frequency Delta Activity in the Human Sleep EEG," *Neuropsychopharmacology,* May 1995; 12(3):229–38.

[34]L. J. Dorfman and M. E. Jarvik, "Comparative Stimulant and Diuretic Actions of Caffeine and Theobromine in Man," *Clinical Pharmacology and Therapeutics,* 1970;11:869–72.

[35]A. Goldstein, R. Warren, and S. Kaizer, "Psychotropic Effects of Caffeine in Man I:

Individual Differences in Sensitivity to Caffeine-Induced Wakefulness," *Journal of Pharmacology and Experimental Therapeutics*, 1965;149:156–59.

[36]H. P. Landolt, E. Werth, A. A. Borbely et al., "Caffeine Intake (200 mg) in the Morning Affects Human Sleep and EEG Power Spectra at Night," *Brain Research*, March 27, 1995;675(1–2):67–74.

[37]V. Wooten, "Sleep Disorders in Geriatric Patients," *Clinics in Geriatric Medicine*, May 1992;8(2):427–39.

[38]N. G. Bliwise, "Factors Related to Sleep Quality in Healthy Elderly Women," *Psychology and Aging*, March 1992;7(1):83–88.

[39]S. L. Brown, M. E. Salive, M. Pahor et al., "Occult Caffeine as a Source of Sleep Problems in an Older Population," *Journal of the American Geriatric Society*, August 1995;43(8):860–64.

[40]J. D. Morrison, "Fatigue as a Presenting Complaint in Family Practice," *Journal of Family Practice*, 1980;10:795.

[41]G. S. Bonham and P. E. Leaverton, "Coffee Use Habits among Adults," in I. S. Scarpa et al. (eds.), *Sourcebook on Food and Nutrition*, vol 2 (Chicago: Marquis Academic Media, 1980), pp. 334–40.

[42]"New Hope for Tired People," *U.S. News & World Report*, October 31, 1988;71–73.

[43]D. M. Graham, "Caffeine: Its Identity, Dietary Sources, Intake, and Biological Effects," *Sourcebook on Food and Nutrition* (Chicago: Marquis Academic Media, 1980).

[44]J. S. Lewis and K. Inove, "Effect of Coffee Ingestion on Urinary Thiamine Excretion," *Federal Proceedings*, 1981;40:914.

[45]D. M. Hilker, K. Chan, R. Chen et al., "Antithiamine Effects of Tea," *Nutrition Reports International*, 1971;4:223–27.

[46]V. Tanphaichitr and B. Wood, "Thiamin," in *Present Knowledge in Nutrition*, fifth edition (Washington D.C.: Nutrition Foundation, 1984), pp. 273–84.

[47]S. L. Vimokesant, S. Kunjara et al. "Beri-beri Caused by Antithiamin Factors in Food and Its Prevention," *Annals of the New York Academy of Sciences*, 1982;378:123–36.

[48]L. Massey and T. Berg, "The Effect of Dietary Caffeine on Urinary Excretion of Calcium, Magnesium, Phosphorus, Sodium, Potassium, Chloride and Zinc in Healthy Males," *Nutrition Research*, 1985;5:1281–84.

[49]Neuhauser-Berthold, S. Beine, C. Verwied et al., "Coffee Consumption and Total Body Water Homeostasis as Measured by Fluid Balance and Bioelectrical Impedance Analysis," *Annals of Nutrition and Metabolism*, 1997;41(1):29–36.

[50]P. Hollingberry and L. Massey, "Effects of Dietary Caffeine and Sucrose on Urinary Calcium Excretion in Adolescents," *Federal Proceedings*, 1986;45:375.

[51]E. A. Bergman, L. K. Massey, K. J. Wise et al., "Effects of Dietary Caffeine on Renal Handling of Minerals in Adult Women," *Life Sciences*, 1990;47(6):557–64.

[52]K. Van Dyck, S. Tas, H. Robberecht et al., "The Influence of Different Food Components on the In Vitro Availability of Iron, Zinc and Calcium from a Composed Meal," *International Journal of Food Science and Nutrition*, November 1996; 47(6):499–506.

[53]G. Wyshak, R. E. Frisch, T. E. Albright et al., "Non-alcoholic Carbonated Beverage Consumption among Women Former Collegiate Athletes," *Journal of Orthopedic Research,* 1989;7:91–99.

[54]G. Wyshak and R. E. Frisch, "Carbonated Beverages, Dietary Calcium, the Dietary Calcium/Phosphorus Ratio, and Bone Fractures in Girls and Boys," *Journal of Adolescent Health,* 1994;15:210–15.

[55]N. Kojima, D. Wallace and G. W. Bates, "The Effect of Chemical Agents, Beverages, and Spinach on the In Vitro Solubilization of Iron from Cooked Pinto Beans," *American Journal of Clinical Nutrition,* 1981;34:1392–1401.

[56]T. A. Morck, S. R. Lynch, and J. D. Cook, "Inhibition of Food Iron Absorption by Coffee," *American Journal of Clinical Nutrition,* 1983;37:416–20.

[57]G. B. Gabrielli and G. De Sandre, "Excessive Tea Consumption Can Inhibit the Efficacy of Oral Iron Treatment in Iron-Deficiency Anemia," *Haematologica,* November 1995;80(66):518–20.

[58]A. C. Bancu, M. Gherman et al., "Regulation of Human Natural Cytotoxicity by IgG. II: Cyclic AMP as a Mediator of Monomeric IgG-induced Inhibition of Natural Killer Cell Activity," *Cellular Immunology,* 1988;114(2):246.

[59]P. T. Paradowski and K. Zeman, "Pentoxifylline," *Postepy Higieny Imedycyny Doswiadczalnej,* 1995;49(2):201–20.

[60]G. Gatti, R. Cavallo, M. L. Sartori et al. "Inhibition by Cortisol of Human Natural Killer (NK) Cell Activity," *Journal of Steroid Biochemistry,* January 1987;26(1):49–58.

[61]H. N. Baybutt and F. Holsboer, "Inhibition of Macrophage Differentiation and Function by Cortisol," *Endocrinology,* July 1990;127(1):476–80.

[62]O. Khorram, L. Vu, and S. S. Yen, "Activation of Immune Function by Dehydroepiandrosterone (DHEA) in Age-Advanced Men," *Journal of Gerontology,* 1997;52A(1):M1–M7.

[63]J. A. McLachlan, C. D. Serkin, and O. Bakouche, "Dehydroepiandrosterone Modulation of Lippolysaccharide-Stimulated Monocyte Cytotoxicity," *Journal of Immunology,* January 1, 1996;156(1):328–35.

[64]R. J. Reiter, D. X. Tan, B. Poeggeler et al., "Melatonin as a Free Radical Scavenger: Implications for Aging and Age-Related Diseases," *Annals of the New York Academy of Sciences,* 1994;719:1–12.

[65]G. J. Maestroni and A. Conti, "Immuno-derived Opiods as Mediators of the Immuno-enhancing and Anti-stress Action of Melatonin," *Acta Neurologica* (Napoli), August 1991;13(4):356–60.

[66]P. Monteleone, A. Fuschino, G. Nolfe et al., "Temporal Relationship between Melatonin and Cortisol Responses to Nighttime Physical Stress in Humans," *Psychoneuroendocrinology,* 1992;17(1):81–86.

[67]G. Heuther, "Melatonin Synthesis in the Gastrointestinal Tract and the Impact of Nutritional Factors on Circulating Melatonin," *Annals of the New York Academy of Sciences,* 1994;719:146–58.

[68]K. P. Wright, Jr., P. Badia, B. L. Myers et al., "Caffeine and Light Effects on Nighttime Melatonin and Temperature Levels in Sleep-deprived Humans," *Brain Research,* January 30, 1997;747(1):78–84.

[69]S. M. Armstrong and J. R. Redman, "Melatonin: A Chronobiotic with Anti-aging Properties?" *Medical Hypothesis,* April 1991;34(4):300–09.

[70]W. Pierpaoli and V. Lesnikov, "The Pineal Aging Clock," *Annals of the New York Academy of Sciences,* 1994;719:461–71.

[71]J. E. Blalock, E. M. Smith, and W. J. Meyer, 3rd., "The Pituitary-adrenocortical Axis and the Immune System," *Clinical Endocrinology and Metabolism,* 1985;14(4):1021.

[72]T. L. Pruett and F. B. Cerra, "The Physiologic and Metabolic Responses to Stress and Sepsis," *Medical Times,* 1985;113(2):98.

Chapter 4

[1]W. R. Lovallo, M. Al'Absi, K. Blick et al., "Stress-like Adrenocorticotropin Responses to Caffeine in Young Healthy Men," *Pharmacology; Biochemistry and Behavior,* November 1996;55(3):365–69.

[2]I. Iancu, O. T. Dolberg, and J. Zohar, "Is Caffeine Involved in the Pathogenesis of Combat-stress Reaction?" *Military Medicine,* April 1996;161(4):230–32.

[3]P. Cotton, "Neurophysiology and Philosophy," *Journal of the American Medical Association,* 1993;269(12):1485–86.

[4]D. J. Roca, G. D. Schiller, and D. H. Farb, "Chronic Caffeine or Theophylline Exposure Reduces Gamma-aminobutyric Acid/Benzodiazepine Receptor Site Interactions," *Molecular Pharmacology,* May 1988;33(5):481–85.

[5]L. N. Robins et al., "Lifetime Prevalence of Specific Psychiatric Disorders in Three Sites," *Archives of General Psychiatry,* 1984;41:949–58.

[6]O. G. Cameron and R. M. Nesse, "Systemic Hormonal and Physiological Correlations in Anxiety Disorders," *Psychoneuroendocrinology,* 1988;13(4):287–307.

[7]F. A. Wiesel, "Positron Emission Tomography in Psychiatry," *Psychiatric Developments,* 1989, Spring;7(1):19–47.

[8]T. Kuboki and H. Suematsu, "Panic Disorder," *Nippon Rinsho,* November 1992;50(11):2773–82.

[9]H. M. van Praag, "Central Monoamine Metabolism in Depression II: Catecholamines and Related Compounds," *Comprehensive Psychiatry,* 1980;21(1):44–54.

[10]J. M. Gorman and M. R. Liebowitz, "Panic and Anxiety Disorders," in R. Michels et al. (eds.), *Psychiatry,* vol. 1 (Philadelphia: J. B. Lippincott, 1985), pp. 1–13.

[11]R. J. Matthew and W. H. Wilson, "Behavioral and Cerebrovascular Effects of Caffeine in Patients with Anxiety Disorders," *Acta Psychiatrica Scandinavica,* July 1990;82(1):17–22.

[12]M. C. McManamy and P. G. Schube, "Caffeine Intoxication," *New England Journal of Medicine,* 1936;215:616–20.

[13]P. P. Roy-Byrne and T. W. Uhde, "Exogenous Factors in Panic Disorder: Clinical and Research Implications," *Journal of Clinical Psychiatry,* February 1988;49(2):56–61.

[14]A. Breier, D. S. Charney, and G. R. Heninger, "Agoraphobia with Panic Attacks:

Development, Diagnostic Stability, and Course of Illness," *Archives of General Psychiatry,* November 1986;43(11):1029–36.

[15]M. A. Lee, P. Flegel, J. F. Greden et al., "Anxiogenic Effects of Caffeine on Panic and Depressed Patients," *American Journal of Psychiatry,* May 1988;145(5):632–35.

[16]J. P. Boulanger et al., "Increased Sensitivity to Caffeine in Patients with Panic Disorder," *Archives of General Psychiatry,* 1984;41:1067–71.

[17]D. S. Charney, G. R. Heninger, and P. I. Jatlow, "Increased Anxiogenic Effects of Caffeine in Panic Disorders," *Archives of General Psychiatry,* March 1985;42(3):233–43.

[18]D. V. Sheehan, J. C. Ballenger, and G. Jacobsen, "Treatment of Endogenous Anxiety with Phobic, Hysterical and Hypochondriacal Symptoms," *Archives of General Psychiatry,* 1980;37:51–59.

[19]J. D. Lane, R. A. Adcock, R. B. Williams et al., "Caffeine Effects on Cardiovascular and Neuroendocrine Responses to Acute Psychosocial Stress and Their Relationship to Level of Habitual Caffeine Consumption," *Psychosomatic Medicine,* May–June 1990;52(3):320–36.

[20]D. C. Mackay and J. W. Rollins, "Caffeine and Caffeinism," *Journal of the Royal Navy Medical Service,* 1989;75(2):65–67.

[21]J. R. Hughes, S. T. Higgins, W. K. Bickel et al., "Caffeine Self-Administration, Withdrawal, and Adverse Effects among Coffee Drinkers," *Archives of General Psychiatry,* July 1991;48(7):611–17.

[22]J. D. Lane, "Effects of Brief Caffeinated-beverage Deprivation on Mood, Symptoms, and Psychomotor Performance," *Pharmacology, Biochemistry and Behavior,* September 1997;58(1).203–08.

[23]K. Silverman, S. M. Evans, E. C. Strain et al., "Withdrawal Syndrome after the Double-blind Cessation of Caffeine Consumption," *New England Journal of Medicine,* October 15, 1992;327(16):1109–14.

[24]"Pharmacology Update," *Internal Medicine Alert,* 1992;14(1):7.

[25]M. Weissman, "Epidemiology of Depression: Frequency, Risk Groups, and Risk Factors," in *Perspectives on Depressive Disorders: A Review of Recent Research* (Washington, D.C.: National Institute of Mental Health, 1986).

[26]D. A. Regier, R. M. A. Hirschfeld, and F. K. Goodwin, "The NIMH Depression Awareness, Recognition and Treatment (D/ART) Program: Structure, Aims and Scientific Basis," *American Journal of Psychiatry,* 1988;145:1351–57.

[27]"Caffeine Can Increase Brain Serotonin Levels," *Nutrition Reviews,* October 1988;46(10):366–67.

[28]K. Silverman, S. M. Evans, E. C. Strain et al., "Withdrawal Syndrome after the Double-blind Cessation of Caffeine Consumption," *New England Journal of Medicine,* October 15, 1992;327(16):1109–14.

[29]R. Caccioatore, A. Helbling, C. Jost et al., "Episodic Headache, Diminished Performance and Depressive Mood" (in German), *Schweizerische Rundschau for Medizin Praxis,* May 28, 1996;85(22):727–29.

[30]L. Tondor, N. Rudhause et al., "Course of Seasonal Bipolar Disorder Influenced by Caffeine," *Journal of Affective Disorders,* 1991;22:249–51.

[31]W. H. Frishman, "Beta-adrenergic Blockers," *Medical Clinics of North America,* 1988;72:37.

[32]*Physicians' Desk Reference,* 44th edition, 1990.

[33]*Pharmacotherapy,* 1987;7:1–15.

[34]M. A. Lee, P. Flegel, J. F. Greden et al., "Anxiogenic Effects of Caffeine on Panic and Depressed Patients," *American Journal of Psychiatry,* May 1988;145(5):632–35.

[35]T. Kuboki and H. Suematsu, "Panic Disorder," *Nippon Rinsho,* May 1994;52(5):1334–38.

[36]J. F. Mortola, J. H. Liu, J. C. Gillin et al., "Pulsatile Rhythms of Adrenocorticotropin (ACTH) and Cortisol in Women with Endogenous Depression: Evidence for Increased ACTH Pulse Frequency," *Journal of Clinical Endocrinology and Metabolism,* November 1987;65(5):962–68.

[37]M. Vollrath, W. Wicki, and J. Angst, "The Zurich Study VIII: Insomnia: Association with Depression, Anxiety, Somatic Syndromes, and Course of Insomnia," *European Archives of Psychiatry and Neurological Sciences,* 1989;239(2):113–24.

[38]D. J. Haleem, A. Yasmeen, M. A. Haleem et al., "24 hour Withdrawal Following Repeated Administration of Caffeine Attenuates Brain Serotonin but Not Tryptophan in Rat Brain: Implications for Caffeine-Induced Depression," *Life Sciences,* September 29, 1995;57(19):PL285–92.

[39]T. C. Neylan, "Treatment of Sleep Disturbances in Depressed Patients," *Journal of Clinical Psychiatry,* 1995;56 supplement 2:56–61.

[40]Anon. "The Impact of Stress on the Recurrence of Bipolar Episodes," *Family Practice Recertification,* 1992;14(2):412.

[41]P. J. O'Connor, W. P. Morgan, J. S. Raglin et al., "Mood State and Salivary Cortisol Levels Following Overtraining in Female Swimmers," *Psychoneuroendocrinology,* 1989;14(4):303–10.

[42]E. Leibenluft, P. L. Fiero, J. J. Bartko et al., "Depressive Symptoms and the Self-reported Use of Alcohol, Caffeine, and Carbohydrates in Normal Volunteers and Four Groups of Psychiatric Outpatients," *American Journal of Psychiatry,* February 1993;150(2):294–301.

[43]T. C. Neylan, "Treatment of Sleep Disturbances in Depressed Patients," *American Journal of Clinical Psychiatry,* 1995;56 supplement 2:56–61.

[44]E. Susman, "Prozac May Rob You of a Good Night's Sleep," Medical Tribune News Service; September 16, 1997.

[45]J. D. Morrison, "Fatigue as a Presenting Complaint in Family Practice," *Journal of Family Practice,* 1980;10:795.

[46]S. Findlay, "New Hope for Tired People," *U.S. News & World Report,* October 31, 1988:71–73.

[47]W. S. Terry and B. Phifer, "Caffeine and Memory Performance on the AVLT," *Journal of Clinical Psychology,* November 1986;42(6):860–3.

[48]R. Gilliland and D. Andress, "Ad Lib Caffeine Consumption, Symptoms of Caffein-

ism, and Academic Performance," *American Journal of Clinical Psychiatry,* April 1981;138(4):512–14.

[49]J. R. Bradley and A. Petree, "Caffeine Consumption, Expectancies of Caffeine-enhanced Performance, and Caffeinism Symptoms among University Students," *Journal of Drug Education,* 1990;20(4):319–28.

[50]C. H. Ashton and F. Kamali, "Personality, Lifestyles, Alcohol and Drug Consumption in a Sample of British Medical Students," *Medical Education,* May 1995;29(3):187–92.

[51]G. A. Pincomb, W. R. Lovallo, R. B. Passey et al., "Caffeine Enhances the Physiological Response to Occupational Stress in Medical Students," *Health Psychology,* 1987;6(2):101–12.

[52]R. T. Cox, and R. J. Walker, "An Analysis of the Adenosine Receptors Responsible for Modulation of an Excitatory Acetylcholine Response on an Identified Helix Neuron," *Comparative Biochemistry and Physiology,* C: Comparative Pharmacology and Toxicology, 1987;88(1):121–30.

[53]O. Nikodijevic, K. A. Jacobson, and J. W. Daly, "Locomotor Activity in Mice During Chronic Treatment with Caffeine and Withdrawal," *Pharmacology, Biochemistry and Behavior,* January 1993;44(1):199–216.

[54]L. Linde, "An Auditory Attention Task: A Note on the Processing of Verbal Information," *Perceptual and Motor Skills,* April 1994;78(2):563–70.

[55]O. G. Cameron, J. G. Modell, and M. Hariharan, "Caffeine and Human Cerebral Blood Flow: A Positron Emission Tomography Study," *Life Sciences,* 1990;47(13):1141–46.

[56]R. J. Matthew and W. H. Wilson, "Substance Abuse and Cerebral Blood Flow," *American Journal of Psychiatry,* March 1991;148(3):292–305.

[57]A. Nehlig, J. L. Daval, and G. Debry, "Caffeine and the Central Nervous System: Mechanisms of Action, Biochemical, Metabolic and Psychostimulant Effects," *Brain Research Reviews,* May–August 1992;17(2):139–70.

[58]J. C. Galduroz and E. A. Carlini, "The Effects of Long-term Administration of Guarana on the Cognition of Normal, Elderly Volunteers," *Revista Paulista de Medicina,* January–February 1996;114(1):1073–78.

[59]J. C. Galduroz and E. de A. Carlini, "Acute Effects of the *Paulinia cupana,* 'Guarana,' on the Cognition of Normal Volunteers," *Revista Paulista de Medicina,* July–September 1994;112(3):607–11.

[60]O. M. Wolkowitz, V. I. Reus, E. Roberts et al., "Dehydroepiandrosterone (DHEA) Treatment of Depression," *Biological Psychiatry,* 1997;41:311–18.

[61]D. M. Diamond, B. J. Branch, M. Fleshner et al., "Effects of Dehydroepiandrosterone Sulfate and Stress on Hippocampal Electrophysiological Plasticity," *Annals of the New York Academy of Science,* 1995;774:304–07.

[62]J. Ferri, "Under Pressure," *Tampa Tribune-Times,* April 27, 1997; p. 1.

[63]S. L. Dubovsky, "Generalized Anxiety Disorder: New Concepts and Psychopharmacologic Therapies," *Journal of Clinical Psychiatry,* January 1990;51 supplement:3–10.

[64]A. Koczapski, J. Paredes, C. Kogan et al., "Effects of Caffeine on Behavior of Schizophrenic Inpatients," *Schizophrenia Bulletin*, 1989;15(2)339–44.

[65]T. J. Crowley, D. Chesluk, S. Dilts et al., "Drug and Alcohol Abuse among Psychiatric Admissions—Multidrug Clinical-toxicologic Study," *Archives of General Psychiatry*, 1974;30:13–20.

[66]M. Rihs, C. Muller, and P. Baumann, "Caffeine Consumption in Hospitalized Psychiatric Patients," *European Archives of Psychiatry and Clinical Neuroscience*, 1996;246(2):83–92.

[67]D. C. Mackay and J. W. Rollins, "Caffeine and Caffeinism," *Journal of the Royal Naval Medical Service*, Summer 1989;75(2):65–67.

[68]A. Kruger, "Chronic Psychiatric Patients' Use of Caffeine: Pharmacological Effects and Mechanisms," *Psychological Reports*, June 1996;78(pt 1):915–23.

[69]P. B. Lucas, D. Pickar, J. Kelsoe et al., "Effects of the Acute Administration of Caffeine in Patients with Schizophrenia," *Biological Psychiatry*, July 1, 1990;28(1):35–40.

[70]G. F. Searle, "The Effect of Dietary Caffeine Manipulation on Blood Caffeine, Sleep and Disturbed Behaviour," *Journal of Intellectual Disability Research*, August 1994;38(pt 4):383–91.

[71]J. F. Greden, "Anxiety or Caffeinism: A Diagnostic Dilemma," *American Journal of Psychiatry*, 1974;131:1089.

[72]K. Nishihara and K. Mori, "The Differences of Self-ratings of Sleep Quality Associated with Epinephrine and Wake Time During 4-Hour Sleep," *Psychiatry and Clinical Neuroscience*, October 1996;50(5):277–83.

[73]M. H. Bonnet and D. L. Arand, "The Consequences of a Week of Insomnia," *Sleep*, July 1996;19(6):453–61.

[74]B. V. Reifler, "Depression, Anxiety, and Sleep Disturbances," *International Psychogeriatrics*, 1996;8 supplement 3:415–18.

[75]T. Q. Miller, T. W. Smith, C. W. Turner et al., "A Meta-analytic Review of Research on Hostility and Physical Health," *Psychological Bulletin*, March 1996;119(2):322–48.

[76]M. Wald, "Violent Aggressive Motorists Account for 28,000 Deaths," New York Times News Service, July 1997.

[77]D. K. Dekker, M. J. Paley, S. M. Popkin et al., "Locomotive Engineers and Their Spouses: Coffee Consumption, Mood, and Sleep Reports," *Ergonomics*, January–March 1993;36(1–3)233–38.

[78]G. V. Hughes and F. J. Boland, "The Effects of Caffeine and Nicotine Consumption on Mood and Somatic Variables in a Penitentiary Inmate Population," *Addictive Behaviors*, September–October 1992;17(5):447–57.

[79]K. Raikkonen, A. Hautanen, and L. Keltikangas-Jarvinen, "Feelings of Exhaustion, Emotional Distress, and Pituitary and Adrenocortical Hormones in Borderline Hypertension," *Journal of Hypertension*, June 1996;14(6):713–18.

[80]P. Jin, "Changes in Heart Rate, Noradrenaline, Cortisol and Mood during Tai Chi," *Journal of Psychosomatic Research*, 1989;33(2):197–206.

[81]A. McGrady, M. Woerner, G. A. Bernal et al., "Effect of Biofeedback-assisted Relax-

ation on Blood Pressure and Cortisol Levels in Normotensives and Hypertensives," *Journal of Behavioral Medicine,* June 1987;10(3):301–10.

[82]G. A. Smith, "Caffeine Reduction as an Adjunct to Anxiety Management," *British Journal of Clinical Psychology,* 1988;27:265–66.

Chapter 5

[1]*American Medical News,* January 27, 1992, p. 20.

[2]W. R. Lovallo, G. A. Pincomb, B. H. Sung et al., "Hypertension Risk and Caffeine's Effect on Cardiovascular Activity during Mental Stress in Young Men," *Health Psychology,* 1991;10(4):236–43.

[3]J. M. MacDougall, L. Musante, S. Castillo et al., "Smoking, Caffeine, and Stress: Effects on Blood Pressure and Heart Rate in Male and Female College Students," *Health Psychology,* 1988;7(5):461–78.

[4]J. P. Henry and J. C. Cassel, "Psychosocial Factors in Essential Hypertension: Recent Epidemiological and Animal Experimental Evidence," *American Journal of Epidemiology,* 1969;90:171–200.

[5]G. A. Pincomb, W. R. Lovallo, R. B. Passey et al., "Effect of Behavior State on Caffeine's Ability to Alter Blood Pressure," *American Journal of Cardiology,* April 1, 1988;61(10):798–802.

[6]W. R. Lovallo, M. al'Absi, G. A. Pincomb et al., "Caffeine and Behavioral Stress Effects on Blood Pressure in Borderline Hypertensive Caucasian Men," *Health Psychology,* January 1996;15(1):11–17.

[7]P. J. Green and J. Suls, "The Effects of Caffeine on Ambulatory Blood Pressure, Heart Rate, and Mood in Coffee Drinkers," *Journal of Behavioral Medicine,* April 1996;19(2):111–28.

[8]J. Ratliff-Crain, M. K. O'Keeffe, and A. Baum, "Cardiovascular Reactivity, Mood, and Task Performance in Deprived and Nondeprived Coffeedrinkers," *Health Psychology,* 1989;8(4):427–47.

[9]P. Smits, T. Thein, and A. van 't Laar, "Coffee and the Human Cardiovascular System," *Netherlands Journal of Medicine,* 1987;31(7):36.

[10]C. R. Lake, G. Zaloga, J. Bray et al., "Transient Hypertension after Two Phenylpropanolamine Diet Aids and the Effects of Caffeine: A Placebo-controlled Follow-up Study," *American Journal of Medicine,* April 1989;86(4):427–32.

[11]S. S. Chua and S. I. Benrimoj, "Non-prescription Sympathomimetic Agents and Hypertension," *Medical Toxicology and Adverse Drug Experience,* September–October 1988;3(5):387–417.

[12]S. C. Dilsaver, N. A. Votolato, and N. E. Alessi, "Complications of Phenylpropanolamine," *American Family Physician,* April 1989;39(4):201–06.

[13]M. A. Sloan, S. J. Kittner, D. Rigamonti et al., "Occurrence of Stroke Associated with Use/Abuse of Drugs," *Neurology,* September 1991;41(9):1358–64.

[14]C. R. Lake, D. B. Rosenberg, S. Gallant et al., "Phenylpropanolamine Increases

Plasma Caffeine Levels," *Clinical Pharmacology and Therapeutics,* June 1990;47(6):675–85.

[15]C. R. Lake, "Manic Psychosis after Coffee and Phenylpropanolamine," *Biological Psychiatry,* August 15, 1991;30(4):401–04.

[16]E. Casiglia, S. Bongiovi, C. D. Paleari et al., "Haemodynamic Effects of Coffee and Caffeine in Normal Volunteers: A Placebo-controlled Clinical Study," *Journal of Internal Medicine,* June 1991;229(6):501–04.

[17]B. H. Sung, W. R. Lovallo, G. A. Pincomb et al., "Effects of Caffeine on Blood Pressure Response during Exercise in Normotensive Healthy Young Men," *American Journal of Cardiology,* April 1, 1990;65(13):909–13.

[18]G. A. Pincomb, M. F. Wilson, B. H. Sung et al., "Effects of Caffeine on Pressor Regulation during Rest and Exercise in Men at Risk for Hypertension," *American Heart Journal,* October 1991;122(pt 1):1107–15.

[19]K. J. Wise, E. A. Bergman, D. J. Sherrard et al., "Interactions between Dietary Calcium and Caffeine Consumption on Calcium Metabolism in Hypertensive Humans," *American Journal of Hypertension,* March 1996;9(3):223–29.

[20]J. D. Kark, Y. Friedlander, N. A. Kaufmann et al., "Coffee, Tea and Plasma Cholesterol: The Jerusalem Lipid Research Clinic Prevalence Study," *British Medical Journal,* 1985;291:699.

[21]B. R. Davis, J. D. Curb, N. O. Borhani et al., "Coffee Consumption and Serum Cholesterol in the Hypertension Detection and Follow-up Program," *American Journal of Epidemiology,* July 1988;128(1):124–136.

[22]J. Tuomilehto, A. Tanskanen, P. Pietinen, et al., "Coffee Consumption Is Correlated with Serum Cholesterol in Middle-aged Finnish Men and Women," *Journal of Epidemiology and Community Health,* 1987;41:237–42.

[23]O. H. Forde, S. F. Knutsen, E. Arnesen et al., "The Tromso Heart Study: Coffee Consumption and Serum Lipid Concentrations in Men with Hypercholesterolemia: A Randomized Intervention Study," *British Medical Journal,* 1985;290:893–95.

[24]B. D'Avanzo, L. Santoro, A. Nobili et al., "Coffee Consumption and Serum Cholesterol," *Preventive Medicine,* 1993;22:219–24.

[25]D. S. Thelle et al., "Effects of Coffee on Serum Cholesterol," *New England Journal of Medicine,* 1983;308(24):1454–57.

[26]E. Arnesen, O. H. Forde, and D. S. Thelle, "Coffee and Serum Cholesterol," *British Medical Journal,* June 30, 1984;288(6435):1960.

[27]J. D. Curb, D. M. Reed, J. A. Kautz et al., "Coffee, Caffeine, and Serum Cholesterol in Japanese Men in Hawaii," *American Journal of Epidemiology,* April 1986;123(4):648–55.

[28]R. E. Fried et al., "The Effect of Filtered Coffee Consumption on Plasma Lipid Levels," *Journal of the American Medical Association,* 1992;267(6):811–15.

[29]M. Wei, C. A. Macera, C. A. Hornung et al., "The Impact of Changes in Coffee Consumption on Serum Cholesterol," *Journal of Clinical Epidemiology,* October 1995;48(10):1189–96.

[30]H. Heckers, U. Gobel, and U. Kleppel, "End of the Coffee Mystery: Diterpene Alcohols Raise Serum Low-density Lipoprotein Cholesterol and Triglyceride Levels," *Journal of Internal Medicine*, 1994;235:192–93.

[31]M. P. Weusten van der Wouw, M. B. Katan, R. Viani et al., "Identity of the Cholesterol-raising Factor from Boiled Coffee and Its Effects on Liver Function Enzymes," *Journal of Lipid Research*, 1994;35:721–33.

[32]P. T. Williams, P. D. Wood, K. M. Vranizan et al., "Coffee Intake and Elevated Cholesterol and Apolipoprotein B Levels in Men," *Journal of the American Medical Association*, 1985;253:1407–11.

[33]P. C. Rosmarin, "Coffee and Coronary Heart Disease: A Review," *Progress in Cardiovascular Disease*, 1989;32:239–45.

[34]D. J. Dobmeyer, R. A. Stine, C. V. Leier et al., "The Arrhythmogenic Effects of Caffeine in Human Beings," *New England Journal of Medicine*, April 7, 1983; 308(14):814–16.

[35]R. J. Thomas, "Caffeine and Arrhythmias: What Are the Risks?" *Your Patient & Fitness*, 1991;5(5):6–8.

[36]M. J. Shirlow and C. D. Mathers, "A Study of Caffeine Consumption and Symptoms: Indigestion, Palpitations, Tremor, Headache and Insomnia," *International Journal of Epidemiology*, June 1985;14(2):239–48.

[37]J. S. Stamler, M. E. Goldman, J. Gomes et al., "The Effect of Stress and Fatigue on Cardiac Rhythm in Medical Interns," *Journal of Electrocardiology*, October 1992;25(4):333–38.

[38]C. M. Pratt et al., "Complex Ventricular Arrhythmias Associated with the Mitral Valve Prolapse Syndrome," *American Journal of Medicine*, 1986;80(4):626–32.

[39]A. M. Costa, I. G. Maia, F. Cruz Filho et al., "Relationship between Mitral Valve Prolapse and Arrhythmogenic Right Ventricular Disease," *Arquivos Brasileiros de Cardiologia*, December 1996;67(6):379–83.

[40]A. Wennmalm and M. Wennmalm, "Coffee, Catecholamines and Cardiac Arrhythmia," *Clinical Physiology*, June 1989;9(3):201–06.

[41]D. Rush, "Caffeine and PAT," *Hospital Practice*, 1992;27(4A):35.

[42]T. Nakanishi and M. Yoshimura, "Recent Progress in Holter Electrocardiography, Focused on Heart Rate Variability" (in Japanese), *Rinsho Byori*, November 1993;41(11):1206–13.

[43]H. R. Hellstrom, "Coronary Artery Vasospasm: The Likely Immediated Cause of Acute Myocardial Infarction," *British Heart Journal*, April 1979;41(4):426–32.

[44]H. Weiner, "Stressful Experience and Cardiorespiratory Disorders," *Circulation*, April 1991;83(4 supplement):II2–8.

[45]B. T. Altura, "Type-A Behavior and Coronary Vasospasm: A Possible Role of Hypomagnesemia," *Medical Hypothesis*, July 1980;6(7):753–57.

[46]K. Tanabe, K. Noda, A. Ozasa et al., "The Relation of Physical and Mental Stress to Magnesium Deficiency in Patients with Variant Angina," *Journal of Cardiology*, 1992;22(2–3):349–55.

[47]V. Legrand, M. Deliege, L. Henrard et al., "Patients with Myocardial Infarction and Normal Coronary Arteriogram," *Chest,* December 1982;82(6):678–85.

[48]O. Nygard, H. Refsum, P. M. Ueland et al., "Coffee Consumption and Plasma Total Homocysteine: The Hordaland Homocysteine Study," *American Journal of Clinical Nutrition,* January 1997;65(1):136–43.

[49]I. M. Graham, L. Daly, H. Refsum et al., "Plasma Homocysteine as a Risk Factor for Vascular Disease: The European Concerted Action Project," *Journal of the American Medical Association,* 1997;277:1775–81.

[50]A. Tawakol, T. Omland, M. Gerhard et al., "Hyperhomocyst(e)inemia is Associated with Impaired Endothelium-dependent Vasodilation in Humans," *Circulation,* 1997;95(5):1119–21.

[51]I. M. Graham, L. Daly, H. Refsum et al., "Plasma Homocysteine as a Risk Factor for Vascular Disease: The European Concerted Action Project," *Journal of the American Medical Association,* 1997;277:1775–81.

[52]O. Vaccaro, D. Ingrosso, A. Rivellese et al., "Moderate Hyperhomocysteinaemia and Retinopathy in Insulin-dependent Diabetes," *Lancet,* April 12, 1997; 349(9058):1102–03.

[53]S. Neugebauer, T. Baba, K. Kurokawa et al., "Defective Homocysteine Metabolism as a Risk Factor for Diabetic Retinopathy," [letter], *Lancet,* February 15, 1997; 349(9050):473–74.

[54]R. Roubenoff, P. Dellaripa, M. R. Nadeau et al., "Abnormal Homocysteine Metabolism in Rheumatoid Arthritis," *Arthritis and Rheumation,* April 1997;40(4):718–22.

[55]E. Joosten, E. Lesaffre, R. Riezler et al., "Is Metabolic Evidence for Vitamin B-12 and Folate Deficiency More Frequent in Elderly Patients with Alzheimer's Disease?" *Journal of Gerontology,* March 1997;52(2):M76–79.

[56]K. Robinson, E. L. Mayer, D. P. Miller et al., "Hyperhomocysteinemia and Low Pyridoxal Phosphate: Common and Independent Reversible Risk Factors for Coronary Artery Disease," *Circulation,* November 15, 1995;92(10):2825–30.

[57]P. Modica, "The Coffee Craze and Your Health," *Medical Tribune,* June 25, 1997.

[58]K. Robinson, "Hyperhomocysteinemia," 2825–30.

[59]L. J. Freeman, P. G. Nixon, P. Sallabank et al., "Psychological Stress and Silent Myocardial Ischemia," *American Heart Journal,* September 1987;114(3):477–82.

[60]M. K. Pope and T. W. Smith, "Cortisol Excretion in High and Low Cynically Hostile Men," *Psychosomatic Medicine,* July–August 1991;53(4):386–92.

[61]M. Abdulla, A. Behbehani, and H. Dashti, "Dietary Intake and Bioavailability of Trace Elements," *Biological Trace Element Research,* July–September 1989;21:173–78.

[62]R. B. Costello, P. B. Moser-Veillon, and R. DiBianco, "Magnesium Supplementation in Patients with Congestive Heart Failure," *Journal of the American College of Nutrition,* February 1997;16(1):22–31.

[63]L. Massey and T. Berg, "The Effect of Dietary Caffeine on Urinary Excretion of Calcium, Magnesium, Phosphorus, Sodium, Potassium, Chloride and Zinc in Healthy Males," *Nutrition Research,* 1985;5:1281–84.

[64]E. A. Bergman, L. K. Massey, K. J. Wise et al., "Effects of Dietary Caffeine on Renal Handling of Minerals in Adult Women," *Life Sciences*, 1990;47(6):557–64.

[65]B. M. Altura, A. Gebrewold, B. T. Altura et al., "Magnesium Depletion Impairs Myocardial Carbohydrate and Lipid Metabolism and Cardiac Bioenergetics and Raises Myocardial Calcium Content In-Vivo: Relationship to Etiology of Cardiac Diseases," *Biochemical and Molecular Biology International*, December 1996;40(6):1183–90.

[66]B. I. Hustler, J. Singh, J. J. Waring et al., "Dietary and Physiological Studies Involving Magnesium Homeostasis in the Heart," *Annals of the New York Academy of Sciences*, September 30, 1996;793:473–78.

[67]R. B. Singh, U. C. Gupta, N. Mittal et al., "Epidemiologic Study of Trace Elements and Magnesium on Risk of Coronary Artery Disease in Rural and Urban Indian Populations," *Journal of the American College of Nutrition*, February 1997;16(1):62–67.

[68]S. Douban, M. A. Brodsky, D. D. Whang et al., "Significance of Magnesium in Congestive Heart Failure," *American Heart Journal*, September 1996;132(3):664–71.

[69]H. G. Henrotte, P. F. Plouin, C. Levy-Leboyer et al., "Blood and Urinary Magnesium, Zinc, Calcium, Free Fatty Acids, and Catecholamines in Type A and Type B Subjects," *Journal of the American College of Nutrition*, 1985;4(2):165–72.

[70]M. Zehender, T. Meinertz, T. Faber et al., "Antiarrhythmic Effects of Increasing the Daily Intake of Magnesium and Potassium in Patients with Frequent Ventricular Arrhythmias: Magnesium in Cardiac Arrhythmias (MAGICA) Investigators," *Journal of the American College of Cardiology*, April 1997;29(5):1028–34.

[71]L. Rosenberg, J. R. Palmer, J. P. Kelly et al., "Coffee Drinking and Nonfatal Myocardial Infarction in Men under 55 Years of Age," *American Journal of Epidemiology*, 1988;128(3):570–78.

[72]A. Gramenzi, A. Gentile, M. Fasoli et al., "Association between Certain Foods and Risk of Acute Myocardial Infarction in Women," *British Medical Journal*, 1990;300(6727):771–73.

[73]L. Rosenberg, D. Slone, S. Shapiro et al., "Coffee-drinking and Myocardial Infarction in Young Women," *American Journal of Epidemiology*, 1980;111:675.

[74]J. E. James, "Is Habitual Caffeine Use a Preventable Cardiovascular Risk Factor?" *Lancet*, January 25, 1997;349(9047):279–81.

[75]C. La Vecchia, A. Gentile, E. Negri et al., "Coffee Consumption and Myocardial Infarction in Women," *American Journal of Epidemiology*, September 1989; 130(3):481–85.

[76]G. A. Pincomb, W. R. Lovallo, R. B. Passey et al., "Effect of Behavior State on Caffeine's Ability to Alter Blood Pressure," *American Journal of Cardiology*, April 1, 1988;61(10)798–802.

[77]A. Wennmalm and M. Wennmalm, "Coffee, Catecholamines and Cardiac Arrhythmia," *Clinical Physiology*, June 1989;9(3):201–06.

[78]D. Ornish, S. E. Brown, L. W. Scherwitz et al., "Can Lifestyle Changes Reverse Coronary Heart Disease? The Lifestyle Heart Trial," *Lancet*, July 21, 1990; 336(8708):129–33.

[79]J. B. Ubbink, W. J. H. Vermaals, A. vander Merwe et al., "Vitamin B-12, Vitamin B-6, and Folate Nutritional Status in Men with Hyperhomocysteinemia," *American Journal of Clinical Nutrition*, 1993;57:47–53.

[80]I. M. Graham, L. Daly, H. Refsum et al., "Plasma Homocysteine as a Risk Factor for Vascular Disease: The European Concerted Action Project," *Journal of the American Medical Association*, 1997;277:1775–81.

[81]E. B. Rimm, M. J. Stampfer, A. Ascherio et al., "Vitamin E Consumption and the Risk of Coronary Heart Disease in Men," *New England Journal of Medicine*, 1993;328:1450–56.

[82]M. J. Stampfer, C. H. Hennekens, J. E. Manson et al., "Vitamin E and the Risk of Coronary Disease in Women," *New England Journal of Medicine*, 1993;328:1444–49.

[83]*New England Journal of Medicine*, April 20, 1997.

[84]"Reversing Heart Disease through Diet, Exercise, and Stress Management: An Interview with Dean Ornish," *Journal of the American Dietetic Association*, February 1991;91(2):162–65.

[85]P. Hill, "It Is Not What You Eat, but How You Eat It: Digestion, Life-style, Nutrition," *Nutrition*, November 1991;7(6):385–95.

[86]B. B. Fredholm, "Gastrointestinal and Metabolic Effects of Methylxanthines," *Progress in Clinical and Biological Research*, 1984;158:331–54.

[87]M. W. Groer, S. Humenick, and P. D. Hill, "Characterizations and Psychoneuroimmunologic Implications of Secretory Immunoglobulin A and Cortisol in Preterm and Term Breast Milk," *Journal of Perinatal and Neonatal Nursing*, March 1994;7(4):42–51.

[88]P. Brauchli, "Comparative Study of the Psychophysiologic Relaxation Effects of an Optic-acoustic Mind Machine with Relaxation Music," *Zeitschrift fur Experimentelle und Angewandte Psychologie*, 1993;40(2):179–93.

[89]M. U. Khanna and P. Abraham, "Determinants of Acid Secretion," *Journal of the Association of Physicians in India*, September 1990;38 supplement 1:727–30.

[90]S. Cohen, "Pathogenesis of Coffee-induced Gastrointestinal Symptoms," *New England Journal of Medicine*, July 17, 1980;303(3):122–24.

[91]E. Turchetto, "Effects of Coffee on Digestion," *Minerva Medica*, September 5, 1972;63(61):3314–18.

[92]H. Glatzel and K. Hackenberg, "Effects of Caffeine Containing and Decaffeinated Coffee on the Digestive Functions: X-ray Studies of the Secretion and Peristalsis of Stomach, Intestines and Gallbladder," *Medizinische Klinik*, April 21, 1967; 62(16):625–28.

[93]C. A. Loehry, J. Kingham, and J. Baker, "Small Intestinal Permeability in Animals and Man," *Gut*, September 1973;14(9):683–88.

[94]K. R. Gardiner, N. H. Anderson, B. J. Rowlands et al., "Colitis and Colonic Mucosal Barrier Dysfunction," *Gut*, October 1995;37(4):530–35.

[95]P. Forget, F. Sodoyez-Goffaux, A. Zappitelli et al., "Permeability of the Small Intestine to [51Cr]EDTA in Children with Acute Gastroenteritis or Eczema," *Journal of Pediatric Gastroenterology and Nutrition*, June 1985;4(3):393–96.

[96]B. O. Eggum, B. Pederson, and I. Jacobsen, "The Influence of Dietary Tea, Coffee and Cocoa on Protein and Energy Utilization of Soya-bean Meal and Barley in Rats," *British Journal of Nutrition*, September 1983;50(2):197–205.

[97]R. R. Babb, "Coffee, Sugars, and Chronic Diarrhea: Why a Dietary History Is Important," *Postgraduate Medicine*, June 1984;75(8):82.

[98]E. Krag, "Irritable Bowel Syndrome: Current Concepts and Future Trends," *Scandinavian Journal of Gastroenterology*, supplement 1985;109:107–15.

[99]R. S. Sandler, M. C. Jordan, and B. J. Shelton, "Demographic and Dietary Determinants of Constipation in the U.S. Population," *American Journal of Public Health*, February 1990;80(2):185–89.

[100]S. R. Brown, P. A. Cann, and N. W. Read, "Effect of Coffee on Distal Colon Function," *Gut*, April 1990;31(4):450–53.

[101]A. Wald, C. Back, and T. M. Bayless, "Effect of Caffeine on the Human Small Intestine," *Gastroenterology*, 1976;71:738.

[102]F. B. Thomas, J. T. Steinbaugh, J. J. Fromkes et al., "Inhibitory Effect of Coffee on Lower Esophageal Sphincter Pressure," *Gastroenterology*, December 1980; 79(6):1262–66.

[103]B. Wendl, A. Pfeiffer, C. Pehl et al., "Effect of Decaffeination of Coffee or Tea on Gastro-oesophageal Reflux," *Alimentary Pharmacology and Therapeutics*, June 1994;8(3):283–87.

[104]S. Cohen, "Pathogenesis of Coffee-induced Gastrointestinal Symptoms," *New England Journal of Medicine*, July 17, 1980;303(3):122–24.

[105]S. R. Brazer, J. E. Onken, C. B. Dalton et al., "Effect of Different Coffees on Esophageal Acid Contact Time and Symptoms in Coffee-sensitive Subjects," *Physiology and Behavior*, March 1995;57(3):563–67.

[106]*American Family Physician*, 1992;45(3):995.

[107]K. Taniyama, "GABAergic Neurons in the Mammalian Intestine," *Nippon Yakurigaku Zasshi*, May 1985;85(5):305–13.

[108]F. Sundler, G. Bottcher, E. Ekblad et al., "The Neuroendocrine System of the Gut," *Acta Oncologica* 1989;28(3):303–14.

[109]G. Gentilini, S. Franchi-Micheli, D. Pantalone et al., "GABAB Receptor-mediated Mechanisms in Human Intestine In Vitro," *European Journal of Pharmacology*, June 24, 1992;217(1):9–14.

[110]D. J. Roca, G. D. Schiller, and D. H. Farb, "Chronic Caffeine or Theophylline Exposure Reduces Gamma-aminobutyric Acid/Benzodiazepine Receptor Site Interactions," *Molecular Pharmacology*, May 1988;33(5):481–85.

[111]P. Demol, H. J. Ruoff, and T. R. Weihrauch, "Rational Pharmacotherapy of Gastrointestinal Motility Disorders," *European Journal of Pediatrics*, April 1989;148(6):489–95.

[112]S. Levenstein, C. Prantera, V. Varvo et al., "Psychological Stress and Disease Activity in Ulcerative Colitis: A Multidimensional Cross-Sectional Study," *American Journal of Gastroenterology*, August 1994;89(8):1219–25.

[113]M. Tatsuta, H. Iishi, M. Baba et al., "Attenuation by the GABA Receptor Agonist Baclofen of Experimental Carcinogenesis in Rat Colon by Azoxymethane," *Oncology,* 1992;49(3):241–45.

[114]M. E. Tucker, "Despite *H. pylori,* Stress Still a Factor in Ulcers," *Family Practice News,* 1994;24(12):17.

[115]R. B. Marotta and M. H. Floch, "Diet and Nutrition in Ulcer Disease," *Medical Clinics of North America,* July 1991; 75(4):967–79.

[116]R. B. Johnson, D. M. McCance, and W. M. Lukash, "Coffee—Treat or Trick?" *American Family Physician,* 1975;11:101–04.

[117]S. Hayashi, T. Sugiyama, K. Hisano et al., "Quantitative Detection of Secretory Immunoglobulin A to *Helicobacter pylori* in Gastric Juice: Antibody Capture Enzyme-linked Immunosorbent Assay," *Journal of Clinical and Laboratory Analysis,* 1996;10(2):74–77.

[118]R. F. Anda et al., "Self-perceived Stress and the Risk of Peptic Ulcer Disease: A Longitudinal Study of U.S. Adults," *Archives of Internal Medicine,* April 1992;152:829–33.

[119]S. Levenstein, C. Prantera, M. L. Scribano et al., "Psychologic Predictors of Duodenal Ulcer Healing," *Journal of Clinical Gastroenterology,* March 1996;22(2):84–89.

[120]A. Ramirez-Ramos, R. H. Gilman, R. Leon-Barua et al., "Rapid Recurrence of *Helicobacter pylori* Infection in Peruvian Patients after Successful Eradication," *Clinical Infectious Diseases,* November 1997;25(5):1027–31.

[121]O. Pieramico, M. V. Zanetti, M. Innerhofer et al., "Omeprazole-based Dual and Triple Therapy for the Treatment of *Helicobacter pylori* Infection in Peptic Ulcer Disease: A Randomized Trial," *Helicobacter,* June 1997;2(2):92–97.

[122]J. M. Ritchie, "Caffeine" in Goodman and Gillman (eds.), *The Pharmacological Basis of Therapeutics,* (4th ed.), 1970:359.

[123]R. C. Pearson and R. F. McCloy, "Preference for Hot Drinks Is Associated with Peptic Disease," *Gut,* September 1989;30(9):1201–05.

[124]G. Friedman, "Nutritional Therapy of Irritable Bowel Syndrome," *Gastroenterology Clinics of North America,* September 1989;18(3):513–24.

[125]G. Heuther, "Melatonin Synthesis in the Gastrointestinal Tract and the Impact of Nutritional Factors on Circulating Melatonin," *Annals of the New York Academy of Sciences,* 1994;719:146–58.

[126]P. C. Konturek, S. J. Konturek, T. Brzozowski et al., "Gastroprotective Activity of Melatonin and Its Precursor, L-tryptophan, Against Stress-induced and Ischaemia-induced Lesions Is Mediated by Scavenge of Oxygen Radicals," *Scandinavian Journal of Gastroenterology,* May 1997;32(5)433–38.

[127]T. Brzozowski, P. C. Konturek, S. J. Konturek et al., "The Role of Melatonin and L-tryptophan in Prevention of Acute Gastric Lesions Induced by Stress, Ethanol, Ischemia, and Aspirin," *Journal of Pineal Research,* September 1997;23(2):79–89.

[128]P. Modica, "The Coffee Craze and Your Health," Medical Tribune News Service, June 25, 1997.

[129]P. A. Nathan, R. C. Keniston, R. S. Lockwood et al., "Tobacco, Caffeine, Alcohol,

and Carpal Tunnel Syndrome in American Industry: A Cross-sectional Study of 1,464 Workers," *Journal of Occupational and Environmental Medicine*, March 1996;38(3):290–98.

[130]J. M. McPartland and J. A. Mitchell, "Caffeine and Chronic Back Pain," *Archives of Physical Medicine and Rehabilitation*, January 1997;78(1):61–63.

[131]S. Seltzer, "Foods, and Food and Drug Combinations, Responsible for Head and Neck Pain," *Cephalalgia*, June 1982;2(2):111–24.

[132]J. P. Savineau and J. Mironneau, "Caffeine Acting on Pregnant Rat Myometrium: Analysis of Its Relaxant Action and Its Failure to Release Ca2+ from Intracellular Stores," *British Journal of Pharmacology*, February 1990;99(2):261–66.

[133]R. C. Small, J. P. Boyle, J. Cortijo et al., "The Relaxant and Spasmogenic Effects of Some Xanthine Derivatives Acting on Guinea-pig Isolated Trachealis Muscle," *British Journal of Pharmacology*, August 1988;94(4):1091–1100.

[134]S. V. Hildebrand, D. Aripin, and G. Cardinet 3d, "Contracture Test and Histologic and Histochemical Analyses of Muscle Biopsy Specimens from Horses with Exertional Rhabdomyolysis," *Journal of the American Veterinary Medical Association*, April 1, 1990;196(7):1077–83.

[135]S. Orimo, M. Araki, H. Ishii et al., "A Case of 'Myopathy with Tubular Aggregates' with Increased Muscle Fibre Sensitivity to Caffeine," *Journal of Neurology*, August 1987;234(6):424–26.

[136]R. Leira and R. Rodriguez, "Diet and Migraine," *Revista de Neurologia*, May 1996;24(129):534–38.

[137]O. G. Cameron, J. G. Modell, and M. Hariharan, "Caffeine and Human Cerebral Blood Flow: A Positron Emission Tomography Study," *Life Sciences*, 1990; 47(13):1141–46.

[138]A. Mauskop, B. T. Altura, R. Q. Cracco et al., "Chronic Daily Headache—One Disease or Two? Diagnostic Role of Serum Ionized Magnesium," *Cephalalgia*, February 1994;14(1):24–28.

[139]H. C. Diener, J. Dichgans, E. Scholz et al., "Analgesic-induced Chronic Headache: Long-term Results of Withdrawal Therapy," *Journal of Neurology*, January 1989;236(1):9–14.

[140]A. H. Elkind, "Drug Abuse and Headache," *Medical Clinics of North America*, May 1991;75(3):717–32.

[141]A. Panconesi, P. L. Del Bianco, C. Curradi et al., "Headache Caused by Analgesic and/or Ergotamine Abuse," *Clinica Terapeutica*, May 15, 1991;137(3):169–83.

[142]J. R. Hughes, S. T. Higgins, W. K. Bickel et al., "Caffeine Self-administration, Withdrawal, and Adverse Effects among Coffee Drinkers," *Archives of General Psychiatry*, July 1991;48(7):611–17.

[143]M. van Dusseldorp and M. B. Katan, "Headache Caused by Caffeine Withdrawal among Moderate Coffee Drinkers Switched from Ordinary to Decaffeinated Coffee: A 12-week Double-Blind Trial," *British Medical Journal*, June 16, 1990; 300(6739):1558–59.

[144]P. L. Cerrato, "Headaches? Change Your Diet," *RN*, May 1993;56(5):69–71.

[145]R. R. Griffiths, "Caffeine Abstinence Effects in Humans," *Nida Research Monograph,* 1989;95:129–30.

[146]M. J. Shirlow and C. D. Mathers, "A Study of Caffeine Consumption and Symptoms: Indigestion, Palpitations, Tremor, Headache and Insomnia," *International Journal of Epidemiology,* June 1985;14(2):239–48.

[147]E. Susman, "'Alarm Clock Headaches' Cured by Coffee," Medical Tribune News Service, June 13, 1997.

[148]H. Jaggy and E. Koch, "Chemistry and Biology of Alkylphenols from *Ginkgo biloba,*" *L. Pharmazie,* October 1997;52(10):735–38.

[149]J. Haase, P. Halama, and R. Horr, "Effectiveness of Brief Infusions with *Ginkgo biloba* Special Extract in Dementia of the Vascular and Alzheimer Type," *Zeitschrift fur Gerontogie und Geriatrie,* July 1996;29(4):302–09.

[150]M. Fennelly, D. C. Galletly, and G. I. Purdei, "Is Caffeine Withdrawal the Mechanism of Postoperative Headache?" *Anesthesia and Analgesia,* April 1991;72(4):449–53.

[151]J. G. Weber, J. T. Klindworth, J. J. Arnold et al., "Prophylactic Intravenous Administration of Caffeine and Recovery after Ambulatory Surgical Procedures," *Mayo Clinic Proceedings,* July 1997;72(7):621–26.

[152]Neuhauser-Berthold, S. Beine, S. C. Verwied et al., "Coffee Consumption and Total Body Water Homeostasis as Measured by Fluid Balance and Bioelectrical Impedance Analysis," *Annals of Nutrition and Metabolism,* 1997;41(1):29–36.

[153]L. M. Burke, "Nutrition for Post-exercise Recovery," *Australian Journal of Science and Medicine in Sport,* March 1997;29(1):3–10.

[154]"Effect of Environmental Temperature on the Toxicity of Caffeine and Dextroamphetamine in Mice," *Journal of Pharmacology and Experimental Therapeutics,* January 1970;171(1):153–58.

[155]P. J. Muller and J. Vernikos-Danellis, "Alteration in Drug Toxicity by Environmental Variables," *Proceedings of the Western Pharmacologic Society,* 1968;11:52–53.

[156]B. K. Park and N. R. Kitteringham, "Assessment of Enzyme Induction and Enzyme Inhibition in Humans: Toxicological Implications," *Xenobiotica,* November 1990;20(11):1171–85.

[157]Y. Ohsaki, S. Ishida, T. Fujikane et al., "Combination Effect of Caffeine and Cisplatin on a Cisplatin Resistant Human Lung Cancer Cell Line," *Gan To Kagaku Ryoho,* July 1990;17(7):1339–43.

[158]J. A. Carrillo and J. Benitz, "CYP1A2 Activity, Gender and Smoking as Variables Influencing the Toxicity of Caffeine," *British Journal of Clinical Pharmacology,* June 1996;41(6):605–08.

[159]N. H. Shear, S. P. Spielberg, D. M. Grant et al., "Differences in Metabolism of Sulfonamides Predisposing to Idiosyncratic Toxicity," *Annals of Internal Medicine,* August 1986;105(2):179–84.

[160]M. Rieder, N. H. Shear, A. Kanee et al., "Prominence of Slow Acetylator Phenotype among Patients with Sulfonamide Hypersensitivity Reactions," *Clinical Pharmacology and Therapeutics,* January 1991;49(1):13–17.

NOTES

[161]J. E. Trosko and H. Y. Chu, "Inhibition of Repair of UV-damaged DNA by Caffeine and Mutation Induction in Chinese Hamster Cells," *Chemico-Biological Interactions,* 1973;6:317–32.

[162]A. Antoccia, R. Ricordy, P. Maraschio et al., "Chromosomal Sensitivity to Clastogenic Agents and Cell Cycle Perturbations in Nijmegen Breakage Syndrome Lymphoblastoid Cell Lines," *International Journal of Radiation Biology,* January 1997;71(1):41–49.

[163]P. J. Donovan and J. A. DiPaolo, "Caffeine Enhancement of Chemical Carcinogen-induced Transformation of Cultured Syrian Hamster Cells," *Cancer Research,* 1974;34:2720–27.

[164]L. L. Anderson, C. C. Lau, E. J. Gracely et al., "Enhancement of 131I-mediated Cytotoxicity by Caffeine," *Gynecologic Oncology,* May 1997;65(2):253–57.

[165]C. Petit, "Wake Up and Smell Health Benefits of Fresh Coffee," *San Francisco Chronicle,* April 14, 1997.

[166]X. Shi, N. S. Dalal, and A. C. Jain, "Antioxidant Behaviour of Caffeine: Efficient Scavenging of Hydroxyl Radicals," *Food and Chemical Toxicology,* January 1991;29(1):1–6.

[167]T. P. Devasagayam, J. P. Kamat, H. Mohan et al., "Caffeine as an Antioxidant: Inhibition of Lipid Peroxidation Induced by Reactive Oxygen Species," *Biochemica et Biophysica Acta,* June 13, 1996;1282(1):63–70.

[168]K. P. Wright, Jr., P. Badia, B. L. Myers et al., "Caffeine and Light Effects on Nighttime Melatonin and Temperature Levels in Sleep-deprived Humans," *Brain Research,* January 30, 1997;747(1):78–84.

[169]P. C. Konturek, S. J. Konturek, T. Brzozowski et al., "Gastroprotective Activity of Melatonin and Its Precursor, L-tryptophan, against Stress-induced and Ischaemia-induced Lesions Is Mediated by Scavenge of Oxygen Radicals," *Scandinavian Journal of Gastroenterology,* May 1997;32(5):433–38.

[170]W. U. Muller, T. Bauch, A. Wojcik et al., "Comet Assay Studies Indicate that Caffeine-mediated Increase in Radiation Risk of Embryos Is Due to Inhibition of DNA Repair," *Mutagenesis,* January 1996;11(1):57–60.

[171]L. J. McIntosh and R. M. Sapolsky, "Glucocorticoids May Enhance Oxygen Radical-mediated Neurotoxicity," *Neurotoxicology,* 1996;17(3–4):873–82.

[172]V. V. Frolkis, "Stress-age Syndrome," *Mechanisms of Ageing and Development,* June 1993;69(1–2):93–107.

[173]S. Hoyer, "Age-related Changes in Cerebral Oxidative Metabolism: Implications for Drug Therapy," *Drugs and Aging,* March 1995;6(3):210–18.

[174]R. M. Sapolsky, "Why Stress Is Bad for Your Brain," *Science,* August 9, 1996;273(5276):749–50.

[175]G. Gatti, R. Cavallo, M. L. Sartori et al., "Inhibition by Cortisol of Human Natural Killer (NK) Cell Activity," *Journal of Steroid Biochemistry,* January 1987;26(1):49–58.

[176]J. E. Blalock et al., "The Pituitary-adrenocortical Axis and the Immune System," *Clinical Endocrinology and Metabolism,* 1985;14(4):1021.

[177]H. J. Naurath, E. Joosten, R. Riezler et al., "Effects of Vitamin B12, Folate, and Vitamin B6 Supplements in Elderly People with Normal Serum Vitamin Concentrations," *Lancet*, July 8, 1995;346(8967):85–89.

[178]H. E. Sauberlich, "Implications of Nutritional Status on Human Biochemistry, Physiology, and Health," *Clinical Biochemistry*, April 1984;17(2):132–42.

[179]G. Schmid-Ott, R. Jacobs, B. Jager et al., "Stress-induced Endocrine and Immunological Changes in Psoriasis Patients and Healthy Controls: A Preliminary Study," *Psychotherapy and Psychosomatics*, 1998;67(1):37–42.

[180]D. Christensen, "Diabetes at All-time High in U.S.," Medical Tribune News Service, October 30, 1997.

[181]L. Vergauwen, P. Hespel, and E. A. Richter, "Adenosine Receptors Mediate Synergistic Stimulation of Glucose Uptake and Transport by Insulin and by Contractions in Rat Skeletal Muscle," *Journal of Clinical Investigation*, March 1994;93(3):974–81.

[182]M. Sachs and H. Forster, "Effect of Caffeine on Various Metabolic Parameters In Vivo," *Zeitschrift für Ernahrungswissenschaft*, September 1984;23(3):181–205.

[183]J. Portugal-Alvarez, A. Zamarron, J. Yanguela et al., "Lipolysis Induced by Coffee and Tobacco: Its Modification by Insulin," *Journal of Pharmacy and Pharmacology*, 1973;25:668–69.

[184]O. Vaccaro, D. Ingrosso, A. Rivellese et al., "Moderate Hyperhomocysteinaemia and Retinopathy in Insulin-dependent Diabetes," *Lancet*, April 12, 1997; 349(9058):1102–03.

[185]S. Neugenbauer, T. Baba, K. Kurokawa et al., "Defective Homocysteine Metabolism as a Risk Factor for Diabetic Retinopathy," *Lancet*, February 1997;349(9050):473–74.

[186]C. Lehman, J. Rodin, B. S. McEwen et al., "Impact of Environmental Stress on the Expression of Insulin-dependent Diabetes Mellitus," *Behavioral Neuroscience*, 1991;105:241–45.

[187]K. Raikkonen, L. Keltikangas-Jarvinen, H. Aldercreutz et al., "Psychosocial Stress and the Insulin Resistance Syndrome," *Metabolism*, 1996;45:1533–38.

[188]J. Tuomilehto, E. Tuomilehto-Wolf, R. LaPorte et al., "Coffee Consumption as Trigger for Insulin Dependent Diabetes Mellitus in Childhood," *British Medical Journal*, 1990;300(6725):642–43.

[189]D. Kerr, R. S. Sherwin, F. Pavalkis et al., "Effect of Caffeine on the Recognition of and Responses to Hypoglycemia in Humans," *Annals of Internal Medicine*, October 15, 1993;119(8):799–804.

[190]P. McAdam, "Caffeine May Trigger Hypoglycemia," *Medical Tribune*, 1993; 34(21):21.

[191]Ibid.

[192]F. K. Goodwin, "Behavioral Stress Reactivity Related to Arthritis Susceptibility?" *Journal of the American Medical Association*, 1992;267(7):910.

[193]J. B. Corcuff, P. Lafranque, P. Henry et al., "Isolated Cortiocotroph Insufficiency Associated to Myasthenia Gravis," *Journal of Endocrinology Investigation*, December 1997;20(11):669–71.

NOTES

[194]D. Buchwald, J. Umali, M. Stene, "Insulin-like Growth Factor-I (Somatomedin C) Levels in Chronic Fatigue Syndrome and Fibromyalgia," *Journal of Rheumatology,* April 1996;23(4):739–42.

[195]R. G. Lahita, "The Connective Tissue Diseases and the Overall Influence of Gender," *International Journal of Fertility and Menopausal Studies,* March–April 1996;41(2):156–65.

[196]R. F. van Vollenhoven, L. M. Morabito, E. G. Engleman et al., "Treatment of Systemic Lupus Erythematosus with Dehydroepiandrosterone: 50 Patients Treated up to 12 Months," *Journal of Rheumatology,* February 1998;25(2):285–89.

[197]M. Kodama, T. Kodama, and M. Murakami, "The Value of the Dehydroepiandrosterone-annexed Vitamin C Infusion Treatment in the Clinical Control of Chronic Fatigue Syndrome (CFS) I: A Pilot Study of the New Vitamin C Infusion Treatment," *In Vivo,* November 1996;10(6):575–84.

[198]S. J. Pollard, S. L. Spector, S. W. Yancey et al., "Salmeterol versus Theophylline in the Treatment of Asthma," *Annals of Allergy, Asthma and Immunology,* May 1997;78(5):457–64.

[199]A. V. Lubischer and L. M. Lucas, "Monitoring Theophylline Therapy to Prevent Toxicity," *American Journal of Health,* June 1, 1996;53(11):1292–94.

[200]J. T. Barr, G. E. Schumacher, D. B. Luks et al., "Mild Theophylline-related Adverse Reactions and Serum Theophylline Concentration," *American Journal of Hospital Pharmacy,* November 1, 1994;51(21):2688–92.

[201]B. C. Bandyopadhyay and M. K. Poddar, "Theophylline-induced Changes in Mammalian Adenosine Deaminase Activity and Corticosterone Status: Possible Relation to Immune Response," *Methods and Findings in Experimental and Clinical Pharmacology,* April 1997;19(3):181–84.

[202]H. Segawa and Y. Iikura, "Clinical Effects of Theophylline in the Therapy of Intractable Asthmatic Children II: Theophylline Therapy and Behavior Problems in Children with Asthma" (in Japanese), *Arerugi,* October 1990;39(10):1427–36.

[203]K. L. Franson, D. P. Hay, V. Neppe et al., "Drug-induced Seizures in the Elderly: Causative Agents and Optimal Management," *Drugs and Aging,* July 1995;7(1):38–48.

[204]L. A. Coskey, J. Bitting, and M. D. Roth, "Inhibition of Natural Killer Cell Activity by Therapeutic Levels of Theophylline," *American Journal of Respiratory Cell and Molecular Biology,* December 1993;9(6):659–65.

[205]T. Caballero, C. Garcia-Ara, C. Pascual et al., "Urticaria Induced by Caffeine," *Journal of Investigational Allergology and Clinical Immunology,* May 1993;3(3):160–62.

[206]L. J. Crofford, S. R. Pillemer, K. T. Kalogeras et al., "Hypothalamic-Pituitary-Adrenal Axis Perturbations in Patients with Fibromyalgia," *Arthritis and Rheumatism,* November 1994;37(11):1583–92.

[207]E. N. Griep, J. W. Boersma, and E. R. de Kloet, "Altered Reactivity of the Hypothalamic-Pituitary-Adrenal Axis in the Primary Fibromyalgia Syndrome," *Journal of Rheumatology,* March 1993;20(3):469–74.

[208]L. J. Crofford, N. C. Engleberg, and M. A. Demitrack, "Neurohormonal Perturbations in Fibromyalgia," *Baillieres Clinical Rheumatology,* May 1996;10(2):365–78.

[209]J. C. van Denderen, J. W. Boersma, P. Zeinstra et al., "Physiological Effects of Exhaustive Physical Exercise in Primary Fibromyalgia Syndrome (PFS): Is PFS a Disorder of Neuroendocrine Reactivity?" *Scandinavian Journal of Rheumatology,* 1992;21(1):35–37.

[210]M. Kennedy and D. T. Felson, "A Prospective Long-term Study of Fibromyalgia Syndrome," *Arthritis and Rheumatism,* April 1996;39(4):682–85.

[211]"Fibromyalgia," in S. Margolis and H. Moses (eds.), *The Johns Hopkins Medical Handbook* (New York: Random House), pp. 371–75.

[212]J. Bearn, T. Allain, P. Coskeran et al., "Neuroendocrine Responses to D-fenfluramine and Insulin-induced Hypoglycemia in Chronic Fatigue Syndrome," *Biological Psychiatry,* February 15, 1995;37(4):245–52.

[213]P. Strickland, R. Morriss, A. Wearden et al., "A Comparison of Salivary Cortisol in Chronic Fatigue Syndrome, Community Depression and Healthy Controls," *Journal of Affective Disorders,* January 1998;47(1–3):191–94.

[214]L. V. Scott and T. G. Dinan, "Urinary Free Cortisol Excretion in Chronic Fatigue Syndrome, Major Depression and in Healthy Volunteers," *Journal of Affective Disorders,* January 1998;47(1–3):49–54.

[215]W. M. Jefferies, "Mild Adrenocortical Deficiency, Chronic Allergies, Autoimmune Disorders and the Chronic Fatigue Syndrome: A Continuation of the Cortisone Story," *Medical Hypothesis,* March 1994;42(3):183–89.

[216]M. Krisiloff, "Solving Urinary Problems," *Let's Live,* October 1997;100.

[217]M. Krisiloff; personal communication.

[218]T. D. Moon, L. Hagen, and D. M. Heisey, "Urinary Symptomatology in Younger Men," *Urology,* November 1997;50(5):700–03.

[219]P. C. Albertsen, "Urologic 'Nuisances': How to Work Up and Relieve Men's Symptoms," *Geriatrics,* February 1997;52(2):46–50.

[220]M. L. Slattery and D. W. West, "Smoking, Alcohol, Coffee, Tea, Caffeine, and Theobromine: Risk of Prostate Cancer in Utah (United States)," *Cancer Causes and Control,* November 1993;4(6):559–63.

[221]S. Tas, R. Lauwerys, and D. Lison, "Occupational Hazards for the Male Reproductive System," *Critical Reviews in Toxicology,* May 1996;26(3):261–307.

[222]M. Cetinkaya, J. von Duszeln, W. Thiemann et al., "Organochlorine Pesticide Residues in Raw and Roasted Coffee and Their Degradation during the Roasting Process," *Zeitschrift fur Lebensmittel Untersuchung und Forschung,* July 1984;179(1):5–8.

[223]L. Friedman, M. A. Weinberger, T. M. Farber et al., "Testicular Atrophy and Impaired Spermatogenesis in Rats Fed High Levels of the Methylxanthines Caffeine, Theobromine, or Theophylline," *Journal of Environmental Pathology and Toxicology,* January 1979;2(3):687–706.

[224]A. R. Ezzat and Z. M. el-Gohary, "Hormonal and Histological Effects of Chronic Caffeine Administration on the Pituitary-gonadal and Pituitary-adrenocortical Axes in Male Rabbits," *Functional and Developmental Morphology,* 1994;4(1):45–50.

[225]G. Potashnik and A. Porath, "Dibromochloropropane (DBCP):A 17-year Reassessment of Testicular Function and Reproductive Performance," *Journal of Occupational and Environmental Medicine*, November 1995;37(11):1287–92.

[226]Ibid.

[227]D. S. Weathersbee, R. L. Ax, and J. R. Lodge, "Caffeine-mediated Changes of Sex Ratio in Chinese Hamsters," *Journal of Reproduction and Fertility*, 1975;43:141–43.

[228]L. Fenster, D. F. Katz, A. J. Wyrobek et al., "Effects of Psychological Stress on Human Semen Quality," *Journal of Andrology*, March 1997;18(2):194–202.

[229]M. Fukuda, K. Fukuda, T. Shimizu et al., "Kobe Earthquake and Reduced Sperm Motility," *Human Reproduction*, June 1996;11(6):1244–46.

[230]M. J. De Souza, J. C. Arce, L. S. Pescatello et al., "Gonadal Hormones and Semen Quality in Male Runners: A Volume Threshold Effect of Endurance Training," *International Journal of Sports Medicine*, October 1994;15(7):383–91.

[231]H. Kentenich, H. Schmiady, E. Radke et al., "The Male IVF Patient—Psychosomatic Considerations," *Human Reproduction*, June 1992;7 supplement 1:13–18.

[232]P. T. Giblin, M. L. Poland, K. S. Moghissi et al., "Effects of Stress and Characteristic Adaptability on Semen Quality in Healthy Men," *Fertility and Sterility*, January 1988;49(1):127–32.

[233]K. K. Harrison, V. J. Callan, and J. R. Hennessey, "Stress and Semen Quality in an In Vitro Fertilization Program," *Fertility and Sterility*, October 1987;48(4):633–36.

[234]K. D. Israel et al., "Serum Uric Acid in Carbohydrate Sensitive Adults," *Annals of Nutrition and Metabolism*, 1983;32:1078–81.

[235]M. M. Callahan, R. S. Robertson, M. J. Arnaud et al., "Human Metabolism of [1-methyl-14C] and [2-14C] Caffeine after Oral Administration," *Drug Metabolism and Disposition*, July 1982;10(4):417–23.

[236]D. M. Grant, B. K. Tang, M. E. Campbell et al., "Effect of Allopurinol on Caffeine Disposition in Man," *British Journal of Clinical Pharmacology*, April 1986;21(4):454–58.

[237]N. R. Scott, D. Stambuk, J. Chakraborty et al., "Caffeine Clearance and Biotransformation in Patients with Chronic Liver Disease," *Clinical Science*, April 1988;74(4):377–84.

[238]R. H. Davis, "Does Caffeine Ingestion Affect Intraocular Pressure?" *Ophthalmology*, November 1989;96(11):1680–81.

[239]E. J. Higginbotham, H. A. Kilimanjaro, J. T. Wilensky et al., "The Effect of Caffeine on Intraocular Pressure in Glaucoma Patients," *Ophthalmology*, May 1989;96(5):624–26.

[240]B. Hinzpeter and M. Diestelhorst, "1, 3, 7-trimethylxanthine: Effects on Circadian Aqueous Humor Dynamics in Probands," *Ophthalmology*, December 1992; 89(6):465–67.

[241]G. Duncan, R. A. Riach, M. R. Williams et al., "Calcium Mobilisation Modulates Growth of Lens Cells," *Cell Calcium*, January 1996;19(1):83–89.

[242]K. Lofti and J. E. Grunwald, "The Effect of Caffeine on the Human Macular

Circulation," *Investigative Ophthalmology and Visual Science,* November 1991; 32(12):3028–32.

[243]Guide to Macular Degeneration. http://www.eyecare.org/consumer/disease/md.html

[244]J. Evans and R. Wormald, "Is the Incidence of Registrable Age-related Macular Degeneration Increasing?" *British Journal of Ophthalmology,* January 1996;80(1):9–14.

Chapter 6

[1]M. J. Arnaud, "Metabolism of Caffeine and Other Components of Coffee," in S. Garattini (ed.), *Caffeine, Coffee & Health,* (New York: Raven Press, 1993), pp. 43–95.

[2]D. W. Yesair, "Human Disposition and Some Biochemical Aspects of Methylxanthines," in G. A. Spiller, *The Methylxanthine Beverages and Foods: Chemistry, Consumption and Health Effects* (New York: Liss, 1984).

[3]L. Linde, "Mental Effects of Caffeine in Fatigued and Non-fatigued Female and Male Subjects," *Ergonomics,* May 1995;38(5):864–85.

[4]J. Ferri, "Under Pressure," *Tampa Tribune-Times,* April 27, 1997, 1.

[5]T. E. Seeman, B. S. McEwen, B. H. Singer et al., "Increase in Urinary Cortisol Excretion and Memory Declines: MacArthur Studies of Successful Aging," *Journal of Clinical Endocrinology and Metabolism,* 1997;82:2458–65.

[6]J. Ferri, "Under Pressure."

[7]A. Gramenzi and A. Gentile et al., "Association between Certain Foods and Risk of Acute Myocardial Infarction in Women," *British Medical Journal,* March 24, 1990;300(6727):771–73.

[8]R. B. Williams, J. C. Barefoot, J. A. Blumenthal et al., "Psychosocial Correlates of Job Strain in a Sample of Working Women," *Archives of General Psychiatry,* June 1997;54(6):543–48.

[9]M. B. Schenker, M. Eaton, R. Green et al., "Self-reported Stress and Reproductive Health of Female Lawyers," *Journal of Occupational and Environmental Medicine,* June 1997;39(6):556–68.

[10]M. E. Tucker, "Despite *H. pylori,* Stress Still a Factor in Ulcers," *Family Practice News,* 1994;24(12):17.

[11]E. A. Bergman, L. K. Massey, K. J. Wise et al., "Effects of Dietary Caffeine on Renal Handling of Minerals in Adult Women," *Life Sciences,* 1990;47(6):557–64.

[12]P. T. Packard and R. R. Recker, "Caffeine Does not Affect the Rate of Gain in Spine Bone in Young Women," *Osteoporosis International,* 1996;6(2):149–52.

[13]D. C. Bauer, W. S. Browner, J. A. Cauley et al., "Factors Associated with Appendicular Bone Mass in Older Women: The Study of Osteoporotic Fractures Research Group," *Annals of Internal Medicine,* May 1, 1993;118(9):657–65.

[14]R. P. Heaney and R. R. Recker, "Effects of Nitrogen, Phosphorus, and Caffeine on Calcium Balance in Women," *Journal of Laboratory and Clinical Medicine,* January 1982;99(1):46–55.

[15] C. Krahe, R. Friedman, J. L. Gross, "Risk Factors for Decreased Bone Density in Premenopausal Women," *Brazilian Journal of Medical and Biological Research*, September 1997;30(9):1061–66.

[16] S. S. Harris and B. Dawson-Hughes, "Caffeine and Bone Loss in Healthy Postmenopausal Women," *American Journal of Clinical Nutrition*, October 1994;60(4):573–78.

[17] L. K. Massey, E. A. Bergman, K. J. Wise et al., "Interactions between Dietary Caffeine and Calcium on Calcium and Bone Metabolism in Older Women," *Journal of the American College of Nutrition*, December 1994;13(6):592–96.

[18] D. P. Kiel, D. T. Felson, M. T. Hannan et al., "Caffeine and the Risk of Hip Fracture: The Framingham Study," *American Journal of Epidemiology*, October 1990;132(4):675–84.

[19] M. Hernandez-Avila, G. A. Colditz, M. J. Stampfer et al., "Caffeine, Moderate Alcohol Intake, and Risk of Fractures of the Hip and Forearm in Middle-aged Women," *American Journal of Clinical Nutrition*, July 1991;54(1):157–63.

[20] D. Michelson, C. Stratakis, L. Hill et al., "Bone Mineral Density in Women with Depression," *New England Journal of Medicine*, 1996;335:1176–81.

[21] J. E. White, "Osteoporosis: Strategies for Prevention," *Nurse Practitioner*, September 1986;11(9):36–46.

[22] C. L. Deal, "Osteoporosis, Prevention, Diagnosis, and Management," *American Journal of Medicine*, January 27, 1997;102(1A):35S–39S.

[23] J. J. Anderson, P. Rondano, and A. Holmes, "Roles of Diet and Physical Activity in the Prevention of Osteoporosis," *Scandinavian Journal of Rheumatology*, 1996;103:65–74.

[24] M. P. Faine, "Dietary Factors Related to Preservation of Oral and Skeletal Bone Mass in Women," *Journal of Prosthetic Dentistry*, January 1995;73(1):65–72.

[25] V. W. Bunker, "The Role of Nutrition in Osteoporosis," *British Journal of Biomedical Science*, September 1994;51(3):228–40.

[26] W. G. Thompson, "Coffee: Brew or Bane?" *American Journal of the Medical Sciences*, July 1994;308(1):49–57.

[27] T. Gillespy, 3d, and M. P. Gillespy, "Osteoporosis," *Radiology Clinics of North America*, January 1991;29(1):77–84.

[28] T. A. Morck, S. R. Lynch, and J. D. Cook, "Inhibition of Food Iron Absorption by Coffee," *American Journal of Clinical Nutrition*, 1983;37(3):416–20.

[29] L. Hallberg, "Iron," in *Present Knowledge in Nutrition*, 5th ed. (Washington D.C.: The Nutritional Foundation, 1984), pp. 459–78. Also E. M. Haymes, "Nutritional Concerns: Need for Iron," *Medicine and Science in Sports and Exercise*, 1987; supplement 19:S197–S200.

[30] G. B. Gabrielli and G. De Sandre, "Excessive Tea Consumption Can Inhibit the Efficacy of Oral Iron Treatment in Iron-deficiency Anemia," *Haematologica*, November–December 1995;80(6):518–20.

[31]J. D. Cook, C. A. Finch, and N. J. Smith, "Evaluation of the Iron Status of a Population," *Blood,* 1976;48:449–55.

[32]T. H. Bothwell, R. W. Charlton et al., *Iron Metabolism in Man* (Oxford, England: Blackwell Scientific Publications, 1979).

[33]I. G. Ances, J. Granados, and M. Baltazar, "Serum Ferritin as an Early Determinant of Decreased Iron Stores in Pregnant Women," *Southern Medical Journal,* May 1979;72(5):591–92.

[34]E. Kaneshige, "Serum Ferritin as an Assessment of Iron Stores and Other Hematologic Parameters during Pregnancy," *Obstetrics and Gynecology,* February 1981;57(2):238–42.

[35]J. Puolakka, "Serum Ferritin in the Evaluation of Iron Status in Young Healthy Women," *Acta Obstetrica et Gynecologica Scandinavica,* 1980; supplement 95:35–41.

[36]G. H. Guyatt, C. Patterson, M. Ali et al., "Diagnosis of Iron-deficiency Anemia in the Elderly," *American Journal of Medicine,* March 1990;88(3):205–09.

[37]G. H. Guyatt, A. D. Oxman, M. Ali et al., "Laboratory Diagnosis of Iron-deficiency Anemia: An Overview," *Journal of General Internal Medicine,* March–April 1992;7(2):145–53.

[38]J. Puolakka, O. Janne, A. Pakarinen et al., "Serum Ferritin in the Diagnosis of Anemia during Pregnancy," *Acta Obstetrica et Gynecologica Scandinavica,* 1980; supplement 95:57–63.

[39]S. Kiechl, J. Willeit, G. Egger et al., "Body Iron Stores and the Risk of Carotid Atherosclerosis: Prospective Results from the Bruneck Study," *Circulation,* November 18, 1997;96(10):3300–07.

[40]A. B. Bruner, "Randomized Study of Cognitive Effects of Iron Supplementation in Non-anemic Iron-deficient Adolescent Girls," *Lancet,* 1996;348 (October 12), 992–96.

[41]A. M. Rossignol, "Caffeine-containing Beverages and Premenstrual Syndrome in Young Women," *American Journal of Public Health,* November 1985;75(11):1335–37.

[42]A. M. Rossignol and H. Bonnlander, "Caffeine-containing Beverages, Total Fluid Consumption, and Premenstrual Syndrome," *American Journal of Public Health,* September 1990;80(9):1106–10.

[43]A. M. Rossignol, H. Bonnlander, L. Song et al., "Do Women with Premenstrual Symptoms Self-medicate with Caffeine?" *Epidemiology,* November 1991;2(6):403–08.

[44]J. F. Mortola, L. Girton, and S. S. Yen, "Depressive Episodes in Premenstrual Syndrome," *American Journal of Obstetrics and Gynecology,* December 1989;161(pt 1):1682–87.

[45]A. M. Rossignol, J. Y. Zhang, Y. Z. Chen et al., "Tea and Premenstrual Syndrome in the People's Republic of China," *American Journal of Public Health,* January 1989;79(1):67–69.

[46]S. London, W. Willett, C. Longcope et al., "Alcohol and Other Dietary Factors in Relation to Serum Hormone Concentrations in Women at Climacteric," *American Journal of Clinical Nutrition,* January 1991;53(1):166–71.

[47]R. L. Ferrini and E. Barrett-Connor, "Caffeine Intake and Endogenous Sex Steroid

Levels in Postmenopausal Women: The Rancho Bernardo Study," *American Journal of Epidemiology,* October 1, 1996;144(7):642–44.

[48]G. Del Rio, R. Menozzi, G. Zizzo et al., "Increased Cardiovascular Response to Caffeine in Perimenopausal Women Before and During Estrogen Therapy," *European Journal of Endocrinology,* November 1996;135(5)598–603.

[49]M. A. Lucerno and W. W. McCloskey, "Alternatives to Estrogen for the Treatment of Hot Flashes," *Annals of Pharmacotherapy,* July 1997;31(7–8):915–17.

[50]G. L. Clementz and J. W. Dailey, "Psychotropic Effects of Caffeine," *American Family Physician,* May 1988;37(5):167–72.

[51]A. Breier, D. S. Charney, and G. R. Heninger, "Agoraphobia with Panic Attacks: Development, Diagnostic Stability, and Course of Illness," *Archives of General Psychiatry,* November 1986;43(11):1029–36.

[52]F. W. Foote and F. W. Stewart, "Comparative Studies of Cancerous versus Noncancerous Breasts," *Annals of Surgery,* 1945;121:197–222.

[53]P. G. Brooks, S. Gart, A. J. Heldfond et al., "Measuring the Effect of Caffeine Restriction on Fibrocystic Breast Disease: The Role of Graphic Stress Telethermometry as an Objective Monitor of Disease," *Journal of Reproductive Medicine,* June 1981;26(6):279–82.

[54]M. C. Hindi-Alexander, M. A. Zielezny, N. Montes et al., "Theophylline and Fibrocystic Breast Disease," *Journal of Allergy and Clinical Immunology,* June 1985;75(6):709–15.

[55]J. P. Minton and H. Abou-Issa, "Nonendocrine Theories of the Etiology of Benign Breast Disease," *World Journal of Surgery,* November 1989;13(6):680–84.

[56]J. P. Minton, M. K. Foecking et al., "Response of Fibrocystic Disease to Caffeine Withdrawal and Correlation of Cystic Nucleotides with Breast Disease," *American Journal of Obstetrics and Gynecology,* 1979;135:157–58.

[57]L. C. Russell, "Caffeine Restriction as Initial Treatment for Breast Pain," February 1989;14(2):36–37.

[58]B. Bullough, M. Hindi-Alexander, and S. Fetouh, "Methylxanthines and Fibrocystic Breast Disease: A Study of Correlations," *Nurse Practitioner,* March 1990;15(3):36–38.

[59]P. Modica, "The Coffee Craze and Your Health," Medical Tribune News Service, June 25, 1997.

[60]S. J. London, J. L. Connolly, S. J. Schnitt et al., "A Prospective Study of Benign Breast Disease and the Risk of Breast Cancer," *Journal of the American Medical Association,* 1992;267(7):941–44.

[61]C. W. Welsch, "Caffeine and the Development of the Normal and Neoplastic Mammary Gland," *Proceedings of the Society for Experimental and Biological Medicine,* October 1994;207(1):1–12.

[62]T. E. Rohan and A. J. McMichael, "Methylxanthines and Breast Cancer," *International Journal of Cancer,* March 15, 1988;41(3):390–93.

[63]C. K. Stanton and R. H. Gray, "Effects of Caffeine Consumption on Delayed Conception," *American Journal of Epidemiology,* December 15, 1995;142(12):1322–29.

[64]A. Wilcox, C. Weinberg, and D. Baird, "Caffeinated Beverages and Decreased Fertility," *Lancet,* December 24–31, 1988;2(8626–8627):1453–56.

[65]F. Bolumar, J. Olsen, M. Rebagliato et al., "Caffeine Intake and Delayed Conception: A European Multicenter Study on Infertility and Subfecundity: European Study Group on Infertility Subfecundity," *American Journal of Epidemiology,* February 15, 1997;145(4):324–34.

[66]B. Watkinson and P. A. Fried, "Maternal Caffeine Use before, during and after Pregnancy and Effects upon Offspring," *Neurobehavioral Toxicology Teratology,* January–February 1985;7(1):9–17.

[67]P. S. Weathersbee, L. K. Olson, and T. R. Lodge, "Caffeine and Pregnancy: A Retrospective Survey," *Postgraduate Medicine,* 1977;62:64–69.

[68]L. Dlugosz, K. Belanger, K. Hellenbrand et al., "Maternal Caffeine Consumption and Spontaneous Abortion: A Prospective Cohort Study," *Epidemiology,* May 1996;7(3):250–55.

[69]C. Infante-Rivard, A. Fernandez, R. Gauthier et al., "Fetal Loss Associated with Caffeine Intake before and during Pregnancy," *Journal of the American Medical Association,* 1993;270(24):2940–43.

[70]W. Srisuphan and M. B. Bracken, "Caffeine Consumption during Pregnancy and Association with Late Spontaneous Abortion," *American Journal of Obstetrics and Gynecology,* January 1986;154(1):14–20.

[71]R. M. Gilbert, "Caffeine as a Drug of Abuse," in R. J. Gibbins et al. (eds.), *Research Advances in Alcohol and Drug Problems,* vol. 3 (New York: John Wiley & Sons), pp. 49–176.

[72]U.S. Department of Health and Human Services Public Health Service, Food and Drug Administration, *Caffeine and Pregnancy* (FDA) 81–1081.

[73]A. Nehlig and G. Debry, "Effects of Coffee and Caffeine on Fertility, Reproduction, Lactation, and Development: Review of Human and Animal Data," *Journal de Gynecologie, Obstetrique et Biologie de la Reproduction,* 1994;23(3):241–56.

[74]W. J. Hueston, G. M. Eilers, D. E. King et al., "Common Questions Patients Ask during Pregnancy," *American Family Physician,* May 1, 1995;51(6):1465–70.

[75]T. R. Martin and M. B. Bracken, "The Association between Low Birth Weight and Caffeine Consumption during Pregnancy," *American Journal of Epidemiology* 1987;126:813–21.

[76]L. Fenster, B. Eskenazi, G. C. Windham et al., "Caffeine Consumption during Pregnancy and Fetal Growth," *American Journal of Public Health,* 1991;81:458–61.

[77]I. Fortier, S. Marcoux, and L. Beaulac-Baillargeon, "Relation of Caffeine Intake during Pregnancy to Intrauterine Growth Retardation and Preterm Birth," *American Journal of Epidemiology,* 1993;137:931–40.

[78]H. Vlajinao, R. R. Petrovic, J. M. Marinkovic et al., "Effect of Caffeine Intake during Pregnancy on Birth Weight," *American Journal of Epidemiology,* 1997;145:335–38.

[79]H. Tanaka, K. Nakazawa, and M. Arima, "Effects of Maternal Caffeine Ingestion on the Perinatal Cerebrum," *Biology of the Neonate,* 1987;51(6):332–39.

[80]R. Matsuoka, H. Uno, H. Tanaka et al., "Caffeine Induces Cardiac and Other Malformations in the Rat," *American Journal of Medical Genetics,* supplement, 1987;3:433–43.

[81]M. J. Rossowska, W. Carvajal, F. Joseph, Jr., et al., "Postnatal Caffeine Effects on Copper, Zinc, and Iron Concentrations in Mammary Gland, Milk, and Plasma of lactating Dams and Their Offspring," *Annals of Nutrition and Metabolism,* 1997;41(1):60–65.

[82]A. Nehlig and G. Debry, "Potential Teratogenic and Neurodevelopmental Consequences of Coffee and Caffeine Exposure: A Review of Human and Animal Data," *Neurotoxicology and Teratology,* November–December 1994;16(6):531–43.

[83]J. D. McGowan, R. E. Altman, and W. P. Kanto, Jr., "Neonatal Withdrawal Symptoms after Chronic Maternal Ingestion of Caffeine," *Southern Medical Journal,* September 1988;81(9):1092–94.

[84]J. T. Sullivan, "Caffeine Poisoning in an Infant," *Journal of Pediatrics,* 1977;90:1022–23.

[85]"Caffeine May Contribute to Infant Deaths," *Los Angeles Times,* January 28, 1998; A-10.

[86]L. J. Benincosa, K. Sagawa, L. K. Massey et al., "Effects of Acute Caffeine Ingestion and Menopause on Sulfate Homeostasis in Women," *Life Science,* September 8, 1995;57(16):1497–1505.

Chapter 7

[1]P. J. Rogers, N. J. Richardson, and N. A. Elliman, "Overnight Caffeine Abstinence and Negative Reinforcement of Preference for Caffeine-Containing Drinks," *Psychopharmacology* (Berlin), August 1995;120(4):457–62.

[2]B. G. Phillips-Bute and J. D. Lane, "Caffeine Withdrawal Symptoms Following Brief Caffeine Deprivation," *Physiology and Behavior,* December 31, 1997;63(1):35–39.

[3]J. M. Peters, "Factors Affecting Caffeine Toxicity: A Review of the Literature," *Journal of Clinical Pharmacology,* 1967;7:131–41.

[4]R. M. Gilbert, "Caffeine as a Drug of Abuse," in R. J. Gibbins et al. (eds.), *Research Advances in Alcohol and Drug Problems,* vol. 3 (New York: John Wiley & Sons, 1976), pp. 49–176.

[5]N. J. Birkett and A. G. Logan, "Caffeine-containing Beverages and the Prevalence of Hypertension," *Journal of Hypertension,* 1988;6 (supplement 4):S620–S622.

[6]F. A. Holloway, R. C. Michaelis, and P. L. Huerta, "Caffeine-phenylethylamine Combinations Mimic the Amphetamine Discriminative Cue," *Life Science,* February 25, 1985;36(8):723–30.

[7]S. M. Mueller, J. Muller, and S. M. Asdell, "Cerebral Hemorrhage Associated with Phenylpropanolamine in Combination with Caffeine," *Stroke,* January 1984; 15(1):119–23.

[8]R. C. Michaelis, F. A. Holloway, D. C. Bird et al., "Interactions between Stimulants:

Effects on DRL Performance and Lethality in Rats," *Pharmacology, Biochemistry and Behavior,* 1987;27:299–306.

[9]D. Delibovi, "Is Coffee Fattening?" *Lear's,* July 1991;13(2):36.

[10]B. Livermore, "Caffeine Boosts Eating Disorders," *Health,* June 1991;16.

[11]T. W. Castonguay, "Glucorcorticoids as Modulators in the Control of Feeding," *Brain Research Bulletin,* September–October 1991;27(3–4):423–28.

[12]"FDA Issues Public Warning Against Ma Huang Product," *Food Labeling News,* 1995;3(22):15.

[13]General Accounting Office (GAO), "Better Regulation of Pesticide Exports and Pesticide Residues in Imported Food is Essential." CED-79-43, Washington, D.C., 1979, pg 11.

[14]S. A. Hearne, *Harvest of Unknowns: Pesticide Contamination in Imported Foods,* Natural Resources Defense Council, New York, 1984, Appendix V.

[15]Ibid.

[16]Ibid.

[17]A. H. el Sebae, "Special Problems Experienced with Pesticide Use in Developing Countries," *Regulatory Toxicology and Pharmacology,* June 1993;17(3):287–91.

[18]J. G. Machado-Neto, T. Matuo, and Y. K. Matuo, "Semiquantitative Evaluation of Dermal Exposure to Granulated Insecticides in Coffee (*Coffea arabica L.*) Crop and Efficiency of Individual Protective Equipment," *Bulletin on Environmental Contamination and Toxicology,* December 1996;57(6):946–51.

[19]D. B. Rama and K. Jaga, "Pesticide Exposure and Cholinesterase Levels among Farm Workers in the Republic of South Africa," *Science of the Total Environment,* July 29, 1992;122(3):315–19.

[20]L. Tangley, *Science,* November 22, 1996.

[21]G. Monbiot, "Land Ownership and the Flight to Amazonia," in M. Colchester and L. Lohmann (eds.), *The Struggle for Land and the Fate of the Forests* (London: Zed Books, 1995), pp. 139–63.

Chapter 8

[1]C. Gerrans, "Soft Drinks Tend to Boost Dietary Aluminum Intake," *Medical Tribune,* 1992;33(4):17.

[2]I. Marci and M. Giannoni, "Effect of Some Low pH Soft Drinks on Enamel," *Prevenzione e Assistenza Dentale,* November–December 1988;14(6):10–14.

[3]A. I. Ismail, B. A. Burt, and S. A. Eklund, "The Cariogenicity of Soft Drinks in the United States," *Journal of the American Dental Association,* August 1984;109(2):241–45.

[4]M. McKinney, "People with Braces Advised to Cut Soda Consumption," Medical Tribune News Service, October 14, 1997.

NOTES

[5]S. Stellman and L. Garfinkel, "Short Report: Artificial Sweetener Use and Weight Changes among Women," *Preventive Medicine*, 1986;15:195–202.

[6]A. Liguori, J. R. Hughes, and A. H. Oliveto, "Caffeine Self-administration in Humans: Efficacy of Cola Vehicle," *Experimental and Clinical Psychopharmacology*, August 1997;5(3):286–94.

[7]E. C. Strain, G. K. Mumford, K. Silverman et al., "Caffeine Dependence Syndrome; Evidence from Case Histories and Experimental Evaluations," *Journal of the American Medical Association*, 1994;272:1043–48.

[8]R. H. Adamson and H. R. Roberts, "Caffeine Dependence Syndrome," (Letter), *Journal of the American Medical Association*, 1995;273(18):1418.

[9]Council on Scientific Affairs, "Caffeine Labeling," *Journal of the American Medical Association*, 1984;252(6):803–06.

[10]P. M. Guenther, "Beverages in the Diets of American Teenagers," *Journal of the American Dietetic Association*, 1986;86:493.

[11]D. M. Graham, "Caffeine: Its Identity, Dietary Sources, Intake, and Biological Effects," *Sourcebook on Food and Nutrition* (Chicago: Marquis Academic Media, 1980).

[12]C. Kawai, A. Wakabayashi, T. Matsumura et al., "Reappearance of Beriberi Heart Disease in Japan: A Study of 23 Cases," *American Journal of Medicine*, September 1980;69(3):383–86.

[13]A. C. Looker, P. R. Dallman, M. D. Carroll et al., "Prevalence of Iron Deficiency in the United States," *Journal of the American Medical Association*, March 26, 1997;277(12):973–76.

[14]M. M. Garriga and D. D. Metcalfe, "Aspartame Intolerance," *Annals of Allergy*, December 1988;61 (pt 2):63–69.

[15]B. J. Kaplan, J. McNicol, R. A. Conte et al., "Dietary Replacement in Preschool-aged Hyperactive Boys," *Pediatrics*, January 1989;823(1):7–17.

[16]M. Maes, M. Vandewoude, C. Schotte et al., "The Decreased Availability of L-tryptophan in Depressed Females: Clinical and Biological Correlates," *Progress in Neuro-Psychopharmacology and Biological Psychiatry*, 1990;14(6):903–19.

[17]J. Tynjala, L. Kannas, and E. Levalahti, "Perceived Tiredness among Adolescents and Its Association with Sleep Habits and Use of Psychoactive Substances," *Journal of Sleep Research*, September 1997;6(3):189–98.

[18] W. S. Terry and B. Phifer, "Caffeine and Memory Performance on the AVLT," *Journal of Clinical Psychology*, November 1986;42(6):860–63.

[19]A. B. Bruner, "Randomized Study of Cognitive Effects of Iron Supplementation in Non-anemic Iron-deficient Adolescent Girls," *Lancet*, 1996;348 (October 12), 992–96.

[20]"You Are What You Drink, Too," *Los Angeles Times*, December 22, 1996, p. E-2.

[21]*Dietary Goals for the United States*, Select Committee on Nutrition and Human Needs, United States Senate. U.S. Government Printing Office, February 1977, pp. 46–47.

[22]*1996 Statistical Abstract of the United States*.

[23]M. L. Arbeit, T. A. Nicklas, G. C. Frank et al., "Caffeine Intakes of Children from a Biracial Population: The Bogalusa Heart Study," *Journal of the American Dietetic Association,* April 1988;88(4):466–71.

[24]G. A. Bernstein, N. Walters, R. Crosby et al., "Caffeine Withdrawal and the Effect on Normal Children," in Scientific Proceedings 43rd Annual meeting of the American Academy of Child and Adolescent Psychiatry, Philadelphia, Penn., 1997.

[25]H. L. Abrams, Jr., "Caffeine: A Paradigm of Subliminal Cultural Drug Habituation," *Journal of Applied Nutrition,* 1976;28:33–40.

[26]L. L. Palmer, "Early Childhood Caffeine and Sugar Habituation," *Journal of Orthomolecular Psychiatry,* 1977;6:248–50.

[27]G. Wyshak and R. E. Frisch, "Carbonated Beverages, Dietary Calcium, the Dietary Calcium/phosphorus Ratio, and Bone Fractures in Girls and Boys," *Journal of Adolescent Health,* May 1994;15(3):210–15.

[28]H. H. Draper and R. R. Bell, "Nutrition and Osteoporosis," in H. H. Draper, (ed.), *Advances in Nutrition Research,* vol 2. (New York: Plenum Press, 1977).

[29]L. K. Massey and M. M. Strang, "Soft Drink Consumption, Phosphorus Intake, and Osteoporosis," *Journal of the American Dietetic Association,* 1982;80:581–83.

[30]K. G. Dewey, M. E. Romero-Abal, J. Quan de Serrano et al., "A Randomized Intervention Study of the Effects of Discontinuing Coffee Intake on Growth and Morbidity of Iron-deficient Guatemalan Toddlers," *Journal of Nutrition,* February 1997;127(2):306–13.

[31]B. Bates, "The Scoop on Soda Pop: Carbonated Beverages No Threat to Bones," *Family Practice News,* April 1996;1:49.

[32]*American Family Physician,* 1994;50(4):830.

[33]D. G. Simons-Morton, S. A. Hunsberger, L. Van Horn et al., "Nutrient Intake and Blood Pressure in the Dietary Intervention Study in Children," *Hypertension,* April 1997;29(4):930–36.

[34]H. Baker, O. Frank, S. Feingold et al., "Vitamins, Total Cholesterol, and Triglycerides in 642 New York City School Children," *American Journal of Clinical Nutrition,* 1987;20(8):850–57.

[35]P. M. Guenther, "Beverages in the Diets of American Teenagers," *Journal of the American Dietetic Association,* 1986;86:493.

[36]C. L. Hays, "Be True to Your Cola, Rah, Rah: Battle for Soft Drink Loyalties Moves to Public Schools," *The New York Times,* March 10, 1998, p. C1–4.

[37]Ibid.

[38]Ibid.

[39]"Sweet Deals for Women's Sports," *Working Woman,* vol. 20, issue 2, February 1995;14.

[40]S. Elliott, "Boys and Girls Clubs in Project with Coke," *The New York Times,* December 6, 1996, p. D4.

[41]D. Barboza, "More Hip, Higher Hop: Caffeinated Drinks Catering to Excitable Boys and Girls," *The New York Times,* Friday August 22, 1997, pp. C1–C5.

[42]Ibid.

Chapter 9

[1]B. D. Page and C. F. Charbonneau, "Headspace Gas Chromatographic Determination of Methylene Chloride in Decaffeinated Tea and Coffee, with Electrolytic Conductivity Detection," *Journal of the Association of Official Analytical Chemists,* July 1984;67(4):757–61.

[2]E. Lynge, A. Anttila, and K. Hemminki, "Organic Solvents and Cancer," *Cancer Causes and Control,* May 1997;8(3):406–19.

[3]R. G. Liteplo, G. W. Long, and M. E. Meek, "Relevance of Carcinogenicity Bioassays in Mice in Assessing Potential Health Risks Associated with Exposure to Methylene Chloride," *Human and Experimental Toxicology,* February 1998;17(2):84–87.

[4]H. R. Superko, W. Bortz, Jr., P. T. Williams et al., "Caffeinated and Decaffeinated Coffee Effects on Plasma Lipoprotein Cholesterol, Apolipoproteins, and Lipase Activity: A Controlled, Randomized Trial," *American Journal of Clinical Nutrition,* September 1991;54(3):599–605.

[5]H. N. Graham, "Tea: The Plant and Its Manufacture: Chemistry and Consumption of the Beverage," in G. A. Spiller (ed.), *The Methrylxanthine Beverages and Foods: Chemistry, Consumption and Health Effects* (New York: Alan R. Liss, 1984), pp. 29–74.

[6]C. Rice-Evans, "Plant Polyphenols: Free Radical Scavengers or Chain-breaking Antioxidants?" *Biochemical Society Symposia,* 1995;61:103–16.

[7]K. Okushio, N. Matsumotot, T. Kohri et al., "Absorption of Tea Catechins into Rat Portal Vein," *Biological and Pharmaceutical Bulletin,* February 1996;19(2):326–29.

[8]Y. Yoshiki, T. Kahara, K. Okuba et al., "Mechanism of Catechin Chemiluminescence in the Presence of Active Oxygen," *Journal of Bioluminescence and Chemiluminescence,* May–June 1996;11(3):131–36.

[9]G. C. Yen and H. Y. Chen, "Relationship between Antimutagenic Activity and Major Components of Various Teas," *Mutagenesis,* January 1996;11(1):37–41.

[10]A. Constable, N. Varga, J. Richoz et al., "Antimutagenicity and Catechin Content of Soluable Instant Teas," *Mutagenesis,* March 1996;11(2):189–94.

[11]K. Goto, S. Kanaya, and Y. Hara, Proceedings of the International Symposium on Tea Science, 314 (Shizuoka, Japan); August 1991.

[12]Y. Hara, T. Matsuzaki, and T. Suzuki, *Nippon Nogeikagaku Kaishi,* 61;803(1987).

[13]Y. Sagesaka-Mitane, M. Miwa, and S. Okada, "Platelet Aggregation Inhibitors in Hot Water Extract of Green Tea," *Chemical and Pharmaceutical Bulletin,* (Tokyo) March 1990;38(3):790–93.

[14]H. L. Gensler, B. N. Timmerman, S. Valcic et al., "Prevention of Photocarcinogenesis by Topical Administration of Pure Epigallocatechin Gallate Isolated from Green Tea," *Nutrition and Cancer,* 1996;26(3):325–35.

[15]P. Simon, P. Charbonneau, B. Vaucel et al., "Iron-deficiency Anemia during Excessive Consumption of Tea," *Nouvelle Presse Medicale,* January 10, 1981;10(1):44.

[16]S. Vimkesant, S. Nakornchai, K. Rungruangsak et al., "Food Habits Causing Thiamine Deficiency in Humans," *Journal of Nutrition Science and Vitaminology,* August 1976;22 supplement:1–2.

[17]R. S. Wang and C. Kies, "Niacin, Thiamin, Iron and Protein Status of Humans as Affected by the Consumption of Tea (*Camellia sinensis*) Infusions," *Plant Foods and Human Nutrition,* October 1991;41(4):337–53.

[18]K. Imai and K. Nakachi, "Cross Sectional Study of Effect of Drinking Green Tea on Cardiovascular and Liver Diseases," *British Medical Journal,* 1995;310:693–96.

[19]"Evaluation of the Carcinogenic Risk to Humans: Coffee, Tea, Mate, Methylxanthines, and Methylglyoxal." *International Agency for Research on Cancer Monograph,* 1991; vol. 51.

[20]I. Oguni et al., *Japanese Journal of Nutrition,* 47;31(1989).

[21]Y. T. Gao, J. K. McLaughlin, W. J. Blot et al., "Reduced Risk of Esophageal Cancer Associated with Green Tea Consumption," *Journal of the National Cancer Institute,* June 1, 1994;86(11):855–58.

[22]E. Giovannucci, A. Ascherio, E. B. Rimm et al., "Intake of Carotenoids and Retinol in Relation to Risk of Prostate Cancer," *Journal of the National Cancer Institute,* December 6, 1995;87(23):1767–76.

[23]L. Kohlmeier, K. G. Weterings, S. Steck et al., "Tea and Cancer Prevention: An Evaluation of the Epidemiologic Literature," *Nutrition and Cancer,* 1997;27(1):1–13.

[24]B. D. Page and C. F. Charbonneau, "Headspace Gas Chromatographic Determination of Methylene Chloride in Decaffeinated Tea and Coffee with Electrolytic Conductivity Detection," *Journal of the Association of Official Analytical Chemists,* July 1984;67(4):757–61.

[25]"Eleutherococcus: Strategy of the Use and New Data," Research Institute of Biological Testing of Chemical Compounds. Academy of Medical Sciences, Moscow, 1987.

[26]H. J. Meyer, "Pharmacology of Kava," in *Ethnopharmacologic Search for Psychoactive Drugs,* D. H. Efron et al. (eds.), Public Health Service Publication no. 1645. Washington, D.C.: U.S. Government Printing Office, 1967, 133–40.

[27]A. von Gadow, E. Joubert, and C. F. Hansmann, "Comparison of the Antioxidant Activity of Rooibos Tea with Green, Oolong and Black Tea," *Food Chemistry,* 1997;vol. 60:(1)73–77.

[28]C. Rabe, J. A. Steenkamp, E. Joubert et al., "Phenolic Metabolites from Rooibos Tea (*Aspalathus linearis*)" *Phytochemistry,* 1994; vol. 35:(6):1559–65.

[29]E. Joubert and D. Ferrera, "Antioxidants of Rooibos Tea—A Possible Explanation for Its Health Promoting Properties?" *South African Journal of Food Science and Nutrition,* 1996;8:79–83.

[30]S. Stellman and L. Garfinkel, "Short Report: Artificial Sweetener Use and Weight Changes among Women," *Prevention Medicine,* 1986;15:195–202.

NOTES

Chapter 10

[1]H. Jaggy and E. Koch, "Chemistry and Biology of Alkylphenols From *Ginkgo biloba* L." *Pharmazie,* October 1997;52(10):735–38.

[2]J. Haase, P. Halama, and R. Horr, "Effectiveness of Brief Infusions with *Ginkgo biloba* Special Extract EGb 761 in Dementia of the Vascular and Alzheimer Type," *Zeitschrift fur Gerontologie and Geriatrie,* July 1996;29:(4):302–09.

[3]M. V. R. Apparao, K. Srinivasan, and R. T. L. Koteswara, "The Effect of *Centella asiatica* on the General Mental Ability of Mentally Retarded Children," *Indian Journal of Psychiatry,* 1977;19:54–59.

[4]K. Nalini et al., "Effect of *Centella asiatica* Fresh Leaf Aqueous Extract on Learning and Memory and Biogenic Amine Turnover in Albino Rats," *Phytotherapia,* 1992;63(3):232–37.

[5]"Caffeine Can Increase Brain Serotonin Levels," *Nutrition Reviews,* October 1988;46(10):366–67.

[6]S. Foster, "Milk Thistle, *Silybum marianum,*" Botanical series no. 305, American Botanical Council, Austin, Texas, 1991.

[7]G. Palasciano et al., "The Effect of Silymarin on Plasma Levels of Malon-dialdehyde in Patients Receiving Long Term Treatment with Psychotropic Drugs," *Current Therapeutic Research,* May 1994;55(5):537–45.

[8]G. P. Littarru, S. Lippa, A. Oradei et al., "Coenzyme Q10: Blood Levels and Metabolic Demand," *International Journal of Tissue Reactions,* 1990;12(3):145–48.

[9]S. Fujimoto, N. Kurihara, K. Hirata et al., "Effects of Coenzyme Q10 Administration on Pulmonary Function and Exercise Performance in Patients with Chronic Lung Diseases," *Clinical Investigation,* 1993;71(8 supplement):S162–S166.

[10]W. J. Koroshetz, B. G. Jenkins, B. R. Rosen et al., "Energy Metabolism Defects in Huntington's Disease and Effects of Coenzyme Q10," *Annals of Neurology,* February 1997;41(2):160–65.

[11]R. Lodi, R. Rinaldi, A. Gaddi et al., "Brain and Skeletal Muscle Bioenergetic Failure in Familial Hypobetalipoproteinaemia," *Journal of Neurology, Neurosurgery and Psychiatry,* June 1997;62(6):574–80.

[12]M. Mizuno, B. Quistorff, H. Theorell et al., "Effects of Oral Supplementation of Coenzyme Q10 on 31P-NMR Detected Skeletal Muscle Energy Metabolism in Middle-aged Post-polio Subjects and Normal Volunteers," *Molecular Aspects of Medicine,* 1997;18 supplement:S291–S298.

[13]M. Kamei and T. Fujita et al., "The Distribution and Content of Ubiquinone in Foods," *International Journal for Vitamin and Nutrition Research,* 1986;56:57.

[14]G. Lenaz, R. Fato, G. Castelluccio et al., "An Updating of the Biochemical Function of Coenzyme Q in Mitochondria," *Molecular Aspects of Medicine,* 1994;15 supplement:S29–S36.

[15]D. A. Porter, D. L. Costill, J. J. Zachwieja et al., "The Effect of Oral Coenzyme Q10 on the Exercise Tolerance of Middle-aged, Untrained Men," *International Journal of Sports Medicine,* October 1995;16(7):421–27.

[16]J. Karlsson, L. Lin, C. Sylven et al., "Muscle Ubiquinone in Healthy Physically Active Males," *Molecular and Cellular Biochemistry,* March 23, 1996;156(2):169–72.

[17]C. Marconi, G. Sassi, and P. Cerretelli, "The Effect of an Alpha-Ketoglutarate-Pyridoxine Complex on Human Maximal Aerobic and Anaerobic Performance," *European Journal of Applied Physiology,* 1982;49(3):307–17.

[18]A. L. Goldberg and T. W. Chang, "Regulation and Significance of Amino Acid Metabolism in Skeletal Muscle," *Federation Proceedings,* 1978;37:2301–07.

[19]R. P. Shank and D. J. Bennett, "2-Oxoglutarate Transport: A Potential Mechanism for Regulating Glutamate and Tricarboxylic Acid Cycle Intermediates in Neurons," *Neurochemical Research,* April 1993;18(4):401–10.

[20]G. F. Karandashova, E. M. Kruptiskii, V. N. Petrov et al., "Study of Gamma-aminobutyric Acid (GABA) Concentration in Blood Plasma of Alcoholism Patients," *Voprosy Meditsinskoi Khimii,* March–April 1993;39(2):36–37.

[21]A. E. Morgan and S. L. Dewey, "Effects of Pharmacologic Increases in Brain GABA Levels on Cocaine-induced Changes in Extracellular Dopamine," *Synapse,* January 1998;28(1):60–65.

[22]T. Kaneko and N. Mizuno, "Glutamate-synthesizing Enzymes in GABAergic Neurons of the Neocortex, A Double Immunofluorescence Study in the Rat," *Neuroscience,* August 1994;61(4):839–49.

[23]C. Marconi, "The Effect of an Alpha-Ketoglutarate-Pyridoxine Complex."

[24]M. H. Williams, "Vitamin Supplementation and Athletic Performance," *International Journal for Vitamin and Nutrition Research,* 1989;30:163–91.

[25]B. Chrisley and J. Driskell, "Vitamin B-6 Status of Adults in Virginia," *Nutrition Reports International,* 1979:19:553–60.

[26]H. Gutherie and A Crocetti, "Implications of a Protein-based Standard for Vitamin B-6," 1983;28:133–38.

[27]A. Stewart, "Clinical and Biochemical Effects of Nutritional Supplementation on the Premenstrual Syndrome," *Journal of Reproductive Medicine,* 1987;32(6):345–41.

[28]R. L. Rizek and K. S. Tippett, "Diets of American Women: 1977 & 1985," *Bulletin of the Michigan Dental Hygiene Association,* 1989;19(2):3–6.

[29]K. Suboticanec et al., "Effects of Pyridoxine and Riboflavin Supplementation on Physical Fitness in Young Adolescents," *International Journal for Vitamin and Nutrition Research,* 1990;60(10):81–88.

[30]W. Bunker, M. M. Lawson et al., "The Uptake and Excretion of Chromium by the Elderly," *American Journal of Clinical Nutrition,* 1984;39:799–802.

[31]P. Koivistoinen, "Mineral Element Composition of Finnish Foods," *Acta Agricultura Scandinavica,* 1980; supplement, 22.

[32]R. A. Anderson and A. S. Kozlovsky, "Chromium Intake, Absorption and Excretion of Subjects Consuming Self-selected Diets," *American Journal of Clinical Nutrition,* 1984;41:1177–83.

[33]R. Riales and M. J. Albrink, "Effect of Chromium Chloride Supplementation on

Glucose Tolerance and Serum Lipids Including High Density Lipoprotein of Adult men," *American Journal of Clinical Nutrition*, 1981;34:2670–78.

[34]R. A. Anderson, M. M. Polansky et al., "Chromium Supplementation of Human Subjects: Effects on Glucose, Insulin and Lipid Parameters," *Metabolism*, 1983;32:894–99.

[35]R. A. Anderson, M. M. Polansky et al., "Effects of Supplemental Chromium on Patients with Reactive Hypoglycemia," *Metabolism*, 1987;36:351–55.

[36]W. H. Glinsmann and W. Mertz, "Effect of Trivalent Chromium on Glucose Tolerance," *Metabolism: Clinical and Experimental*, 1966;15:510.

[37]R. A. Anderson, M. M. Polansky et al., "Effects of Chromium Supplementation on Insulin, Insulin Binding and C-peptide Values of Hypoglycemic Human Subjects," *American Journal of Clinical Nutrition*, 1985;41:841.

[38]J. Clausen, "Chromium Induced Clinical Improvement in Symptomatic Hypoglycemia," *Biological Trace Element Research*, 1988;17:229–36.

[39]J. T. Hicks, "Treatment of Fatigue in General Practice: A Double Blind Study," *Clinical Medicine*, 1964;71:85–90.

[40]D. L. Shaw et al., "Management of Fatigue, A Physiological Approach," *American Journal of Medical Science*, 1962;243:98–109, 758–69.

[41]I. Franz and H. Paradies, "Potassium-magnesium Aspartate as a Positive Homotropic Effector," *Arzneim Forsch*, 1979;29:1676–80.

[42]V. Tyler, *The Honest Herbal*, 3rd ed. (New York: Pharmaceutical Product Press, 1993), p. 155.

[43]I. Wiklund, J. Karlberg, and B. Lund, "Improved Quality of Life with Ginseng Preparations? Positive Effects in Healthy Working People," *Lakartidningen*, September 6, 1995;92(36):3196–3200.

[44]K. A. Wesnes, R. A. Faleni, N. R. Hefting et al., "The Cognitive, Subjective, and Physical Effects of a *Ginkgo biloba*/Panax Ginseng Combination in Healthy Volunteers with Neurasthenic Complaints," *Psychopharmacology Bulletin*, 1997;33(4):677–83.

[45]T. K. Yun and S. Y. Choi, "Preventive Effect of Ginseng Intake Against Various Human Cancers: A Case-control Study on 1987 Pairs," *Cancer Epidemiology, Biomarkers and Prevention*, June 1995;4(4):401–08.

[46]X. Chen, S. Salwinski, and T. J. Lee, "Extracts of *Ginkgo biloba* and Ginsenosides Exert Cerebral Vasorelaxation via a Nitric Oxide Pathway," *Clinical and Experimental Pharmacology and Physiology*, December 1997;24(12):958–59.

[47]*Eleutherococcus: Strategy of the Use and New Data*, Research Institute of Biological Testing of Chemical Compounds, Academy of Medical Sciences, Moscow, 1987.

[48]*Pharmacology and Application of Chinese Materia Medica*, Chinese Medicinal Material Research Center, Chinese University of Hong Kong, 1984.

[49]Y. Y. Cui and M. Z. Wang, "Aspects of Schizandrin Metabolism In Vitro and In Vivo," *European Journal of Drug Metabolism and Pharmacokinetics*, April–June 1993;18(2):155–60.

[50]L. Zhang and X. Niu, "Effects of Schizandrol A on Monoamine Neurotransmitters in the Central Nervous System," *Acta Academiae Medicinae Sinicae*, February 1991;13(1):13–16.

[51]P. Laukkanen, E. Heikkinen, M. Schroll et al., "A Comparative Study of Factors Related to Carrying Out Physical Activities of Daily Living (PADL) among 75-Year-Old-Men and Women in Two Nordic Localities," *Aging*, August 1997;9(4):258–67.

[52]M. P. van Boxtel, F. G. Paas, P. J. Houx et al., "Aerobic Capacity and Cognitive Performance in a Cross-sectional Aging Study," *Medicine and Science in Sports and Exercise*, October 1997;29(10):1357–65.

[53]M. S. Albert, K. Jones, G. R. Savage et al., "Predictors of Cognitive Change in Older Persons: MacArthur Studies of Successful Aging," *Psychology and Aging*, December 1995;10(4):578–89.

[54]R. Manber, R. R. Bootzin, C. Acebo et al., "The Effects of Regularizing Sleep-wake Schedules on Daytime Sleepiness," *Sleep*, June 1996;19(5):432–41.

[55]H. J. Meyer, "Pharmacology of Kava," in *Ethnopharmacologic Search for Psychoactive Drugs*, D. H. Efron et al. (eds.), Public Health Service Publication no. 1645. Washington, D.C.: U.S. Government Printing Office, 1967:133–40.

[56]E. Lehmann, E. Kiszler, and J. Friedemann, "Efficacy of a Special Kava Extract (*Piper methysticum*) in Patients with States of Anxiety, Tension and Excitedness of Non-mental Origin—A Double Blind, Placebo Controlled Study of Four Weeks Treatment," *Phytomedicine*, 1996;3:113–19.

Conclusion

[1]C. Cohen, W. B. Pickworth, E. B. Bunker et al., "Caffeine Antagonizes EEG Effects of Tobacco Withdrawal," *Pharmacology, Biochemistry and Behavior*, April 1994;47(4):919–36.

INDEX

CPSIA information can be obtained at www.ICGtesting.com
Printed in the USA
LVOW11s0514021015

456588LV00001B/36/P